AN INTRODUCTION TO
VETERINARY PHARMACOLOGY

An Introduction to

VETERINARY PHARMACOLOGY

BY

FRANK ALEXANDER

Ph.D., D.Sc., M.R.C.V.S., F.R.S.E.

Professor of Veterinary Pharmacology in the
University of Edinburgh

SECOND EDITION

E. & S. LIVINGSTONE LTD.

EDINBURGH AND LONDON

1969

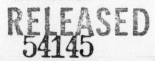

© E. & S. Livingstone Limited, 1969

SBN 443 00640 7

FIRST EDITION 1960
SECOND EDITION 1969

Printed in Great Britain

PREFACE TO THE SECOND EDITION

THE object of the Second Edition of this book is the same as that of the First Edition—namely, to provide the veterinary undergraduate with a concise account of the pharmacological properties of the principal drugs used in veterinary therapeutics. However, the book has grown substantially, partly because a large number of new therapeutic agents have been introduced into veterinary medicine, and partly from an expansion of the material. This has entailed a complete revision of the text and some rearrangement of the contents. The number of illustrations has been increased and where possible these have been taken from experiments involving domesticated animals. A selection of chemical formulae has been included; these are not intended to be memorised by the student and, indeed, any such attempt would be an unfortunate waste of time and effort. They are given to draw attention to certain relationships between chemical structure and pharmacological action. A new feature of this Edition is the appendage to each chapter of a short list of selected references chosen to introduce the interested reader to a fuller account of the particular topics of the chapter.

The rate at which new drugs are being marketed makes it essential for the veterinarian to adopt a critical approach to the clinical use of drugs and thus be able to resist some of the less well substantiated claims sometimes made for new drugs. This depends, to a large extent, upon his acquiring a sound grasp of pharmacological principles.

In the decade since the writing of the First Edition there has been a substantial increase in knowledge about the fate of drugs in the body and some interesting differences have been discovered about the way in which various species metabolise drugs. This has, to some extent, provided an explanation for certain of the variations which exist between the domesticated species in their pharmacology. Moreover, the potential toxicity to man of drug residues in the tissues of the food-producing animals lends an additional importance to this aspect of veterinary pharmacology.

The author desires to acknowledge his indebtedness to his colleagues in this school and especially to the members of the Department for their comments and criticism.

F. ALEXANDER

Edinburgh, 1969.

PREFACE TO THE FIRST EDITION

THE purpose of this book is to provide the veterinary undergraduate with a concise account of the pharmacological properties of the principal drugs used in veterinary therapeutics. If therapy is to be scientifically based such knowledge is essential and the main reason veterinary pharmacology is included in the veterinary curriculum is to provide this basis. Moreover, it is hoped that by indicating the kind of information required for a drug to be used to best advantage, the post-graduate reader may be helped to resist the flood of unsubstantiated claims often made for new drugs.

Since the domestic animals differ from man in anatomy, physiology and pathology, the pharmacology of the different drugs has to be studied in relation to the different domestic species. This has given rise to a special branch of pharmacology namely veterinary pharmacology, and the rate of production of new remedies for the diseases of domestic animals makes it essential for this subject to develop and provide the necessary information for the best utilisation of these remedies.

Readers seeking more detailed information than is provided in this text are given an introduction in the Bibliography to the literature in which these details may be found.

The author desires to thank Professors Geo. F. Boddie and Andrew Wilson for their advice, criticism and encouragement and his wife for her tolerance and help in preparing the index.

F. ALEXANDER

Edinburgh, 1960.

CONTENTS

ix

CHAPTER I

INTRODUCTION AND GENERAL PRINCIPLES OF DRUG ADMINISTRATION

INTRODUCTION

PHARMACOLOGY may be defined as the study of the action of drugs on living tissues. It is difficult, however, to separate this from the effects produced by living tissues on drugs, as sometimes it is only after a drug has entered the body, been acted on by the tissues and the drug changed into a different substance that its characteristic pharmacological action is produced. Therefore, it is necessary to study also what happens to the drug in the body, generally termed its fate in the body.

Veterinary pharmacology is concerned with the action of drugs on the tissues of the domesticated animals and the fate of drugs in these species. This information is essential to rational treatment of disease in these animals. Veterinary pharmacology, therefore, provides the scientific basis of veterinary therapeutics.

The action of a drug usually depends upon an adequate concentration being present in the fluids bathing the tissues or in the tissues for a time long enough to produce the effect desired. The concentration and persistence of the drug in these fluids depend upon its absorption, distribution, metabolism and clearance. All these processes involve the passage of the drug across various cell membranes.

There are three main ways by which substances can cross the cell membrane: by simple diffusion, by passage through pores in the membrane, or by means of a specific mechanism. The first of these is the commonest for drugs. This is because the majority of drugs are weak organic electrolytes and in the body are present as ionised and non-ionised molecules. The non-ionised molecules are lipid soluble, whereas the ionised molecules are insoluble in lipids. The cell membrane acts like a lipid membrane and since only the non-ionised molecules are soluble in lipids it follows that the non-ionised molecules will dissolve most readily in the lipids of the cell wall. Thus they will penetrate the cell membrane. Hence the rate at which a drug penetrates a biological membrane depends principally on two physical factors; firstly the solubility of the non-ionised drug molecule in lipids, and secondly, the degree of ionisation of the parent drug.

The lipid insoluble drugs which cross membranes by passing through spaces between the membrane cells are small molecules such as water and urea, and one of the main differences between various anatomical membranes is in the size of these spaces. Hence there are differences between the membranes through which a particular molecule will pass; an example of this is shown in the spaces between the cells of the capillaries and those of the glomeruli. The former are comparatively large and will allow relatively large molecules to pass from the blood plasma to the extracellular fluid, whereas only relatively small molecules can pass through the glomeruli; the usual limiting size of the latter being regarded as that of the hæmoglobin molecule.

Specialised transport mechanisms are usually involved in the movement of naturally occurring compounds across the cell membrane. Sodium ions and glucose are examples of substances transported in this way. These transport mechanisms often involve special carrier substances or special enzyme systems, for example iron is transported by a special carrier protein.

Absorption

The rate and completeness with which a drug enters the body is termed the absorption. It depends not only on the drug itself and on the factors already mentioned but also on the route by which the drug is given. In veterinary practice it is often convenient to give drugs by subcutaneous or intramuscular injection. Absorption from these sites varies from a few minutes in the case of substances like morphine and atropine to several weeks for stilbœstrol diproprionate. The concentration of the drug at the site and the circulation also influence absorption, another important factor is the area of absorbing surface to which the drug is exposed. An example of the latter is shown by the fact that drugs are rapidly absorbed from large absorptive areas such as the intestinal mucosa and pulmonary endothelium. Absorption from an intramuscular injection is usually more rapid than from a subcutaneous injection, and the former route is preferred for the injection of substances which are slightly irritant and might cause pain. However, the subcutaneous space being much greater in the domesticated animals than in man allows greater volumes of fluid to be injected in these species subcutaneously without causing undue discomfort. This route can only be used for drugs which do not cause irritation otherwise a slough may be produced.

As a general rule drugs are not absorbed from the stomach although the epithelium of the rumen is permeable to many substances. The absorption of drugs given by mouth does not usually begin until they pass the pyloric sphincter. This is because the acid conditions in the stomach cause most drugs to ionise and as the ionised drug is insoluble in lipids it does not enter the cell wall. However, a lipid soluble non-electrolyte such as ethanol is rapidly absorbed through the gastric mucous-membrane. Drugs which are weak acids such as the salicylates and barbiturates which are mainly non-ionised in the gastric contents are absorbed from the stomach. The activity of the stomach can greatly influence the rate of absorption. The quickest passage through the stomach in simple stomached animals occurs when this organ is empty and the drug given in a large volume of water. Absorption is delayed when a drug is given in a small volume of water and the stomach is full. Drugs given in a large volume of water when the stomach is full may be absorbed fairly quickly as under these conditions the fluid may pass along the lesser curvature into the duodenum and not mix with the food mass in the stomach.

The absorption of drugs given by mouth to the ruminant presents a special problem. Certain drugs such as atropine can be absorbed through the rumen epithelium, although most substances given by this route are diluted in the large volume of rumen liquor and slowly passed through the abomasum and into the intestine. It may take forty-eight hours for a single dose of a drug to leave the rumen. It is usual to give by mouth to ruminants only those drugs which are required to act within the alimentary tract, such as drugs to change the surface tension of the rumen liquor or to kill parasites in the gastro-intestinal tract.

Absorption time is reduced to a minimum when drugs are given by intravenous injection. This route is chosen therefore, when an immediate effect is desired as when certain anæsthetic agents are given. The intravenous route also allows drugs which are irritant and therefore cannot be given subcutaneously to be administered parenterally with safety. It is essential when administering such a substance to take every precaution to ensure that none of the solution containing the drug is allowed to leak around the vein.

Volatile agents such as the various gaseous anæsthetics are usually given by inhalation. Absorption from the lungs of a volatile drug is very rapid due both to the large absorptive surface available and the good blood flow through the lungs. Drugs may also be given by local application or inserted in a suitable form into the rectum or vagina. These routes are usually employed when a local effect is desired although a few agents are absorbed systemically from these various local applications.

The Distribution of Drugs in the Body

After absorption most substances diffuse through the various fluid compartments of the body. Some drugs cannot penetrate certain cell membranes and are therefore restricted in distribution, whereas others can pass freely into all the fluid compartments.

In the main drugs are distributed as follows :—

(a) through the extracellular fluid, i.e. bromides, thiocyanate, and iodides; (b) through the whole of the body water, i.e. urea, antipyrine; (c) fixed by cells, i.e. digitalis. Sometimes there is an obvious relationship between the distribution of a drug and its site of action, as for example, the high concentration of the aliphatic narcotics in certain parts of the central nervous system as compared with their concentration in blood.

Some drugs may accumulate in various regions as a result of their dissolving in fat or binding with protein. A good example of the latter phenomena which is made use of in experimental and clinical investigations is the very firm binding which takes place between the blue dye, Evans blue, and protein. When a known amount of Evans blue is injected intravenously it binds firmly with the plasma proteins and is thus retained in the circulation. Determinations, at intervals after intravenous injection, of the concentration of Evans blue in plasma and extrapolation of the resulting curve allows an estimate of the theoretical concentration of the drug at zero time to be made. This procedure avoids artifacts due to the initial mixing of the dye with the blood. If the concentration at zero time is divided into the amount of drug given, one obtains the volume of fluid through which the drug is distributed, and in this case it represents very nearly the volume of plasma in the body.

It is possible to measure the volume of extracellular fluid by estimating in a similar fashion the distribution volume of substances such as sodium thiocyanate or thiosulphate. The values obtained by these methods do not agree completely with determination of extracellular fluid by isotope dilution techniques, and it is more correct to speak of thiocyanate or thiosulphate space. Nonetheless, they give values which are useful particularly in clinical investigations.

Clearance of Drugs

Drugs are removed from the body either unchanged or after conversion into some other substance. These conversions usually take place in the liver. The kidney and intestinal epithelium can also metabolise drugs. The unchanged drug or its metabolites usually are excreted by the kidneys, although volatile substances are excreted largely through the lungs. The bile is an excretory route for some substances, but not a very efficient one as many of these substances are re-absorbed from the small intestine. A few drugs are excreted by the alimentary tract.

In most cases the removal of a drug from the body resembles a " wash out " process. That is a constant proportion of the drug is removed in a unit of time, a similar process to washing out a bucket full of a dye by allowing water from a tap to run into the bucket and the coloured liquid to overflow. It is also

B

called exponential clearance. An example of this is shown in Figure 1.1.

Excretion through the kidney involves three processes; a passive filtration through the glomerulus, active secretion in the tubules and passive diffusion in the tubules. The amount of drug entering the tubules in the glomerular filtrate depends not only on the rate of filtration but also on the degree of protein binding of the drug. Many drugs bind to a greater or

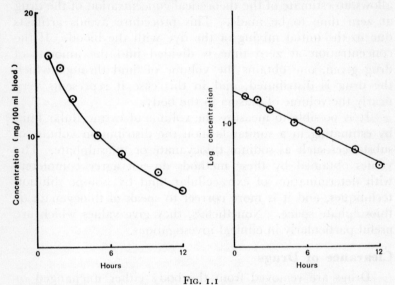

FIG. 1.1

The concentration of sulphanilamide in blood, following the intravenous injection of 160 mg/kg to a sheep, plotted on an arithmetic and a semi-logarithmic scale. The linear nature of the latter curve shows the exponential form of the clearance.

lesser extent with the plasma proteins. The degree of binding influences their glomerular filtration, and their activity. Generally speaking when a drug is bound to protein it is pharmacologically inactive. The binding may be very firm, as for example with Evans blue, or loose, in which case the drug is readily separated. The bound drug is not filtered at the glomerulus.

DETOXICATION

This term is applied to the changes which a drug undergoes after absorption. It is not an entirely satisfactory term as these changes do not always make the substance less poisonous; they may in fact increase toxicity. An example of toxicity being increased by metabolism is shown by the fate in the body of the chemical compound 2-naphthylamine. This compound which is an important substance in the chemical industry, will produce a tumour of the bladder in man and dogs, but not in rats. The reason for this species difference is that although 2-naphthylamine itself is not carcinogenic it forms a metabolite in man and dog which is tumour forming. Since the rat does not form this metabolite, it does not develop bladder tumours. It is probably better to refer to this process as Biometabolism or Biotransformation and to avoid the term detoxication.

The principal reactions involved in Biometabolism or Biotransformation are (1) **combination with sulphuric acid,** for example phenol; (2) **combination with glucuronic acid**, for example steroid compounds; (3) **oxidation,** this is carried out by a group of enzymes which appear to be situated in the microsomes of the liver. These oxidations usually involve hydroxylation reactions; the enzymes responsible being termed hydroxylases, NADPH being an essential co-factor. Certain oxidations take place by dehydrogenation, for example ethyl alcohol is oxidised in the first instance to acetaldehyde by ethanol dehydrogenase; (4) **reduction,** for example, chloral hydrate, which is reduced to trichlorethanol. This latter compound is in fact the substance to which chloral hydrate owes its pharmacological activity; (5) **methylation,** this transformation occurs with a number of pharmacologically active substances, such as adrenaline, noradrenaline and histamine; (6) **acetylation,** certain drugs with an amino group such as sulphanilamide are acetylated by some species; (7) **dehalogenation,** this transformation occurs with a number of halogenated hydrocarbons, such as certain insecticides; (8) **hydrolysis,** a number of drugs such as procaine and various choline esters are de-esterified by esterases which are widespread in the body.

In the main, detoxication reactions transform the drug into a form which is more readily excreted. For example, by forming a glucuronide a drug is usually made more water soluble, hence when the glucuronide passes through the renal tubules it is less likely to be re-absorbed by entering the lipid membranes of the tubular epithelial cells whereas the more fat soluble parent compound would be absorbed at this site. The oxidation of ethanol ultimately results in the transformation of ethanol into carbon dioxide and water, substances which can be completely removed from the body, one being expired through the lungs and the other being excreted in the urine.

The manner in which drugs are metabolised varies in a number of important ways in the different domesticated species. Cats, for example, lack the enzyme which enables certain drugs to form a glucuronide, hence drugs which are usually detoxicated by glucuronide formation, such as acetylsalicylic acid may be more toxic in the cat than in other species. Similarly the cat lacks various oxidative enzymes. Since these hydroxylases are important in the detoxication of various barbiturates, the cat is less able to metabolise such compounds; hence great care must be used when administering these drugs to the cat. Adult ruminants and horses appeared to be well endowed with oxidative enzymes, and can, therefore, deal with larger amounts of drugs which are metabolised by oxidation, than can other species. The dog lacks the enzyme involved in acetylating drugs, hence sulphonamides when given to the dog are not metabolised by acetylation. On the other hand the dog in common with other species has a de-acetylating enzyme, and sometimes in this species a toxic compound is formed from a drug which is non-toxic in other species, this occurs in the case of the analgesic phenacetin which forms a toxic compound on de-acetylation. This toxic compound persists in the dog because of the lack of an acetylating enzyme.

Cumulation

Drugs which are slowly excreted or slowly detoxicated tend to accumulate in the body. When such substances are given at frequent intervals the amount retained in the body may be sufficient to produce signs of poisoning. This process is called cumulation.

A cumulative effect can be avoided by adjusting the maintenance dose so as to balance the rate at which the drug is inactivated or excreted.

Tolerance

This may be described as the state in which increasing doses are required to produce the same pharmacological or therapeutic effect. Sometimes by administering one drug, the animal becomes tolerant to a second drug; this is referred to as cross-tolerance. Although there is no ready explanation of this condition, some facts are available which may partly account for the phenomenon. It is known, for example, that prior treatment with phenobarbitone has an effect on the liver microsomes so that their oxidative enzyme activity is increased causing subsequent doses of phenobarbitone to be metabolised at an increasing rate. This increased metabolism affects not only phenobarbitone but other drugs which are metabolised by these oxidative enzymes. **Idiosyncrasy** to a drug may be said to exist when the response of an individual animal to a single dose of the drug produces an unexpected or untoward effect.

Summation

This is the addition of the effect of one drug to that of one or more other drugs with similar properties, as for example, in certain mixtures of sulphonamides.

Synergism

This is a term applied to the combined action of two drugs with similar pharmacological properties, when the effect produced is greater than the sum of the effect of each drug given singly. For example, both ammonium chloride and mersalyl are diuretics, which when given together produce a much greater diuresis than when an equiactive dose of either drug is given separately.

Potentiation

This is a term applied to the enhancement of the action of one drug by another with dissimilar properties, for example, the action of penicillin can be prolonged when probenecid is given either before or along with the penicillin. Probenecid delays the urinary excretion of penicillin.

Knowledge of a drug's absorption, distribution, detoxication and clearance are essential for the veterinary surgeon to decide by which route and how often he will need to give the substance.

SUGGESTIONS FOR FURTHER READING

BINNS, T. B. ed. (1964). *The Absorption and Distribution of Drugs.* Edinburgh: Livingstone.

SCHANKER, L. S. (1962). The passage of drugs across body membranes. *Pharmac. Rev.*, **14**, 501.

WEINER, I. M. (1967). Mechanisms of drug absorption and excretion. *A. Rev. Pharmac.*, **7**, 39.

WILLIAMS, R. T. (1959). *Detoxication Mechanisms*, 2nd ed. London: Chapman & Hall.

CHAPTER II

WATER, ELECTROLYTE METABOLISM AND REPLACEMENT FLUIDS

UNLIKE the chemist in a laboratory the body cannot utilise strong acids and alkalis or high temperatures in order to carry out the chemical processes essential to life. It has, therefore, to employ more roundabout methods by which it performs similar reactions at body temperature, and at neutrality. This is brought about by special catalysts called enzymes. Many drugs produce their effects by interfering with these enzymatic reactions and because of this it is easier to understand how such comparatively small amounts of drugs can produce such marked effects.

The chemical reactions of the body are for the most part carried out in water which is itself the largest single constituent of the body. The preservation of a constant internal environment is essential to life; Claude Bernard described this environment as the *"milieu intérieur"* and was the first to appreciate its importance. Many of the body functions are directed to preserve this constancy of the internal environment whilst at the same time permitting these chemical reactions to take place.

BODY WATER

The body water is distributed into the intra- and extracellular water and the blood plasma. Intracellular water in man comprises about 50 per cent of the fat-free body weight, extracellular water 15–24 per cent, and plasma 5 per cent. These values for intra- and extracellular water are probably rather high for adult ruminants because of the large weight of alimentary tract contents in these animals, and in sheep the fleece is an additional factor in increasing body weight without affecting body water.

Total body water may be measured by determining the distribution volume of a drug which is evenly distributed throughout the whole body water. The substance which answers best this requirement is deuterium or tritium oxide. Unfortunately the determination of these substances requires special facilities which are not generally available, hence the antipyretic, antipyrine or what is considered a better substance the acetylated derivative, n-acetyl antipyrine, have been used extensively for the determination of total body water. The technique employed for a determination of antipyrine space is similar to that described in the first chapter for the determination of plasma volume with Evans blue. Determinations of the total body water of cows using n-acetyl antipyrine

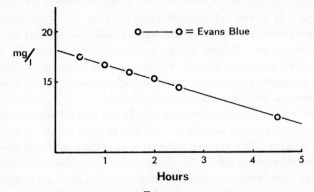

FIG. 2.1

The distribution volume of Evans blue.

A pony weighing 145 kg was given 100 mg Evans blue by intravenous injection. Extrapolation of the clearance curve gave an initial concentration of 18 mg/litre. The distribution volume was 5.5 litres representing 3.8 per cent of the body weight. The packed cell volume (PCV) was 30 per cent, hence the blood volume was 5.4 per cent of the body weight.

gave values between 42 and 51 per cent and that of horses measured by tritiated water 55–64 per cent of their body weight.

Sodium thiocyanate and sodium thiosulphate, inulin and radio-active chloride are substances which are distributed through the extracellular fluid; hence the determination of the thiocyanate space gives an indication of the extracellular water. By subtracting the value obtained for the extracellular water from that obtained for the total body water, a value for the intracellular water may be obtained. Plasma volume may be determined by measuring the distribution volume of the dye Evans blue, which because of its high affinity for plasma protein when injected intravenously stays in the circulation for a substantial period of time. Since, as with most drugs, the clearance from the blood of the substances used for determining these various fractions of the body follow an exponential course, it is preferable to plot the logarithm of the concentration against time which gives a nearly straight line. This can be extrapolated back to zero more easily than the arithmetic curve: an example of the use of Evans blue in the determination of the plasma volume in the horse is shown in Figure 2.1.

The constancy of composition of the extracellular fluid has been referred to already; the mechanisms by which it is maintained are very complex and by no means fully understood. They include the synthesis and release of plasma protein, respiratory reflexes for the excretion and retention of carbon dioxide, absorptive functions of the alimentary tract, cellular activity in maintaining ionic equilibrium and the functions of the renal tubule.

The water content of the body is regulated mainly by the kidneys, absorption of water by the distal tubule being controlled by the antidiuretic hormone (ADH). This hormone is formed in the supra-optic nucleus and passes down to the pars-nervosa of the pituitary gland. Its release is determined by osmoreceptors in the central nervous system which respond to changes in osmotic pressure and by volume receptors in the heart and great blood vessels which respond to changes in circulating volume of blood. If any of these mechanisms fail, chemical changes result which, if uncorrected, will be fatal. A calf with scours loses considerable quantities of water and electrolytes because the absorptive functions of the colon are disturbed. Death in such cases is due to cardiac failure which is produced in part by the hæmoconcentration consequent on the loss of fluid and electrolytes. It follows, therefore, that therapeutic measures should include replacement of fluid and electrolytes in addition to measures aimed at restoring normal function to the bowel.

It follows from the above that the internal environment can be changed by drugs acting on any of the mechanisms described.   For example, since the main organ involved in maintaining the volume and electrolyte composition of the body fluids is the kidney, drugs acting on the kidney affect the volume and composition of the body fluids.

The main drugs affecting water and electrolyte balance are various replacement fluids, certain hormones of the adrenal cortex and of the posterior pituitary gland and diuretics.

REPLACEMENT FLUIDS

The main cation of the extracellular fluid is sodium, whereas the main cations of the intracellular fluid are potassium and magnesium.   The main anions of the extracellular fluid are bicarbonate and chloride and of the intracellular fluid phosphate and protein.   The respective concentrations of these various electrolytes depends on the integrity of the cell membranes. If, for example, the cell membranes disintegrate to any great extent enough potassium may be released to affect the heart, and could stop the heartbeat.

When body fluids have been lost, treatment should be directed at (a) restoring and maintaining an adequate volume of blood in circulation, (b) at arresting the loss of fluid and (c) at restoring the disturbance of the body fluids by giving water and electrolytes.   The circulating blood volume is usually restored by the transfusion of whole blood, plasma or plasma substitute.   The replacement of water and electrolytes is secondary to this.   It should be appreciated that the redistribution of water and electrolytes subsequent to a serious disturbance takes time.   Sodium deficiencies may require 2–3 days before an equilibrium is obtained and in potassium deficiency a week or more may be required.   When replacement fluids are administered it is important to take account of acid-base balance.

Glucose

It is sometimes desirable to supply water without electrolytes.   This is most conveniently done during intravenous fluid therapy by injecting a solution of 5.5 per cent glucose. The glucose is removed either by oxidation or converted into glycogen leaving the water.   Glucose solutions are also used to supply a source of energy and to spare protein; in such cases the glucose concentration may be increased to 10 per cent.

Lactate

In severe acidosis solutions of sodium lactate, one-sixth molar, are injected intravenously because about half the lactate is converted to bicarbonate. The remainder forms liver glycogen which in turn is converted into bicarbonate after a period. Severe acidosis is a complicating factor in starvation and diarrhœa.

Electrolytes

Isotonic solutions of sodium chloride are often given parenterally to replace these ions which are lost in considerable amounts in diarrhœa or persistent vomiting. Such treatment is, of course, ancillary to efforts to remove the cause of the diarrhœa or vomiting. Sometimes the chlorides of potassium and calcium are included with sodium chloride, as in Ringer's solution, to make the injected solution more like the extra-cellular fluid it is replacing.

It should be appreciated that replacement fluids either of electrolytes or non-electrolytes can be given in excess. A syndrome called " water intoxication " can be produced in dogs, and presumably other species by giving too much water; this may happen with the parenteral administration of fluids. Amongst the main features of this syndrome are muscle tremors, convulsions and cerebral œdema; hæmoglobinuria may also occur.

Isotonic solutions of sodium chloride are only distributed in the extracellular fluid, therefore when injected in large volumes œdema may be produced. Where the cardiac function is good the fluid will pass the capillary bed and peripheral œdema occur. If the cardiac function is impaired hydrostatic pressure in the pulmonary circulation may rise and pulmonary œdema be produced. This is usually fatal.

Blood, plasma and synthetic substitutes

When blood or plasma has been lost from the circulation the various saline solutions mentioned are of little value in restoring the blood volume, because they pass very quickly from the circulation into the extracellular fluid. Loss of whole blood as occurs in hæmorrhage from various causes, is best replaced by whole blood. Blood is collected from a donor animal under aseptic conditions with an anticoagulant such as sodium citrate. It is injected intravenously into the recipient, after matching the serum of the recipient with the red cells of the donor to eliminate the possibility that the donor blood is incompatible and likely to produce a transfusion reaction.

Loss of blood plasma occurs during shock which may be produced by trauma, burning or surgery and is due mainly to an increase in permeability of the capillaries to plasma, allowing it to pass into the interstitial fluid. Blood plasma can be used to restore this loss but may not be readily available and the plasma volume is most conveniently replaced by a synthetic substitute. A plasma substitute should have a viscosity similar to that of plasma and an osmotic pressure similar to that of the plasma proteins. It should be stable over a wide range of temperature, easily sterilized and free from pyrogens. It should be non-toxic and not give rise to the formation of antibodies when injected. Plasma substitutes should be retained long enough in circulation for the plasma proteins to be restored, but ultimately the plasma substitute should be completely excreted or metabolised.

The retention of a substance in the capillaries depends on its physical properties and in particular, on the size and shape of the actual molecules. The molecular weight of plasma protein ranges between that of albumin which is 69,000 to that of fibrinogen which is of the order of 400,000. Albumin which is normally retained in the capillaries leaves them during inflammation because in this condition they become permeable to larger molecules. It follows then that for plasma substitutes to be retained in the circulation they should have a molecular weight greater than 70,000. It is also obvious that the only route of administration by which plasma substitutes may be given is by intravenous injection.

No plasma substitute is entirely free from drawbacks. *Dextran*, a polysaccharide made by the bacterial fermentation of sucrose is probably the most popular. This polymer of glucose is injected intravenously as a 6 per cent solution in isotonic saline. Preparations of dextran vary in molecular size, the average size being 75,000. After injection the molecules of smaller molecular weight are excreted by the kidney. This may account for as much as half the dose. However, the remainder persist in the circulation being slowly oxidised over a period of weeks. Dextran has no harmful effects on the liver or kidneys. The chief objection to dextran is that it may act as an antigen and produce sensitivity reactions.

Polyvinyl pyrrolidine is a polymer of acetylene and has been used as a plasma substitute. It has not proved popular and may, by releasing histamine from the tissues, produce a fatal fall in blood pressure, particularly in dogs.

PARENTERAL FEEDING

As well as maintaining the volume and composition of the body fluids, it is sometimes necessary to supply the energy and nitrogen requirements of a sick animal by injection, as after injury both the water excretion and nitrogen metabolism are disturbed. Energy is usually supplied as glucose. Maintenance of nitrogen balance is more difficult and as yet it is not practicable to supply all the essential amino acids by injection. However, casein, which has been hydrolysed by enzymes to amino-acids and short chain peptides is available in 5 per cent solution with or without 5 per cent glucose. Calories can sometimes be supplied by the administration of ethanol but it is important to remember the narcotic actions of this drug. Parenteral feeding of fat may be accomplished by injecting intravenously an emulsion of 15 per cent cotton-seed oil together with 4 per cent glucose.

SUGGESTIONS FOR FURTHER READING

BLACK, D. A. K. (1964). The alimentary tract and body-fluids. In *The Scientific Basis of Medicine Annual Reviews*, p. 291. University of London: Athlone Press.

PITTS, R. F. (1964). *The Physiology of the Kidney and Body Fluids*. Chicago: Year Book of Medicine Publications.

WILKINSON, A. W. (1969). *Body Fluids in Surgery*, 3rd ed. Edinburgh: Livingstone.

CHAPTER III

DRUGS AFFECTING FLUID AND ELECTROLYTE BALANCE

Adrenal-cortical hormones; diuretics

THE constant composition of the body fluids and the importance of their remaining so has been discussed. Certain endocrine organs secrete substances which are responsible to a large extent for maintaining this. The anterior pituitary gland secretes a substance which stimulates the secretions of the adrenal cortex and the adrenal cortex secretes a number of substances which include, amongst other properties, that of regulating the re-absorption of sodium, potassium and chloride ions by the renal tubule. The posterior pituitary gland secretes a substance which by acting on the renal tubule regulates the excretion of water. This substance is called the **antidiuretic hormone** (ADH) and so far has not found a place in therapeutics. In the absence of ADH the collecting tubules are impermeable to water, hence a very dilute urine is produced.

THE ADRENAL CORTEX

The hormones secreted by this gland are essential to maintain homeostasis. For ease of understanding they are divided into two groups, the mineralocorticoids and the glucocorticoids. However, it is essential to appreciate that such a division is quite arbitrary, as the glucocorticoids possess some mineralocortical activity and *vice versa*. Electrolyte and water metabolism is influenced mainly by the mineralocorticoids, the principal representative being **aldosterone**. The synthetic hormone **deoxycortone acetate** has similar but weaker actions. In the absence of aldosterone the renal tubule appears to be unable to distinguish between sodium and potassium ions. As a consequence large amounts of sodium chloride and corresponding quantities of water are lost by the body whilst the re-absorption of potassium by the kidney produces a sodium/potassium imbalance in the tissues. The loss of water causes hæmoconcentration, a fall in blood pressure and in metabolism. Animals deficient in adrenal cortical hormones may be kept alive by giving large quantities of sodium chloride, but such animals are easily killed by cold, shock and infection. There are, however, marked differences between species in respect to the ease with which adrenalectomized animals may be kept alive by administration of sodium chloride. Adrenalectomized rabbits, for example, resist the effects of restriction of their sodium chloride intake. This is presumably because their renal and possibly intestinal absorption of sodium is particularly efficient. Adrenalectomized rabbits, moreover, do not appear to require mineralocorticoids excepting when the sodium loss is forced by the use of diuretics. Adrenalectomized rats can be maintained by the administration of sodium chloride, but adrenalectomised dogs are less easily maintained.

Aldosterone is secreted by the zona glomerulosa. The secretion of aldosterone is governed by the plasma levels of sodium and potassium, renin from the kidneys and ACTH from the anterior pituitary. There is some evidence that a glomerulotrophin from the pineal area of the brain may be involved in regulating aldosterone secretion. Aldosterone has about 2,000 times the sodium retaining activity of the glucocorticoid cortisone and 40 times that of deoxycortone acetate

Renin is an enzyme present in the kidneys, which reacts with a plasma globulin called hypertensinogen to form a polypeptide with vasoconstrictor properties. The polypeptide is called angiotensin, it has been found to contain ten amino acid residues and a polypeptide with similar properties has been synthesized.

Aldosterone Antagonists

A number of steroids have been synthesized which reverse the action of the mineralocorticoids on the renal transport of sodium. These substances are potentially useful diuretics. **Spironolactone** is probably the best known member of this group. Spironolactone resembles aldosterone in structure; it decreases the potassium excretion and increases the excretion

of sodium, chloride and water in the presence of either exogenous
or endogenous mineralocorticoids. Clinically Spironolactone
has been of use only in subjects in which mercurial and other
diuretics have caused an excessive excretion of potassium.

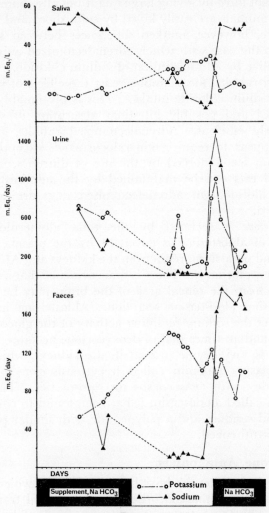

FIG. 3.1

The effect of sodium depletion in the horse on the
excretion of sodium and potassium in the saliva, urine
and faeces. Pony in negative sodium balance unless
receiving supplement.

Evidence that the antagonism of spironolactone with aldosterone is a direct one and concerned with the action of aldosterone on the renal tubule is as follows : spironolactone has little or no effect on the electrolytes in the urine in adrenalectomized animals unless mineralocorticoids are administered. The electrolyte excretion pattern produced by spironolactone in normal animals resembles that produced by the sudden withdrawal of aldosterone. Spironolactone does not act by interfering with aldosterone synthesis because it does not cause changes in either the rate of secretion of aldosterone or the amount of aldosterone in the urine.

Evidence of the action of aldosterone on sodium retention can be shown in sodium deplete animals. This situation can be produced without undue difficulty in both sheep and horses, since these animals secrete large volumes of saliva containing substantial amounts of sodium. Therefore, if they are prepared with fistulae of the parotid duct so that the saliva is lost and not swallowed and their diet adjusted to contain minimal amounts of sodium, they soon show a marked decrease in the sodium content of not only urine, but also fæces and saliva. This is accompanied by a commensurate increase in the secretion of potassium, and is brought about by an increased secretion of aldosterone, which is stimulated by the sodium loss so that the animal makes every effort to retain a maximum amount of sodium. An illustration of this is shown in Figure 3.1.

DRUGS AFFECTING ELECTROLYTE
METABOLISM

The kidneys are essential in the maintenance of a constant internal environment. By regulating the excretion of water they maintain the osmotic pressure of blood and the ratio between the blood proteins and the other constituents of blood. They maintain the alkali reserve by excreting nonvolatile acids and forming ammonia to neutralise excess acid. In essence the glomerulus provides a large volume of protein-free filtrate of plasma, which is mostly re-absorbed during the progress of the fluid through the renal tubule. The remaining small volume of liquid is modified in composition and pH to

C

emerge as urine. The proximal convoluted tubule reduces the volume of glomerular filtrate to about 20 per cent. This is accomplished for the most part by an active re-absorption of sodium, which in order to maintain isosmotic conditions is accompanied by passive re-absorption of both water and chloride. There is also in this region the re-absorption of potassium by an active process, and bicarbonate by a special mechanism involving the enzyme carbonic anhydrase. Glucose and amino acids are actively re-absorbed in this region.

The fluid then passes through the loop of Henle, where the volume is unchanged but the osmolality profoundly modified. Osmolality is the osmotic concentration in a kilogram of water, and osmotic concentration refers to the number of particles in solution. The size of the particle does not affect osmotic concentration. The osmolality of the glomerular filtrate is practically that of plasma, and since re-absorption in the proximal tubule is isosmotic, the fluid has still the same osmolality (285 mOsm/kg). However, in the loop of Henle this changes, osmolality increasing in the descending limb and decreasing in the ascending limb until the fluid which enters the distal convoluted tubule is appreciably hypotonic to plasma (140 mOsm/kg).

The increase in osmolality in the loop of Henle enables the animal to produce a concentrated urine. This is accomplished by the active transport of sodium from the ascending limb against a concentration gradient into the interstitium, whilst at the same time the ascending limb is impermeable to water. This leads to a high sodium concentration in the interstitium. Since the flow in the ascending limb is in the opposite direction to that in the descending limb, i.e. countercurrent, and sodium can enter the descending limb by free diffusion because this limb is freely permeable to sodium and water, the concentration of sodium increases towards the turn of the loop. This is facilitated by the two limbs of the loop being close together, and by this process the osmolality at the turn of the loop is increased to something of the order of 1200 mOsm/kg.

The removal of sodium during the flow through the ascending loop is continued in the distal convoluted tubule giving an osmolality of about 150 mOsm/kg. In the absence of ADH both the distal convoluted tubule and the collecting duct are impermeable to water, and a very dilute urine is produced. When ADH is present the fluid in the distal convoluted tubule becomes isotonic with plasma because the permeability to water

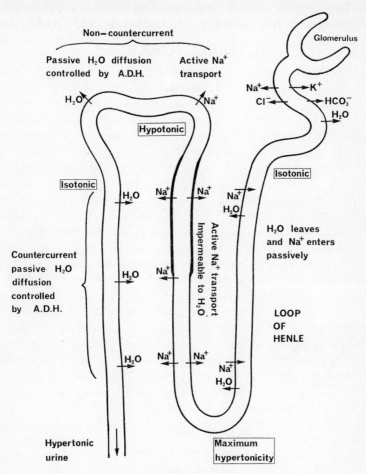

FIG. 3.2
A diagrammatic representation of factors controlling the tonicity of urine.
(*Courtesy P. Eyre.*)

is increased. This allows a small volume of fluid to enter the collecting tubules which themselves are permeable to water in the presence of ADH. Water, therefore, passes from the collecting duct because of the osmotic gradient in the medullary interstitium which is produced by the high osmolality in and around the loops of Henle, which are present in this region.

The variable osmotic concentration of urine is due largely to changes in the quantity of ADH released. ADH also

RENAL TUBULE

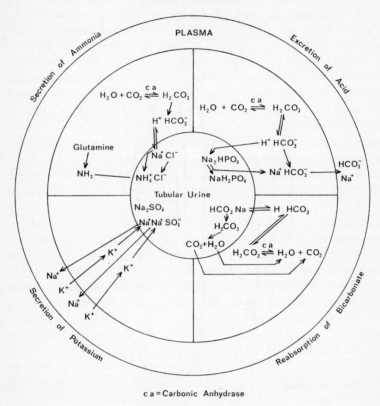

c a = Carbonic Anhydrase

FIG. 3.3
A diagrammatic representation of the factors involved in regulating urinary pH.

increases the permeability of the collecting tubule to urea; this increases the concentration of urea in the medullary interstitium and so contributes to the hypertonicity of this region produced by the countercurrent mechanism.

In the distal convoluted tubule the re-absorption of sodium is associated with an exchange of sodium ions for either potassium ions or hydrogen ions. Aldosterone and other mineralocorticoids increase the exchange of potassium for sodium. The exchange of hydrogen for sodium regulates the excretion of acid, ammonium and bicarbonate ions. These processes are indicated diagrammatically in Figure 3.2.

Acid is produced within the cells of the renal tubule from the reaction between water and carbon dioxide of metabolic origin. This reaction is catalysed by the enzyme carbonic anhydrase, and gives rise to carbonic acid which ionizes into hydrogen ions and bicarbonate ions. The hydrogen ions exchange with sodium ions, which are present in the lumen of the tubule in the form of disodium hydrogen phosphate. After the exchange has taken place the hydrogen ions in the lumen combine to form sodium dihydrogen phosphate, thus lowering the pH of the fluid in the tubule. This exchange gives rise theoretically and transiently to hydrochloric acid, which stimulates the amino acid glutamine to be deaminated forming ammonia which diffuses from the tubular cell into the lumen of the tubule and combines with the hydrochloric acid to form ammonium chloride. The body can conserve bicarbonate by utilising the reaction between CO_2 and water catalysed by carbonic anhydrase, but in this case the hydrogen ions exchange with sodium ions existing in the lumen of the tubule as sodium bicarbonate. This exchange results in the production of carbonic acid in the lumen which breaks down to form water and CO_2. The CO_2 diffuses back into the renal tubular cell and can under the influence of carbonic anhydrase combine again with water to form carbonic acid and in turn more hydrogen ions. Potassium ions in the tubular cell can exchange directly with sodium ions in the lumen, the mechanism for the exchange of sodium for potassium being similar to that involved in the exchange of sodium for hydrogen (Fig. 3.3.)

DIURETICS

Diuretics are drugs which increase the net excretion of sodium and water by the kidney. They are used to reduce the amount of water in the body when this is excessive, as in œdema, or to help in the removal of toxic substances from the body. In veterinary practice diuretics are rarely used because chronic disease is not often treated. However, they are employed in the treatment of œdema of cardiac or renal origin as well as certain other kinds of œdema. Diuretics are used also to supplement an antibacterial drug in treatment of infections of the urinary tract or to make the pH of the urine such that an antibacterial agent can exert its greatest effect.

Drugs may increase the excretion of water by the kidneys in two ways (a) by increasing glomerular filtration; (b) by decreasing tubular re-absorption. Most diuretics act in the latter way, although some act on both mechanisms.

OSMOTIC DIURETICS

A solute which is filtered by the glomerulus and is not re-absorbed to any great extent in the tubules acts as an osmotic diuretic.

Neutral salts and urea are substances which, when given to animals by mouth are easily absorbed from the gut, have no undesirable pharmacological effects and are excreted by the kidney, carrying with them a large volume of water. These substances are not re-absorbed from the tubules to any great extent and increase the excretion of sodium and chloride as well as water. This latter effect is important in the treatment of œdema. Potassium nitrate is the most important osmotic diuretic for horses and cattle, although potassium acetate may be used for the same purpose. Nitrates given to ruminants by mouth are reduced to nitrites by the rumen bacteria. Urea has to be given in such large amounts as to be somewhat impractical. Moreover, given by mouth to ruminants, it is used as a source of nitrogen to manufacture bacterial protein. Potassium salts are preferable to sodium salts as diuretics, because they have a lower renal threshold. However, when the kidneys are functioning abnormally they may be dangerous, as, if they are retained by the body, the excess potassium ions may cause irregularities of the heart beat or even stop the beat. Sodium sulphate is sometimes given by intravenous injection to increase urine flow. This effect is produced by the sulphate ions which pass in the glomerular filtrate and are not re-absorbed in the tubules. Therefore, an increased amount of sulphate will be present within the tubule together with an equivalent amount of cation and water, thus an equivalent amount of water together with sulphate and cation will be excreted into the bladder.

ACIDIFYING DIURETICS

Large doses of **ammonium chloride** or **calcium chloride** reduce the alkaline reserve and this is accompanied by diuresis. The calcium chloride given by mouth forms calcium carbonate by reacting with the carbonates and bicarbonates of the gut contents. The calcium carbonate is insoluble and, therefore, is not absorbed. This immobilisation of the calcium ions frees the chloride ions which are absorbed in excess producing an acidosis. The excess chloride ions take sodium from the alkaline reserve and are excreted with it in solution in water, thus increasing urine flow. The chloride ions from ammonium chloride behave in the same way, the difference lying in the way the drug is metabolised. Ammonium chloride is a water soluble salt which is absorbed from the gut; the ammonium ions are converted into urea in the liver, liberating chloride ions. In ruminants the ammonia through secretion in the saliva may be converted into microbial protein in the rumen.

Since there is only a limited amount of fixed base the administration of these drugs would soon produce a severe acidosis were it not for the fact that acidifying drugs stimulate the kidney to produce ammonia from amino-acids. This ammonia neutralises the excess acid which is excreted in combination with ammonia. Thus acidifying drugs only produce diuresis during the time it takes to reduce the fixed base enough to stimulate ammonia production. The acidifying diuretics are used to supplement the mercurial diuretics, which they potentiate.

XANTHINE DIURETICS

The chief derivatives of xanthine used as diuretics are **caffeine, theophylline** and **theobromine.** Caffeine and theophylline are stimulants of the central nervous system; theobromine is not. Therefore, although theophylline is the most active diuretic of these three drugs, theobromine is preferable because it can be given in very large doses without producing cerebral effects.

These drugs produce their diuretic effect by decreasing the tubular absorption of water, and, by increasing the blood flow through the kidney, increase the rate of glomerular filtration. This latter effect is due to the action of the xanthines on the heart and blood vessels. The xanthine diuretics are usually administered as double salts, theobromine and sodium salicylate, theophylline and sodium acetate. This is because such compounds are more soluble in water. The xanthines are rarely used for their diuretic actions because of the availability of the more active mercurial diuretics and derivatives of the carbonic anhydrase inhibitor diuretics.

MERCURIAL DIURETICS

Mercury in the form of calomel has been used as a diuretic since the sixteenth century. Nowadays organic compounds of mercury are preferred because they are largely and quickly excreted by the kidney and have a low dissociability. This allows them to interfere with tubular function without producing any pathological changes. The mercurial diuretics prevent the active re-absorption in the renal tubule of sodium and chloride and probably act by inhibiting certain enzyme systems with active thiol (SH) groups. This probability is supported by the fact that dimercaprol, an organic compound with SH groups, inhibits the action of mercurial diuretics. **Mersalyl** is the official name of a mercurial diuretic which is given by intramuscular injection.

CARBONIC ANHYDRASE INHIBITORS

The conservation of fixed cation depends on the exchange of H^+ in the renal tubule cell with Na^+ in the tubule urine. The source of H^+ is carbonic acid. This is formed from the reaction between CO_2 and H_2O which is catalysed by carbonic anhydrase. The enzyme carbonic anhydrase was discovered in 1932 by Meldrum and Roughton, and five years later it was observed that the administration of sulphanilamide produced acidosis, a loss of base and an alkaline urine. A few years later it was found that the nitrogen of the amide in sulphanilamide could be substituted and these substituted sulphonamides inhibited carbonic anhydrase. About the same time carbonic anhydrase was found in the kidney, and shortly afterwards the important part played by this enzyme in the tubular re-absorption of electrolytes was discovered. The importance of the substituted sulphonamides was appreciated and in the early 1950's a number of heterocyclic sulphonamides were synthesized, one of which acetazolamide was sufficiently potent and non-toxic to be introduced as an effective diuretic.

Acetazolamide is a drug whose actions are due to the inhibition of carbonic anhydrase. When carbonic anhydrase is inhibited hydrogen ions are no longer available within the renal tubular cell for exchange with sodium ions present in the lumen of the renal tubule where they exist as disodium hydrogen phosphate or sodium bicarbonate; hence not only is the re-absorption of bicarbonate reduced but titrable acid and ammonia disappear from the urine. The kidney thus produces an increased volume of alkaline urine. The net result is the removal of sodium bicarbonate and an isosmotic equivalent of water from the extracellular fluid via the kidney. Acetazolamide can be given by mouth as it is well absorbed from the gut and completely excreted within 24 hours.

Since carbonic anhydrase is involved in the production of aqueous humor, acetazolamide can be given either orally or parenterally to reduce intra-ocular pressure. The disease glaucoma is characterised by an increased intra-ocular pressure and can be treated by either the administration of a myotic such as eserine or with acetazolamide; sometimes both drugs are given.

BENZOTHIADIAZIDES

Chlorothiazide was discovered during the course of the synthesis of a series of carbonic anhydrase inhibitors. Although this drug is a much less potent inhibitor of carbonic anhydrase than acetazolamide, it is a more active diuretic. Its administration causes a marked increase in the urinary excretion of sodium, potassium and chloride. It has been suggested that chlorothiazide may be secreted in the proximal tubule and act at this site. The actual mechanism of action is not understood and probably does not involve carbonic anhydrase inhibition to any great extent because in contrast to acetazolamide the main anion in the urine after chlorothiazide treat-

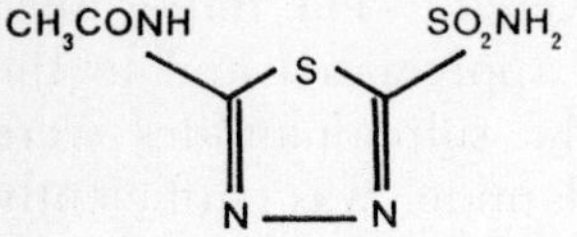

Acetazolamide

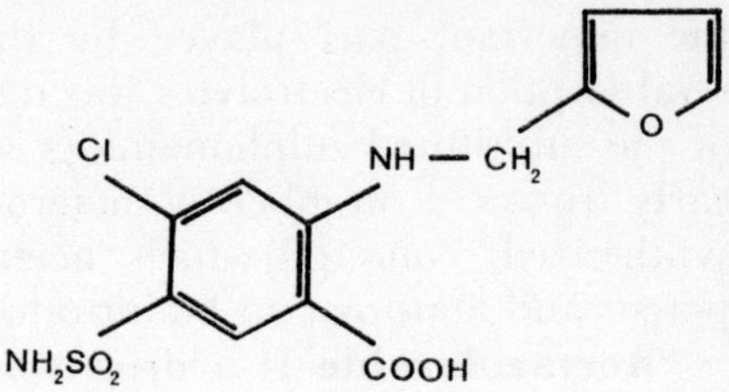

Frusemide

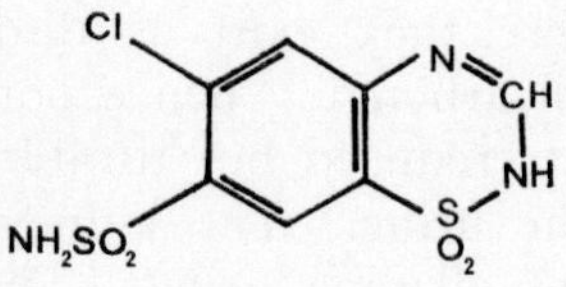

Chlorothiazide

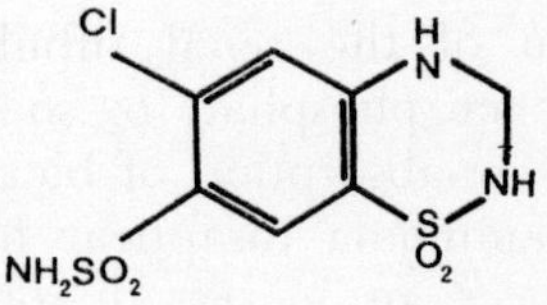

Hydrochlorthiazide

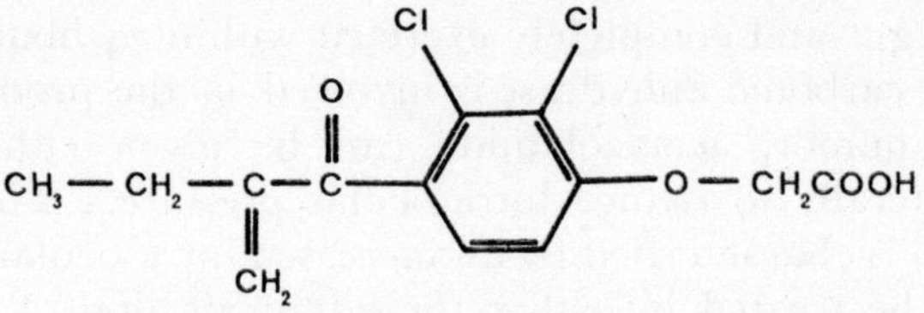

Ethacrynic Acid

FIG. 3.4
The formulae of certain diuretics.

ment is chloride not bicarbonate. The usual route of administration is by mouth and, as with all potent diuretics, chlorothiazide can cause a hypokalæmia because of the excessive loss of potassium.

Hydrochlorothiazide is chemically closely related to chlorothiazide but is about ten times as potent a diuretic and even less active as an inhibitor of carbonic anhydrase. Therapeutically hydrochlorothiazide is used in preference to chlorothiazide.

OTHER DIURETICS

Frusemide can be regarded as a benzene sulphonamide derivative and appears to act by inhibiting the re-absorption of sodium from the renal tubules. It is a more potent diuretic than the thiazides and resembles in activity ethacrynic acid. Its prompt action when given by intravenous injection has made it a useful drug in the treatment of pulmonary œdema; as with other potent diuretics excessive dosage can lead to dehydration, hyponatræmia, hypokalæmia and hypochloræmia. Figure 3. 4 shows the formulæ of a selection of diuretics.

Ethacrynic acid was discovered as the result of a search for compounds which would react with SH groups in the kidney in a similar fashion to the organic mercurials. This drug resembles the organomercurials in certain respects excepting it appears to have no pharmacological activity other than on the kidney. It acts directly on the renal tubules and appears to inhibit the transport of sodium out of the ascending limb of the loop of Henle The resemblance in activity to the organomercurial diuretics is that the main anion in urine after its administration is chloride. It is dissimilar from these compounds in being independent of the acid/base balance. In this latter respect it resembles chlorothiazide but is dissimilar to this compound in neither inhibiting carbonic anhydrase nor increasing the urinary excretion of bicarbonate.

SUGGESTIONS FOR FURTHER READING

BAER, J. E. and BEYER, K. H. (1966). Renal pharmacology. *A. Rev. Pharmac.*, **6**, 261.
BERLINER, R. W. (1966). Use of modern diuretics. *Circulation*, **33**, 802.
BEYER, K. H. and BAER, J. E. (1961). Physiological basis for the action of newer diuretic agents. *Pharmac. Rev.*, **13**, 517.
FLUCKIGER, U. and HOPER, A. (1960). The control of œdematous states in livestock. *Schweizer Arch. Tierheilk.*, **102**, 27.

CHAPTER IV

INORGANIC METABOLISM

SODIUM, POTASSIUM, CALCIUM, MAGNESIUM

SEVERAL inorganic ions are essential components of the *"milieu intérieur"*, principally sodium, potassium, calcium and magnesium. Disturbances in the metabolism of these ions are associated with certain diseases of domestic animals; for example " milk fever ", a disease of parturient cows, is characterised by a fall in the blood calcium which may be rectified by the administration of an appropriate preparation of calcium.

SODIUM

Sodium is the main cation present in the extracellular fluid, and this fluid represents about one-third of the body weight. Of all the sodium in the body, about 47 per cent is present in bone, of which nearly half is fairly readily exchangeable. Disturbances of sodium metabolism are due either to a depletion of sodium or to an excess intake or retention. The commonest cause of sodium depletion is by an animal having vomiting or persistent diarrhoea. Under these conditions sodium together with water and other electrolytes present in the gastro-intestinal secretions are lost. A common cause of sodium excess arises from a too enthusiastic administration of parenteral saline solutions. Depletion of sodium is rarely caused by a reduction of intake because of the efficient sodium conservation shown by the kidneys and bowel, regulated to a considerable extent by aldosterone. However, sodium deficiency may occur when a low sodium intake is combined with the administration of drugs such as diuretics, as may happen in the treatment of liver and cardiac disease. In these circumstances, the renal conservation mechanism is to some extent inhibited.

Although under resting conditions the cell membrane

functions so as to keep the sodium ions in the extracellular fluid and potassium ions in the cell, the permeability of the membrane to these ions alters when the cell is excited. When the permeability changes as when an action potential develops sodium ions enter the cell. This movement of sodium is accompanied by the extrusion of potassium, and is considered in more detail in the discussion of potassium. Small amounts of divalent ions such as calcium and magnesium decrease the permeability of all membranes and this effect may be antagonised by sodium ions.

POTASSIUM

Potassium is the principal intra-cellular cation, 95 per cent of the ion in the body being present within cells. Three-quarters of the total potassium is present in skeletal muscle and only 2 per cent in the extracellular fluid. Potassium accounts for about two-thirds of the intracellular cation; most of the remaining cation inside the cell is magnesium. Like sodium ions, potassium ions are readily absorbed from the ileum, but in contrast have a lower renal threshold, and hence are more readily excreted by the kidneys. This accounts for the preference of potassium salts rather than sodium salts as osmotic diuretics. The fate of potassium in the body is controlled largely by the secretions of the adrenal cortex.

Potassium is involved in the establishment of the membrane potential of cells. The outer surface of an excitable cell carries a positive charge, and the inner surface a negative charge. An exciting impulse causes an alteration in the permeability of a cell membrane which allows sodium ions to pass from the outside of the cell to within the cell, depolarising the cell membrane. The cell membrane is immediately repolarised by potassium ions passing from within the cell to the outer surface. This exchange of potassium ions for sodium ions is then slowly reversed by the sodium pump mechanism which uses energy to extrude the sodium ions which have entered the cell and so restores the original state. Potassium ions applied to the outer membrane of the cell cause depolarisation and the conduction of impulses which is followed by a depression of the tissue. On heart muscle cells the action of potassium is to produce a depression. This depressant effect of potassium ions on the heart is a practical reason for not injecting solutions of potassium salts parenterally.

During the periods of starvation or after injury the catabolism of protein causes the release of large quantities of potassium. This is shown by an increased renal excretion of potassium. In anuria which sometimes accompanies injury there is a rise in the potassium level of the extracellular fluid which may reach toxic concentrations, and can in fact cause death. Survival of all animals depends on their kidneys being able to retain sodium and excrete potassium.

Although potassium deficiency is unlikely to occur in grazing animals because of the wide distribution of the element in forage plants, potassium deficiency can occur when potassium is lost, together with nitrogen and other cellular constituents, in injury. If, because of inadequate water intake or a loss of gastro-intestinal secretions, there is loss of extracellular fluid, this loss can be disproportionate. In the kidney, potassium ions which pass through the glomerulus are completely re-absorbed in the proximal tubule. In the distal tubule sodium ions in the lumen of the tubule are exchanged with potassium ions in the tubule cells resulting in the excretion of potassium and the absorption of sodium. It appears that there is some competition between potassium ions and hydrogen ions for the same transport system, excess of one reducing the exchange of the other; for example, neutral salts such as potassium chloride produce an alkaline urine by depressing the hydrogen ion exchange. Moreover, when hydrogen ion exchange is inhibited, as for example, by carbonic anhydrase inhibitors, an increased output in urine of potassium is produced.

The loss of excess potassium in the urine by diuretic action is brought about by several factors. To promote potassium loss it is essential for there to be sodium ions in the renal tubule at the site at which these ions are exchanged with potassium, because if all the sodium filtered through the glomerulus were re-absorbed there would be none available for exchange with potassium ions, therefore the loss of potassium ions would be prevented. The loss of potassium is increased when the potassium ions are accompanied by a less diffusible anion; for example, the loss is increased when there is more bicarbonate in the urine rather than chloride. Potassium loss is increased by high levels of aldosterone such as is produced when œdema is formed, for example, during heart failure or in cirrhosis of the liver. Other factors which increase the excretion of potassium in the urine are the adrenocorticotrophic hormone, adrenal cortical hormones, certain diuretics and the intravenous injection of sodium salts.

The main use of potassium salts in veterinary medicine is as diuretics in the horse and cow, *potassium nitrate* and *potassium acetate* being the salts of choice. *Potassium chloride* is used also in replacement therapy as the potassium ions form a small though nonetheless essential component of most replacement fluids.

CALCIUM

Most of the calcium in the body is present in the bones where it forms about 20 per cent of the body weight. The plasma usually contains about 10 mg of calcium per 100 ml, and this value is very constant; a fall in the plasma calcium level in a number of species is associated with characteristic clinical signs. The calcium in the extracellular fluids exists partly ionised and partly in combination with protein; only the ionised portion is physiologically active.

Calcium salts given by mouth are only slowly absorbed in the first part of the small intestine. Absorption from the gut is reduced when the intestinal contents are alkaline, because insoluble salts of calcium are then formed. The caudal part of the small intestine usually contains high concentrations of bicarbonate, and hence in this region calcium absorption is further impaired. The absorption of calcium from the gut is increased by the presence of vitamin D or a high protein diet However, for normal calcium metabolism, vitamins D and C in adequate amounts and properly functioning parathyroid glands are essential. After absorption, the calcium may be laid down in bone, an equilibrium being established between the plasma calcium and bone calcium—this equilibrium being controlled by the parathyroid glands. The retention of calcium by the body depends in part on the presence of phosphate; a deficiency of either calcium or phosphate produces bone disease. In ruminants, it has been shown by the use of radio-active isotopes that calcium is secreted into the gut at all levels and this is an important excretory route; in the horse, approximately half of the calcium is excreted in the urine and half in the gut.

The first demonstration of the necessity for calcium ions for the functioning of most tissues was that of Dr Sidney Ringer who found that an isolated frog's heart showed a stronger beat for a longer time when calcium ions were added to the isotonic saline solution with which the heart was perfused. It is now known that probably the most important function of calcium is the effect on the permeability of cell membranes. Calcium ions decrease the permeability of cell membranes to both ions and water—in particular sodium and potassium; this effect is especially important in excitable tissues such as muscles and nerves.

There is evidence that calcium ions enter the muscle cell during or immediately after depolarisation, and leave the muscle cell during contraction. It has been suggested that in some way this movement of calcium ions may link depolarisation of the membrane and contraction of the muscle.

In the absence of calcium, the sodium pump mechanism cannot cope with the increased entry of sodium into the cell through the more permeable membrane. A fall in the ionised calcium level of the plasma increases the irritability and spontaneous discharge of sensory and motor nerves producing tetanic spasms of the muscles. A decrease in the concentration of calcium ions decreases the amount of acetylcholine released by nerve stimulation. Calcium is involved in connecting the stimulus and secretion of certain endocrine glands such as the release of ADH from the pituitary and that of catechol amines from the adrenal gland by acetylcholine.

An increase in the level in plasma of ionised calcium, as for example when this rises above 12 mg per 100 ml, produces the opposite effect resulting in hypotonia and muscular weakness due to decreased excitability and contractility. Hypercalcæmia causes a decreased activity of smooth muscle, causing constipation, loss of appetite and, in some species, vomiting. An increased concentration of calcium ions increases the release of acetylcholine at the neuro-muscular junction. An increase in calcium concentration also reduces the amplitude of the end-plate current produced by acetylcholine, and reduces conductance at the end-plate. Hence, an excess of calcium ions will block both transmission at ganglia and the neuromuscular junction.

Calcium ions are essential for the clotting of blood and milk. However, the parenteral administration of calcium does not encourage the coagulation of blood.

Probably the greatest use of calcium in veterinary therapeutics is in the treatment of hypocalcæmia " milk fever " in cows. This condition which occurs at the time of calving is considered to be brought about by heavy demands on the cow's calcium reserves at a time when the cow is unable to mobilise calcium from the bones, hence there arises a condition when the level of ionised calcium in the blood is too low to maintain neuro-muscular transmission, and the cow develops a tetany. This condition is treated by the parenteral administration of calcium. The **calcium** is usually given as a **borogluconate** because this salt is only slightly irritant, and can, therefore, be injected subcutaneously. Although the clinical signs of milk fever can be rapidly cured by the intravenous injection of a soluble salt of calcium; injected calcium is quickly removed from the blood. Hence it is usual to supplement the intravenous injection of calcium with the subcutaneous administration of a similar amount. The calcium injected subcutaneously forms a depot from which absorption can take place over a period. It has been suggested that *calcium levulinate* would be a better salt to use because it is more soluble in water, contains one-third more calcium per unit weight and is less irritant than the borogluconate; however, the levulinate has not proved popular. A calcium chloride solution is very irritant and unsuitable for parenteral administration. Hypocalcæmia can arise from causes other than those giving rise to milk fever. For example, prolonged deprivation of calcium may produce hypocalcæmia and this condition may occur in vitamin D deficiency, pregnancy, and during periods of rapid growth. The administration of certain poisons, such as carbon tetrachloride, may cause hypocalcæmia.

D

SUBSTANCES AFFECTING CALCIUM METABOLISM

Parathyroid

The hormones secreted by this gland are responsible for maintaining the concentration of calcium in the blood. When the parathyroid gland is removed from dogs the concentration of calcium in the blood falls and tetanic contractions of the voluntary muscles occur and eventually death may result. This effect of parathyroidectomy is less readily shown in some other domesticated animals, possibly because of the distribution of parathyroid tissue and the difficulty of removing it all. In recent years, peptides have been extracted from parathyroid tissue and have been shown to possess pharmacological activity similar to that of the whole parathyroid gland. The isolation and identification of these peptides is not easy because every step in the extraction has to be checked by assaying an extract for parathyroid activity. Such assays are carried out using either dogs or rats. Parathyroid extracts injected into dogs cause a rise in the serum calcium and this effect can be used as a measure of activity; however, dogs are expensive to maintain in large numbers, and many workers prefer to use parathyroidectemised rats for this assay. Rats are easier to maintain in large numbers and are much less expensive than dogs.

Six hours after parathyroidectemy, the serum calcium of the rat has usually fallen to about 6 mg per 100 ml. The degree to which the serum calcium concentration can be maintained above this level is proportional to the dose of parathyroid hormone; in fact, if the level of serum calcium above 6 mg per cent is plotted graphically against the logarithm of the dose of parathyroid hormone, a straight line is obtained.

Evidence has been obtained recently to suggest that the thyroparathyroid glands secrete a hormone which lowers the serum calcium level, and it has been suggested that this hormone be called Calcitonin. Calcitonin is secreted in response to hypocalcæmia. The exact relationship of the thyroid and parathyroid to the formation and release of Calcitonin is not clear.

The parathyroid hormone maintains the concentration of

calcium in the blood independent of any effect the hormone may have on the kidney or on the level of inorganic phosphate in the blood. It is probable that the hormone exerts a direct effect on bone. The parathyroid hormone causes an increased excretion of phosphate in the urine, this effect is independent of the effect on the calcium in bone. The parathyroid hormone also causes an increased re-absorption of calcium by the kidney tubules, and stimulates the absorption of calcium from the gut. Since it is now known that the parathyroid hormone is a peptide, clearly it can be given only by injection, since if it were given by mouth, it would be digested in the same manner as any other peptide.

Dihydrotachysterol

When ergosterol is irradiated with ultra-violet light, tachysterol is produced. Dihydrotachysterol is made by the reduction of tachysterol. This compound will raise the concentration of calcium in the blood, and will cure tetany due to hypocalcæmia. Although it is chemically related to the D vitamins, it will not cure rickets. It has been suggested that dihydrotachysterol acts by increasing the urinary excretion of phosphate, hence lowering the level in the blood and causing the re-absorption of calcium from the bones. However, this theory was the same as that suggested in the action of parathyroid hormone and has since proved incorrect, hence it may also be incorrect in the case of dihydrotachysterol. Dihydrotachysterol increases the absorption of calcium from the gut, but in this respect it is much less active than vitamin D. In contrast to the parathyroid hormone, dihydrotachysterol can be given orally. It is slowly destroyed in the gut and its effect on the blood calcium lasts several days; however, its effect is too slow to be of value in treating hypocalcæmic tetany, and hence clinical cases of milk fever. It has been used prophylactically to prevent an occurrence of milk fever, but there is no clear evidence that it is effective for this purpose.

Vitamin D

There are several steroids which have the common property of curing rickets. This is a disease of young animals in which the bones become abnormally soft due to a lack of calcium.

The steroids which prevent rickets are stable chemicals, soluble in fat and fat solvents and known as the D vitamins. Those present in cod liver oil, a naturally-occurring rich source of these vitamins, will keep for several years. They are absorbed from the intestine only in the presence of bile, hence any interference with the secretion of bile as may occur in disease of the liver will also interfere with the absorption of vitamin D. Vitamin D cures and prevents rickets by increasing the absorption of calcium and phosphate from the intestine. It also maintains a substance in the serum which is necessary in the calcification of bone. Although both vitamin D and parathyroid hormone produce an increase in the concentration of both calcium and phosphate in the blood, the way in which this is produced is entirely different; the parathyroid mobilises calcium from the bone, and vitamin D increases the absorption of calcium from the gut.

The usual signs of vitamin D deficiency include soft bones, because of the lack of calcium and phosphate, badly formed teeth and, when the calcium in the blood is very low, tetanic convulsions may occur. There is usually an increased concentration of phosphatase in the blood. The administration of vitamin D decreases the excretion of calcium and phosphate in the fæces; this reflects the increased absorption from the gut. The main effect is on calcium; the vitamin D appears to prevent the formation of insoluble calcium phosphates in the gut. The increased absorption of calcium increases the concentration in the extracellular fluid, and if the renal threshold is exceeded there may be an increased excretion of calcium in the urine. The increase in the plasma calcium level decreases the secretion of the parathyroid hormone. The absorption of calcium from the gut appears to take place in two stages: there is first a rapid uptake of calcium from the intestinal lumen followed by a slower transfer of calcium ions from the gut mucosa to the serosal side of the gut.

Whilst the effects of vitamin D deficiency are now widely appreciated by stock breeders and other animal owners, it is by no means fully realised that an excessive administration of vitamin D can have very serious consequences. When large amounts of this vitamin are given, there is an excessive absorption of calcium and phosphate and a rise in the concentration in the blood of both these substances. This excess may then be deposited in the aorta, liver and kidneys as calcium phosphate. Animals suffering from an excess of vitamin D usually show a loss of appetite and diarrhœa. In pigs muscular tremors and ataxia have been observed and when death has occurred the lesions in the liver and skeletal muscle have resembled those produced by vitamin E deficiency; vitamin E has been used in the treatment of excess vitamin D.

The usual form in which vitamin D is given is in the form of cod liver or halibut liver oil. It is present in both these oils together with vitamin A. A more expensive form is calciferol or vitamin D_2, which is sometimes used for administration to dogs and cats.

Calcium metabolism is also affected by œstrogens, androgens, adrenalcortical hormones, and substances such as carbon tetrachloride which damage the liver.

MAGNESIUM

Magnesium deficiency produces a definite clinical syndrome in both sheep and cattle which is fairly common and requires treatment by the parenteral administration of a soluble magnesium salt; hence it is important that a practising veterinary surgeon understands what is known about the pharmacology of this cation.

Magnesium is very slowly absorbed from the gut, resembling calcium in this respect. The region of the gut where most magnesium is absorbed is the mid-ileum and it is probable that there is a common mechanism for the absorption from the gut of both calcium and magnesium. There is evidence that the absorption of magnesium is inhibited by the thyroid and parathyroid hormones, aldosterone and deoxycortone.

Magnesium also resembles calcium in having a concentration in the plasma which in health remains remarkably constant. The concentration of magnesium in the extracellular fluid is probably regulated by the kidney, and may be related to the excretion of calcium. The regulation of plasma magnesium is as yet poorly understood, and it appears that magnesium continues to be excreted in the urine even after the plasma magnesium has fallen below the normal level. Another source of magnesium loss which may be involved in the development of hypomagnesæmia arises from the observation that ruminants secrete substantial amounts of endogenous magnesium into the gut. The amount of magnesium lost by this route may equal that lost in the urine. When magnesium is given to ruminants by injection about 20 per cent is excreted into the gut. The skeletal magnesium is labile and hence can be drawn on to replace extracellular magnesium, but the replacement of magnesium in the bone is much slower.

Magnesium ions inhibit the release of acetylcholine at the neuro-muscular junction, and depress the sensitivity of the motor end-plate to acetylcholine. In high concentrations, magnesium may block the neuro-muscular junction unless sufficient calcium ions are present to antagonise this effect. The activity of the enzyme choline-acetylase is influenced by both magnesium and calcium; magnesium increases synthesis of acetylcholine, and calcium reduces the synthesis. Magnesium is also concerned in maintaining contractility in plain muscle and excitability in nervous tissue.

High concentrations of both magnesium and calcium depress the oxygen consumption of cells, and this effect may be associated with their action in decreasing the permeability of the cell membrane, as a decrease in permeability is antagonised by increasing the concentration of potassium. Magnesium is concerned in the activation of a variety of enzymes involved in the transfer and utilisation of energy; hence the presence of this cation in the mitochondria. Amongst the enzymes involved are, ATPase, pyruvic phosphatase and fructokinase.

Probably the main use of magnesium in Veterinary Medicine is in the treatment of hypomagnesæmia for which purpose the sulphate of magnesium is usually employed as it is very soluble in water and relatively non-irritant. It is given usually by subcutaneous injection, although occasionally in acute cases the drug may be injected intravenously. If the latter route is chosen, very great care is needed because of the depressant effect of magnesium ions on the central nervous system, and especially the respiratory centres. This depressant effect is antagonised by calcium and more commonly mixtures of calcium borogluconate and magnesium sulphate are used. The central depression produced by magnesium and by mixtures of magnesium and chloral hydrate have been used for their anæsthetic properties. They are unsafe, and there is no justification for any continuance of their employment. Solutions of magnesium sulphate are sometimes injected intravenously to destroy dogs.

Manganese is a minor element which is, however, essential to living tissue. It is slowly absorbed from the gut and rapidly fixed by tissues, especially the liver. Manganese is slowly excreted in the urine and bile. Chickens deficient in this element develop " slipped tendons" due to osteoporosis of the bones.

SUGGESTIONS FOR FURTHER READING

CARE, A. D. (1965–6). Nutritional and metabolic disorders. *Vet. A.*, **7**, 208.
STEVENSON, D. E. and WILSON, A. A. (1963). *Metabolic Disorders of Domestic Animals*. Oxford: Blackwell.
WILSON, A. A. (1964). Hypomagnesæmia and magnesium metabolism. *Vet. Rec.*, **76**, 1382.

CHAPTER V

DRUGS AFFECTING TISSUE METABOLISM

THYROID

THE active principles of the thyroid, **thyroxine** and **tri-iodothyronine,** are present in the gland incorporated in the protein thyroglobulin. These hormones are made from tyrosine and iodine. The first stage in their manufacture involves the uptake of iodide by the thyroid gland, in the second stage iodide is oxidised, tyrosyl groups are iodinated and the iodotyrosyl is converted to iodothyroglobulin. Tri-iodothyronine and thyroxine are then released into the blood. Disturbances of the thyroid by disease or drugs can be brought about by the interference with the synthesis or release of the hormone.

A series of daily doses of these active substances have more effect than a single large dose which is excreted mainly in the bile. Thyroglobulin or the crude gland is readily but irregularly absorbed from the digestive tract. The half-life of thyroxine in man is more than six days whereas for tri-iodothyronine it is about two days. This is probably because the tri-iodothyronine is loosely bound to protein and it is of interest to note that the protein binding is inhibited by salicylates and dicoumarin. The thyroid hormones are conjugated in the liver and the conjugates are excreted in the bile.

The main effect of these active substances is to produce a general increase in metabolism which lasts several weeks. This effect is shown by an increase in oxygen consumption, increased production of CO_2 and a slight rise in temperature. The urinary excretion of calcium and nitrogen is increased, the blood sugar increased, liver glycogen decreased and water excretion increased. These changes produce a loss in body weight.

The excitability of sympathetic receptors is increased, leading to an increased pulse rate and disturbance of the rhythm. The thyroid hormone produces a change in the tissues themselves as is shown by the fact that an isolated heart from a hyperthyroid animal beats quicker than one from an untreated animal.

Iodinated proteins have been made from casein, egg albumen and soya bean protein, and they have an action similar to that of the thyroid hormone. These substances have been used to stimulate milk production in cows. Within a limited range the increase in milk yield is proportional to the dose; however, extra food has to be given to prevent the loss in body weight and the use of these drugs is of doubtful economic value. They increase the percentage of fat in the milk and cause a slight fall in the milk nitrogen. The iodinated protein is not transmitted in the milk. Iodinated protein may be beneficial in improving the fertility of sluggish bulls, increasing the growth rate of young pigs and preventing the decline in egg-laying which occurs in hens with age and in the summer. Their use is very limited.

ANTI-THYROID SUBSTANCES

When studying the effect of sulphaguanidine on the intestinal flora of rats, it was noticed that the animals so treated showed a marked gain in body weight and hyperplasia of the thyroid glands. A similar effect was produced in separate experiments which involved the use of phenylthiourea. This is a very bitter substance and was used in these experiments to study taste in rats. An investigation into the hyperplastic effect of compounds related to these led to discovery of **thiourea** and **thiouracil.** The thyroid gland of animals treated with these drugs showed an increase in size and weight whilst the animals' metabolic rate fell. These thyroid glands when examined histologically had irregular follicles devoid of colloid. It is clear that the antithyroid drugs do not affect the peripheral actions of the thyroid hormones and that the changes in the thyroid gland are due to hyperactivity of the anterior pituitary, because their administration does not cause hyperplasia after hypophysectomy, and the effects of these antithyroid agents are prevented by the administration of thyroid. These substances act by interfering with the combination of iodine and tyrosine. Thiouracil is readily absorbed from the gut and about 60 per cent is destroyed within 24 hours.

Thiouracil and related substances have been given to chickens and turkeys in the last three to four weeks of fattening, and to pigs in the last four to six weeks to produce a gain in weight. Feeding these substances to sheep and beef cattle has given inconsistent results. These drugs depress milk production and egg-laying.

Œstrogens, antibiotics and some arsenical compounds are also used to increase carcase weight and are discussed elsewhere.

VITAMIN A

This substance is essential for tissue metabolism. It is an unsaturated alcohol which oxidises readily. The body converts carotenes into vitamin A, and, as carotenes are widely distributed in plants, deficiency is rare in herbivores. Vitamin A and the carotenes depend on fat and bile salts being present before they can be absorbed from the gut. After absorption the vitamin is stored in the liver and this organ can retain sufficient to last for several months. Vitamin A is involved in the synthesis of glucocorticoids—for example, the conversion of deoxycorticosterone to corticosterone requires this vitamin.

The domestic animals most likely to suffer from vitamin A deficiency are pigs, dogs and fowls. As with most vitamin deficiencies, growing animals are stunted in growth when they lack vitamin A. There are, however, more characteristic signs of A deficiency; mucous membranes degenerate and change to stratified squamous epithelium. This is the cause of xerophthalmia. The sheaths of peripheral nerves degenerate due to changes in the bones, especially around foramina through which nerves pass. The central nervous system becomes more sensitive to poisons, such as ergot and Lathyrus sativa, an Indian pea. Very large doses of vitamin A prevent the loss in weight and increased metabolism produced by thyroxine. However, chronic poisoning can occur from the prolonged administration of excessive amounts of vitamin A. Signs of this condition include premature closure of the epiphyses, spontaneous fractures and anorexia. The condition can be treated by the administration of vitamin K. The usual sources of vitamin A are **cod** or **halibut liver oil.**

VITAMIN E

Seven separate tocopherols have been isolated from wheat germ oil and shown to have vitamin E activity. Alpha (a) tocopherol is the most active member of this group and probably acts as an antioxidant. This property allows it to protect certain metabolites and prevent the formation of toxic oxidation products such as arise from unsaturated fatty acids. Tocopherol may prevent the development of an unphysiological oxidation-reduction potential in certain tissues and may act as a co-factor or prosthetic group in one or more enzyme systems. Evidence in support of the view that the action of vitamin E is due to its antioxidant actions lies in the fact that feeding methylene blue produces similar effects in vitamin E deficiency to feeding the vitamin. Vitamin E is necessary for the normal reproductive process in rats, mice and guinea-pigs, and probably in pigs and poultry.

Muscular dystrophy in lambs, calves and dogs is due probably to a deficiency of vitamin E. In this disease the muscle fibres are degenerate but show an increased consumption of oxygen; similar degenerations affect the cardiac muscle. Encephalomalacia in chickens (crazy chick disease) is a disease which is characterised by ataxia, muscular tremors, inco-ordination and tonic convulsions which can be prevented by adding antioxidants to the feed. A nutritional steatitis (yellow fat disease) which occurs in mink, pigs and cats can be prevented by the administration of vitamin E. Wheat germ oil is the naturally occuring source of vitamin E, but it is usually given as **tocopherol acetate.**

THE VITAMIN B COMPLEX

The members of this group of vitamins are essential for normal tissue metabolism. The adult ruminant has a microbial population which can synthesise all the B vitamins. It seems that the horse also can synthesise these substances, but there is little experimental evidence about the extent of this synthesis. Rats and rabbits obtain some of their B vitamins by eating their fæces, which contain B vitamins produced by microbial action in the large intestine.   This process is termed "refection ".   Young ruminants and the other domestic animals require B vitamins in their diet.

Aneurine

This vitamin, which is also known as Thiamine or B_1, contains pyrimidine and a thiazole ring.   Aneurine diphosphate is the co-enzyme which enables the enzyme carboxylase to oxidise pyruvic acid.   Aneurine-deficient animals accumulate pyruvic acid since they lack the enzyme to oxidise it.   This causes lactic acid to accumulate since lactic acid is normally converted to pyruvic acid, thus deranging carbohydrate metabolism.   The main effects produced by lack of aneurine are polyneuritis, cardiac disturbances and disorders of the stomach and intestines.

Bracken, raw carp, and raw herring contain an enzyme which destroys aneurine, and as a consequence animals eating these substances often develop aneurine deficiency.   Mink fed on raw herring or dogs similarly fed have shown this disease. Bracken poisoning in horses is due entirely to this enzyme depriving the horse of aneurine and can be cured by injecting aneurine.   In cattle, however, bracken poisoning is only partly due to the aneurine-destroying enzyme and cannot be cured by aneurine.   While the vitamin is available as aneurine chloride hydrochloride, the cheapest and most convenient form is as dried yeast.   Aneurine is not usually stored in the body although pigs appear to be able to store two months' supply.

Riboflavine

This substance is known also as Vitamin B_2 and exists as an orange pigment lumiflavin combined with ribose.   It can be synthesised and is stable.   Alkalis and light destroy it.

Riboflavine phosphate combines with a protein to form the yellow co-enzyme which is concerned with cell respiration. Only adult ruminants can synthesise enough for their requirements.   Deficiency signs can occur in all the other domestic animals. Chickens are stunted in growth and develop a paralysis of the legs; the eyes, skin and hooves of swine show lesions; dogs die of inanition, and horses show an iritis. This vitamin is also present in dried yeast.

Nicotinic acid

This substance forms part of the co-hydrogenases which are concerned with tissue oxidation, in particular, the dehydrogenation of glucose to form triose phosphate. The horse and newborn ruminant convert dietary tryptophane into nicotinic acid, and most animals can store nicotinic acid in their liver.

The domestic animals which are most liable to suffer nicotinic acid deficiency are dogs and pigs. Pigs lose weight and have diarrhœa and dermatitis; dogs develop " black tongue ". This disease in dogs is due to the oral mucous membrane failing to resist infection which allows large necrotic areas to develop. A clinically similar and more common disease of dogs is due to *Leptospira canicola* which, of course, is unaffected by nicotinic acid.

PYRIDOXINE is also a derivative of pyridine and is concerned in protein metabolism. Dermatitis and neurological signs of disease occur in pigs and dogs deficient in this vitamin.

BIOTIN, a member of the B complex, is concerned with growth. Biotin-deficient chickens show in addition dermatitis.

PTEROYLGLUTAMIC ACID is also called Folic Acid because it was isolated from a leafy vegetable. It is essential for the growth of dogs, pigs, and some bacteria and is widely distributed in green leaves. Lack of folic acid causes the normoblastic process of blood formation to cease at the megaloblastic stage.

The administration of sulphaguanidine, a sulphonamide which acts mainly in the gut, to rats will produce folic acid deficiency. The rats develop an anæmia which can be cured by folic acid. Sulphaguanidine causes this deficiency by destroying bacteria normally present in the gut which produce folic acid. Folic acid deficiency can also be produced by the administration of specific antagonists such as 4-amino pteroylglutamic acid. These antagonists produce a syndrome similar to the acute radiation syndrome which is characterised by leucopenia and bloody diarrhœa with pathological lesions in the gut and bone marrow.

Cyanocobalamin

This substance is also known as vitamin B_{12} and is a red compound containing cobalt. It has been isolated from the liver and is a product of the metabolism of various micro-organisms, *Streptomyces griseus* being used as commercial source. This vitamin is essential for normal growth, nutrition and hæmatopoiesis since it is essential for nucleoprotein synthesis. It is rapidly absorbed after subcutaneous or intramuscular injection, but its absorption from the gut depends on two different mechanisms. The more important of these mechanisms is governed by the gastric intrinsic factor. After absorption it is transported to the various tissues and in particular the liver, which is the main store. Cyanocobalamin is necessary for the maturation of epithelial cells, and the functional integrity of the myelinated fibres of the central and peripheral nervous system. It prevents certain types of liver damage, probably by affecting transmethylation. Cyano-cobalamin is concerned also in the metabolism of protein, carbohydrate and fat. B_{12} is secreted in the bile and re-absorbed from the intestine; the re-absorbing mechanism is very efficient. There is a group of natural and semi-synthetic cobalamins depending on various groups replacing the CN group of cyanocobalamin. Vitamin $B_{12}b$ is aquocobalamin in which H_2O replaces CN; $B_{12}a$, hydroxocobalamin, is the anhydrous form of $B_{12}b$, both these cobalamins are converted to vitamin B_{12} by treatment with cyanide and have been used therapeutically with success in cyanide poisoning. B_{12} is essential for egg-laying and the hatchability of eggs. Deficiency occurs in pigs and when the diet of ruminants is lacking in cobalt. The rumen bacteria when supplied with cobalt can make enough cyanocobalamin for the animal. Cobalt deficiency in ruminants can be cured either by adding cobalt to the diet or by giving cyanocobalamin.

IRON

The most essential element for tissue metabolism is oxygen, deprivation of which produces death within minutes. The oxygen-carrying power of the blood depends on its hæmoglobin content. When this is deficient the animal is said to be suffering from anæmia. Anæmia may be due to a failure of the body to make enough red blood cells or a failure to make enough hæmoglobin. Anæmias can be classified thus :—

(1) Anæmias due to a deficiency of factors needed for blood formation. These include deficiency of iron, the extrinsic factor B_{12}, thyroxine and ascorbic acid.

(2) Anæmias due to bone marrow poisoning such as produced by benzene, bacterial poisons, X-rays and bracken.

(3) Anæmias due to an excessive destruction of red cells as occurs with certain protozoal parasites, worms and snake venoms.

One of the commonest of these is the anæmia due to iron deficiency. The iron in the body exists in combination with protein as, for example, transferrin, ferritin or in hæme; about 60 per cent circulates as hæmoglobin.

Iron deficiency anæmia is common in suckling piglets due to the poor supply of iron in sow's milk. It also occurs in disease where there is a chronic blood loss. It is remedied by giving iron in a suitable form. **Iron sulphate** is given by mouth to cattle and horses, and the scale preparation, **iron and ammonium citrate**, is suitable for all species.

Piglets are often given capsules containing **reduced iron,** a mixture of metallic iron and ferric oxide, **soluble iron pyrophosphate**, or an injection of a **saccharated iron oxide.** This latter form is rather expensive but is said to ensure that a piglet receives an adequate amount of iron. **Iron-Dextran Complex** is a less irritant preparation containing 5 per cent iron and which is given by intramuscular injection.

Ferrous salts are converted in the stomach into ferrous chloride and are partly absorbed as such from the small intestine. Experiments on dogs and rats show that ferric salts are not absorbed to the same extent as ferrous salts. The amount of iron absorbed depends on the state of the iron reserves and not on the level of hæmoglobin. Although increasing the dose of orally administered iron increases the amount absorbed, the proportion of the dose absorbed decreases. This is because a " mucosal block " mechanism operates which does so by converting a small excess of ferrous iron in the epithelium to ferric iron which combines with the protein apoferritin. A quantity of the epithelial cells containing this ferritin are exfoliated and the iron thus excreted in the fæces. In healthy animals most of an orally administered dose of iron is excreted in the fæces without having been absorbed. The absorption of iron from the intestine appears to depend on the presence of apoferritin in the cells of the mucous membrane. This substance acts as an iron acceptor and combines with iron to form ferritin which, in turn, yields iron to the plasma in which it is transported attached to the protein transferrin, and so is carried to the tissue stores.

The absorption of iron may be inhibited by excess phosphate in the diet since iron forms insoluble or undissociated compounds with inorganic or organic phosphates, an example of the latter being phytic acid. Absorption is favoured by acid conditions and is therefore more likely to take place in the first part of the small intestine. Moreover, lack of gastric acid will decrease absorption.

The body conserves iron very effectively; only minute amounts are excreted in the urine and a little more in the colon. Most of the iron excreted into the gut is from the exfoliated epithelial cells to which reference has already been made. Traces of iron are excreted in the bile.

The most important action of iron is in curing iron deficiency anæmia. However, iron salts are astringent to the mucosa of the bowel and may cause constipation. The scale preparations do not have this disadvantage. Iron deficiency also appears to increase an animal's susceptibility to disease.

THE COAGULATION OF BLOOD

Small hæmorrhages arising from slight injuries would cause death and operative surgery be impossible were it not for the mechanism which produces the clotting of blood. The clot is formed from fibrin which is produced by the interaction of thrombin with fibrinogen. Fibrinogen is a globulin normally present in blood whereas thrombin is formed by the reaction between prothrombin, thromboplastin and calcium; prothrombin and calcium occur in plasma and thromboplastin is present in the tissues.

The control of hæmorrhage is usually a mechanical problem which involves the use of tourniquets and artery forceps. However, small hæmorrhages may be controlled by substances, acting locally, which are called **hæmostatics.** These include **adrenaline** which acts by producing an intense local vasoconstriction, and **alum, tannic acid, ferric chloride,** which act by precipitating proteins. Several more

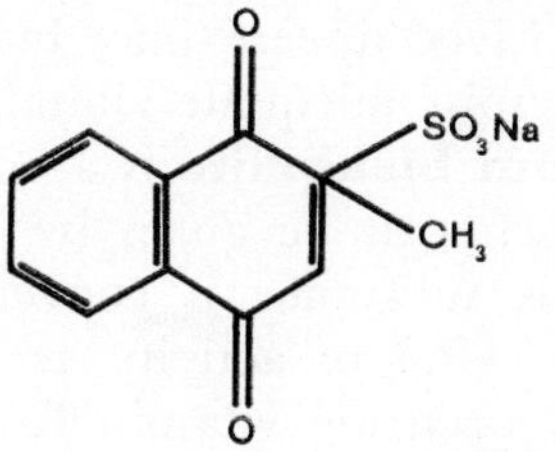

Menaphthone Sodium Bisulphite

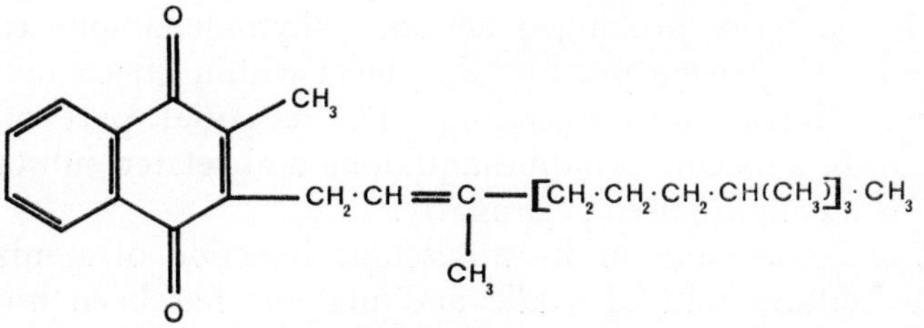

Phytomenadione (Vitamin K₁)

Fig. 5.1
The formulæ of some vitamin K analogues.

physiological hæmostatics are now available. A preparation of **thrombin** is available which can be applied locally either as a powder or in isotonic saline; **fibrin foam** can be obtained as a sterile preparation suitable for application to surfaces from which capillary hæmorrhage is proceeding. The foam forms a basis for clot formation. Absorbable *gelatin sponge* provides a non-antigenic preparation which can be used either within or on the surface of the body to form a base for the formation of a coagulum. *Oxidised cellulose* is used as a hæmostatic and depends for its effect on the acidic affinity for hæmoglobin. A disadvantage to the use of oxidized

E

cellulose on the surface of the body is that it may inhibit epithelialisation of the surface.

Vitamin K is essential for the liver to make prothrombin, and chickens deficient in this vitamin develop fatal hæmorrhages. It is synthesised in the large intestine of mammals by bacteria; bile is necessary for the absorption of this vitamin. Hypoprothrombinæmia may occur in liver disease, where biliary flow has stopped and when the colon bacteria have been interfered with by drugs. Liver disease may interfere with prothrombin manufacture despite adequate vitamin K in the diet. **Menaphthone sodium bisulphite** is a water-soluble analogue of vitamin K which can be given by intravenous injection. In the body this substance is converted into a compound having the same kind of activity as vitamin K. *Phytomenadione* is a naturally occuring vitamin K (K_1) which can be given by intravenous injection or by mouth. It is more rapid in action than menaphthone, is more potent and has a more prolonged action. Phytomenadione causes a rise in the plasma prothrombin level within fifteen minutes after an intravenous injection. The essential part of the vitamin K molecule is naphthaquinone and related substances such as menaphthone act similarly.

The intravenous or intramuscular injection of a mixture of the sodium salts of oxalic and malonic has been used to decrease the coagulation time. The evidence of the effectiveness of this preparation is not convincing. The mode of action is not understood, but it may act by suddenly releasing prothrombin from combination with calcium or by increasing thromboplastin activity.

n-Butyl alcohol has been given to prevent and treat hæmorrhage, but there is no good evidence of its efficacy. A solution of prothrombin and thrombokinase is sometimes injected subcutaneously for the same purpose.

Anticoagulants are substances which inhibit the coagulation of blood. Many drugs have this property, but most are too toxic to give to animals. However, it is sometimes necessary to prevent blood taken from an animal from clotting.

The *in vitro* clotting of blood is delayed by measures which reduce the destruction of platelets such as coating the syringe and needles with silicones or liquid paraffin. This provides a smoother surface and reduces " wetting " of the surface. Clotting is also prevented by substances which remove calcium ions, a 0·1 per cent solution of **oxalate** or **fluoride** is effective as is a 0·6 per cent solution of sodium citrate. Fluorides have the added property of inhibiting certain enzymes which is sometimes useful. Disodium edetate is a useful anticoagulant removing calcium by forming a chelate (see p. 271). Oxalates and fluorides are toxic when injected into animals, citrates are much less toxic and are used in collecting blood for transfusions. An effective antithrombin is present in extracts of leeches called **Hirudin.** Only very pure specimens are safe to use and these are very costly.

Heparin is a complex polysaccharide with anticoagulant properties whose presence in liver extracts was first noticed by a second-year medical student named McLean. It is concentrated in the mast cells round capillaries and small blood vessels. It is released along with histamine in anaphylactic shock in some species, so that clotting is delayed. Heparin is very stable and can be boiled without losing activity. It is an acidic substance, being combined with a large amount of sulphuric acid making it strongly electro-negative; therefore basic substances such as proteins which are electro-positive, inactivate heparin. Protamine and similar substances act in this way as antidotes to heparin. Heparin inhibits the conversion of prothrombin to thrombin, antagonizes thromboplastin and prevents thrombin reacting with fibrinogen to form fibrin. It has no other pharmacological actions. In man it is used to prevent thrombus formation and the risk of embolism. In veterinary medicine it is used mainly to prevent blood clotting *in vitro* when the use of oxalate or fluoride is unsuitable.

Hexadiamethrine bromide is a highly basic polymer which acts as an antagonist to heparin in a similar way to protamine by forming a stable salt with heparin. However, this polymer may release histamine.

Synthetic substitutes for heparin exist but most are too toxic to use in animals. The least toxic is *dextran sulphate*.

Bishydroxycoumarin or **dicoumarol** was first isolated as the toxic principle in spoiled sweet clover hay which caused a hæmorrhagic disease in cattle. It acts by preventing the formation of prothrombin and other factors necessary for coagulation.

It is readily absorbed from the intestine, slowly lowering the prothrombin level—the maximum effect occurring 2–4 days after administration. Its fate in the body is unknown but some is excreted in the urine. The best antidote to dicoumarol is vitamin K in large doses, menaphthone and like substances are not sufficiently powerful. A related coumarin is widely used as the rodenticide **Warfarin,** and sometimes causes poisoning in domestic animals. Large doses of salicylates and liver damage make animals more suceptible to poisoning with dicoumarol or Warfarin. Salicylates inhibit the synthesis of prothrombin in the liver.

COPPER

This element is widely distributed in animals and plants yet its full significance to the animal is not known. Copper deficiency causes a wasting condition of cattle which occurs in Holland, Australia and some parts of Great Britain; also associated with deficiency of this element is a demyelination of the central nervous system of sheep—a disease known as "Sway-back". An excess of molybdenum in grass will produce copper deficiency. Copper is also essential for the folding of the keratin molecule to form wool.

Copper is absorbed only from the first part of the jejunum, and absorption seems to be more efficient in deficiency although the mechanism is poorly understood. Unlike iron, which is lost only in minute amounts, copper is lost continually and appears in the fæces even after intravenous administration. Probably the main excretory route is in the bile.

Calcium copper edetate is a copper preparation suitable for administration by injection in cases of copper deficiency. It should be given only by subcutaneous injection when copper deficiency has been positively confirmed by analysis of both blood and liver.

In sheep a 1 per cent solution of **copper sulphate** stimulates nerve endings in the pharynx which initiate the œsophageal groove reflex, closing the groove so that fluids pass from the mouth into the omasum and abomasum, by-passing the rumen. This reflex in cattle is stimulated more readily by a 10 per cent solution of sodium bicarbonate. These drugs are useful to give with other medicaments such as certain anthelmintics which are required to enter the abomasum. Copper sulphate is itself an anthelmintic against stomach worms of sheep and cattle. In dogs a 1 per cent solution of copper sulphate acts as a reflex emetic (see p. 160). Copper sulphate has also antiseptic, fungicidal and molluscidal activity. The latter property is utilised in treating marshy areas where the snails which act as an intermediate host for the sheep liver fluke live, and it is also used in the treatment of certain infectious conditions of the feet of sheep; for this purpose it is used as a footbath.

Sheep which ingest excessive amounts of copper can accumulate it in their tissues until values 10–20 times normal are reached. They may be poisoned by grazing after horticultural sprays containing copper have been used or if given badly prepared mineral supplements to the diet. Poisoning is shown when the accumulated copper is suddenly liberated into the blood, causing hæmolysis. The animal becomes jaundiced and dies from renal failure. Cattle do not show this syndrome so readily. The ingestion of grass with a high molybdenum content produces depletion of the copper reserves of the liver and so precipitates copper deficiency.

COBALT

This element is essential for growth and nutrition in ruminants. These animals require cobalt for the microorganisms of their digestive tract to manufacture cyanocobalamin of which it forms part of the molecule. Cobalt deficiency has been recognised as a wasting or " pining " disease of cattle. This disease can be cured by giving cobalt by mouth or by injecting cyanocobalamin. Sheep are often given cobalt in solid form, the " cobalt bullet ", which lies in the rumen and allows the slow solution of small amounts over a long time. Sometimes the effectivity of the cobalt depot tablet is limited by the tablet becoming coated by various insoluble substances which prevent the slow solution of the tablet. Whether the sole function of cobalt in the body is as part of the B_{12} molecule is not certain. It is, however, interesting that horses and rabbits can graze cobalt-deficient pastures without showing any ill effects.

Experiments with radio-active cobalt have shown it to be readily absorbed from the intestine. Excretion is through the bile and the kidney.

DRUGS AFFECTING CARBOHYDRATE METABOLISM

A number of drugs affecting metabolism have been discussed already such as the various vitamins and certain hormones from the thyroid gland. There are other hormones

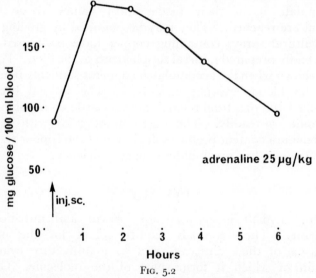

FIG. 5.2
The effect of adrenaline on the blood sugar of the horse.

such as adrenaline and insulin which produce a more rapid effect on metabolism; various diseases of domesticated animals also involve a disturbance of carbohydrate metabolism. Examples of these diseases are: post-parturient indigestion of cattle usually called ketosis; hypoglycæmia in piglets; and diabetes in dogs. In former years it was unusual to treat diabetes but with the standards of small animal practice constantly rising an increasing number of cases of this disease are now treated, hence it is necessary to consider various hypoglycæmic agents of which the oldest is insulin.

Insulin is the hormone obtained from the islet tissue of the pancreas. It is protein which consists of two polypeptide chains linked by the di-sulphide bonds of cystine residues. There are slight differences in the amino acids which form the polypeptide chains in the insulins obtained from different species. Because of its polypeptide nature insulin has to

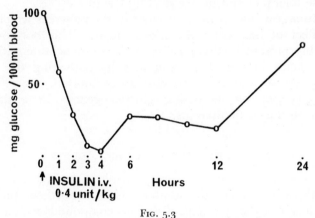

Fig. 5.3

The effect of insulin on the blood sugar of the horse.

be given parenterally. Absorption from the injection can be prolonged by using insulin precipitated with zinc protamine. A number of preparations are available which give varying durations of action depending on the rate of absorption.

Glucose is converted to glucose 6-phosphate through the action of the enzyme hexokinase. The glucose 6-phosphate is then used to form fat, glycogen and energy. The reaction glucose to glucose 6-phosphate appears to be stimulated by insulin, and this gives rise to increased deposits of glycogen in the liver and muscles. This is probably brought about by the insulin increasing the movement of sugar through the cell membrane into the cell. In the absence of insulin glycogen is made from protein and after the injection of insulin more glycogen is made from sugar and less from protein. As part of the body's homeostatic mechanism hypoglycæmia such as that produced by the injection of insulin causes the release of adrenaline and the released adrenaline stimulates the conversion of glycogen into glucose and thus tends to compensate for the fall in blood sugar by adding sugar from the glycogen to the blood. Hypoglycæmia produced experimentally by injecting insulin will cause convulsions in rabbits and mice, but not in sheep, horses or calves of up to 48 hours old. Insulin is used in the treatment in diabetes in dogs and it is useful in such cases to carry out a glucose tolerance test before starting treatment.

Glucagon is a hormone present in the pancreas which has the effect of increasing the blood sugar. This hormone is probably present in the a cells; it is a polypeptide with 29 amino acids in the chain and acts by activating the liver phosphorylase and so increasing glycogenolysis. It restores liver glycogen by increasing gluconeogenesis in a similar fashion to the corticosteroids.

Synthetic Hypoglycæmic Agents

It was noted that a hypoglycæmia occurred after the administration of certain sulphonamides. Further study of this effect and the synthesis of various compounds which gave rise to it led eventually to the development of the sulphonyl-ureas of which tolbutamide and chlorpropamide are important members. These drugs produce a marked hypoglycæmia on oral administration but lack both the anti-bacterial action and toxic action on the bone marrow of the sulphonamides.

Tolbutamide is partly metabolised by carboxylation into an inactive form, and both the active and inactive forms are excreted in the urine. **Chlorpropamide** is excreted in the urine. The sulphonylureas probably act as hypoglycæmic agents by stimulating the secretion of insulin. Hence after the administration of these drugs the level of insulin in the plasma is raised; moreover, these drugs do not lower the blood sugar in animals from which the pancreas has been removed.

The biguanides were introduced as a result of a search for a new oral anti-diabetic drug. At first these compounds were rejected as being too toxic for therapeutic use. However, on re-examination certain members of the series were discovered which were reasonably safe. **Metaformin** is an important member of this group. This drug produces a hypoglycæmic effect within two hours of oral administration, and the effect

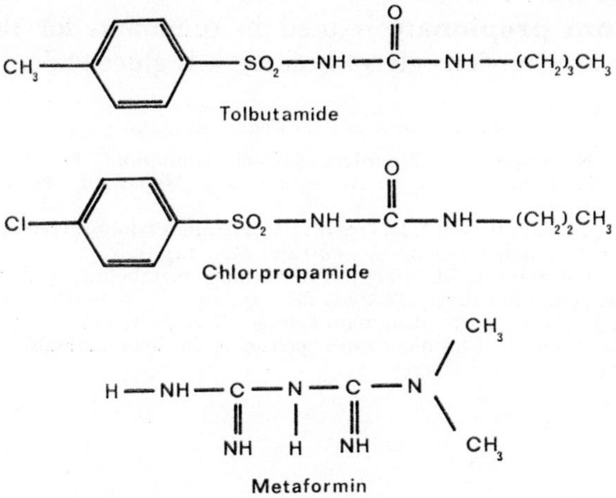

$$CH_3 \text{---} \bigcirc \text{---} SO_2 \text{---} NH \text{---} \overset{\overset{\displaystyle O}{\|}}{C} \text{---} NH \text{---} (CH_2)_3 CH_3$$

Tolbutamide

$$Cl \text{---} \bigcirc \text{---} SO_2 \text{---} NH \text{---} \overset{\overset{\displaystyle O}{\|}}{C} \text{---} NH \text{---} (CH_2)_2 CH_3$$

Chlorpropamide

$$H \text{---} NH \text{---} \overset{\overset{\displaystyle }{\|}}{\underset{\underset{\displaystyle NH}{}}{C}} \text{---} \overset{\overset{\displaystyle }{|}}{\underset{\underset{\displaystyle H}{}}{N}} \text{---} \overset{\overset{\displaystyle }{\|}}{\underset{\underset{\displaystyle NH}{}}{C}} \text{---} N \overset{CH_3}{\underset{CH_3}{<}}$$

Metaformin

FIG. 5.4
The formulæ of some synthetic hypoglycaemic agents.

lasts 6–12 hours. Unlike the sulphonylureas the magnitude and duration of the fall in blood sugar produced by metaformin increases as the dose of the drug is increased. The biguanides probably act by augmenting the action of insulin.

GLUCOGENIC AGENTS

The glucocorticoids are an important group of drugs which have the property of increasing gluconeogenesis and are sometimes used for this property in the treatment of ketosis in dairy cows. They are discussed elsewhere (p. 138).

$$CH_3 CH(OH) CH_2 OH$$

Propylene Glycol

FIG. 5.5

Propylene glycol is also used in the treatment of ketosis in cattle and pregnancy toxæmia in sheep because it increases the concentration of glucose in the blood. After propylene glycol has been absorbed two molecules are combined to form one molecule of glucose and hence the rise in blood sugar is produced. It is given as a drench. Propylene glycol is occasionally used as a vehicle for drugs which are not readily soluble in water.

Sodium propionate is used in ruminants for the same purposes as propylene glycol because it is glucogenic.

SUGGESTIONS FOR FURTHER READING

ARCHER, R. K. (1965–67). Disorders of blood coagulation. *Vet. A.*, **7**, 238.
BOTHWELL, T. H. and FINCH, C. A. (1962). *Iron Metabolism.* Boston: Little, Brown & Co.
DUNCAN, L. J. P. and BAIRD, J. D. (1960). Compounds administered orally in the treatment of diabetes mellitus. *Pharmac. Rev.*, **12**, 91.
MALOOF, F. and SOODAK, M. (1963). Intermediary metabolism of thyroid tissue and the action of drugs. *Pharmac. Rev.*, **15**, 43.
PEARCE, P. J. (1965–67). Ruminant ketosis. *Vet. A.*, **7**, 212.
TODD, J. R. (1962). Chronic copper poisoning in farm animals. *Vet. Bull.*, **32**, 573.

CHAPTER VI

PHARMACOLOGY OF THE AUTONOMIC NERVOUS SYSTEM

ONE of the main homeostatic mechanisms of the body is the autonomic nervous system, which controls in part or entirely respiration, circulation, digestion, body temperature, metabolism, sweating and the secretions of certain endocrine glands. This control is effected by the nervous impulse releasing at the nerve ending a chemical which elicits the response in the gland or muscle. The response of voluntary muscle to the nervous impulse is mediated in a similar fashion.

Evidence for the involvement of a chemical substance in the transmission of the nervous impulse had been accumulating for about 100 years before clear proof was obtained. Schmiedeberg, a pioneer of modern pharmacology, showed in 1896 that muscarine, an alkaloid obtained from a toadstool (*Amanita muscaria*), produced effects similar to those produced by vagal stimulation. However, clear evidence of the release of a chemical substance in nervous transmission was obtained first by Loewi (1921) who studied the effect of vagal stimulation on the isolated frog heart. In this preparation stimulation of the nerve not only slowed the heart to which the nerve was attached but, if the perfusion fluid was allowed to flow over a second isolated frog heart, this heart also slowed whilst the nerve was being stimulated. In the early years of this century Dale, studying extracts of ergot, found that they contained a depressor substance which was identified as acetylcholine. Pharmacologically, acetylcholine resembled the alkaloid muscarine. Loewi then showed that the "vagusstuff" was probably acetylcholine because it was potentiated by physostigmine.

An important technique in the identification of the transmitter substance was that of the use of parallel quantitative assays. In a parallel quantitative assay several pharmacological preparations are used to assay a pharmacologically active substance against a standard. If the substance being assayed is the same as the standard then the results of assays on each preparation will be quantitatively similar. This technique was devised by the late Sir John Gaddum and used to show the presence of acetylcholine in the perfusate from a variety of tissues when the parasympathetic nerve to the particular tissue was stimulated. For example: stimulation of the hypoglossal nerve produced acetylcholine in the perfusate from the tongue. Similarly acetylcholine was shown to appear in the perfusate from the gastrocnemius muscle and superior cervical ganglion when the respective efferent nerves were stimulated.

Evidence of the presence in the body of acetylcholine as a normal constituent was obtained by the actual isolation of the chemical from horse spleen. The evidence of acetylcholine being the transmitter in vagal stimulation to the frog's heart was extended to mammalian preparations, and a mammalian heart-lung preparation was used in confirmation of Loewi's experiments with similar results.

Acetylcholine causes a fall in blood pressure in the cat and if the dose is big enough, stops the heartbeat. The fall in blood pressure is due mainly to vaso-dilation since small amounts of acetylcholine increase the flow of saline through the perfused blood-vessels of the isolated rabbit's ear. These effects resemble those of the alkaloid muscarine and like them are abolished by atropine. The actions of acetylcholine which are antagonised by atropine are called **muscarinic.**

When the muscarinic effects of acetylcholine are abolished by atropine a big dose of acetylcholine produces a rise in blood pressure. This is due to the action of acetylcholine at ganglia of the sympathetic nervous system and in the adrenal medulla which are stimulated. These effects of acetylcholine resemble those produced by the alkaloid nicotine. The similarity between some actions of acetylcholine and nicotine can be further illustrated by an experiment in which it is shown that an injection of nicotine produces a rise in blood pressure, but when the injections of this alkaloid are repeated the size of the increase in blood pressure diminishes until finally it is no longer produced. If the animal is then given atropine and a subsequent large dose of acetylcholine, the acetylcholine no longer causes a rise in blood pressure. The effects of acetylcholine produced after the muscarine actions have been antagonised by atropine are called **nicotinic** because of the similarity with the actions of nicotine.

Acetylcholine probably acts by combining with chemical groups on the surface of cell membranes. These groups are referred to as receptors. Acetylcholine on combination with a

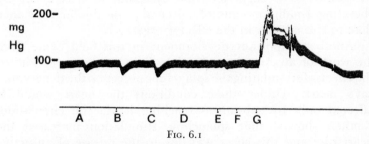

FIG. 6.1

A record of the carotid blood pressure of a sheep given respectively at A, B and C, 1·0, 2·5 and 5 μg/kg acetylcholine. At D, 0·25 mg/kg atropine was followed by 10 μg/kg acetylcholine at E, 0·25 mg/kg atropine at F and 25 μg/kg acetylcholine at G.

The hypotension produced by small doses of acetylcholine was antagonised by atropine and the effect of a big dose of acetylcholine converted into a pressor action, illustrating respectively muscarine and nicotine actions of acetylcholine.

receptor affects the permeability of the cell membrane. If the change in permeability is such that sodium ions which are normally in high concentration outside the cell enter the cell the membrane is depolarised. Whereas an increase in the permeability to ions such as potassium produces a state of hyperpolarisation. Depolarisation usually increases cellular activity, for example, in muscle it initiates propagating action potentials which result in contraction. Hyperpolarisation depresses activity by inhibiting the production of such propagating action potentials. Acetylcholine may depolarise one type of cell but hyperpolarise another hence the smooth muscle of the bronchi may contract but that of certain blood vessels relax.

The presence in the body of a substance which produced effects similar to those obtained by stimulation of post-ganglionic sympathetic nerves had been known since 1894 when Oliver and Shæffer showed the presence of adrenaline in the adrenal medulla. In further perfused frog heart experiments Loewi showed that stimulation of the vago-sympathetic trunk released a transmitter which he called "Acceleranstuff". However, one of the most important developments in this field was made by T. R. Elliot, who in 1904 whilst still a student was struck by the similarity between the effects of stimulating sympathetic nerves and injecting adrenaline. He suggested that sympathetic nerves act by liberating small amounts of adrenaline or similar substance close to special sites in the effector organs.

Another important development in this field came from the work of an American physiologist, Cannon, who studied the effects of stimulating the splanchnic nerves on the denervated cat's heart. Under these conditions the heart would be affected only by substances reaching it via the circulation. Cannon showed that splanchnic stimulation increased the heart rate and this effect was due to the release of an active substance which he called " sympathin ". Sympathin was shown to have effects very similar to, but not identical with, those produced by adrenaline and later work showed that sympathin, that is the substance liberated from sympathetic nerves on stimulation, is **noradrenaline**.

As was described with acetylcholine an increase in the activity of a tissue is a consequence of depolarisation of the cell membrane and inhibition with hyperpolarisation. With the active amines adrenaline and noradrenaline the change in membrane potential may in some cases be due to the reaction of the amine with a particular receptor site whilst in others it may be due to changes in the tissue carbohydrate metabolism.

It is convenient, especially having regard to the way in which various drugs affect the responses of these glands and muscles, to classify the nerves supplying them according to the chemical nature of the transmitter rather than anatomically. This is possible as the principal transmitting agents are recognised to be acetylcholine and a mixture of adrenaline and noradrenaline. On this basis, nerves are referred to as cholinergic or adrenergic and expressions such as cholinergic responses are employed.

CHOLINERGIC NERVES

These nerves release acetylcholine and include nerve fibres arising from cells in the central nervous system and in autonomic ganglia. The fibres arising centrally are connected directly to striated muscle or autonomic ganglia. The effect produced is local and has a short latent period. It is of short duration and there is no summation. Close intra-arterial injections of acetylcholine will imitate these effects of nerve stimulation.

Motor nerves to skeletal muscles end at sites on the muscle surface called end-plates which are very sensitive to acetylcholine. The terminals of these nerves extend beyond the myelin sheath and appear as vesicles from which acetylcholine is released. Although small amounts of acetylcholine are constantly liberated, stimulation of the nerve causes the release of a large quantity, making the surface of the end-plate permeable to sodium ions. Sodium ions move across the membrane causing a spike potential which spreads over the muscle fibres and is followed by contraction. Disturbances of this mechanism are involved in certain pathological conditions; for example, in botulism, the *Botulinus* toxin appears to interfere with the release of acetylcholine and thus paralyses cholinergic nerves. This toxin is produced by *Clostridium botulinum*, an organism which is sometimes involved in food poisoning.

Post-ganglionic cholinergic fibres arise in the peripheral parasympathetic ganglia and are very short. This group of nerve fibres includes some which anatomically are post-ganglionic sympathetic fibres e.g. the vaso-dilator nerves to voluntary muscle.

The effect of stimulating these fibres is less localised compared with the effect of stimulating the central fibres. The latent period is longer, the effect more lasting and summation occurs readily. These effects are mimicked by the injection of acetylcholine and this is antagonised by atropine. The effects of nerve stimulation are usually antagonised by atropine but there are some exceptions to this. The exceptions include the vaso-dilator fibres in the *chorda tympani*, and parasympathetic fibres to the urinary bladder.

Antidromic stimulation of certain sensory fibres causes vaso-dilatation in the skin.   These fibres are also cholinergic.

Understanding the way in which the effects of acetyl-choline may be modified by other drugs is made easier by considering the action of two drugs which themselves are of little therapeutic importance but produce typical effects. They are nicotine and muscarine.

Nicotine

This is an alkaloid obtained from tobacco and is absorbed from mucous membranes more readily than through the skin or after subcutaneous injection.   It is partly destroyed in the body and partly excreted in urine.   Nicotine produces both central and peripheral effects.   It stimulates the cerebrospinal tract and is followed by depression, the action being most marked on the medullary centres.   The respiratory, vagal, vomiting and vasomotor centres are first stimulated and then depressed, hence salivation and, in some species, vomiting are the early signs of nicotine poisoning.

Peripherally the drug produces stimulation and subsequent inhibition of synapses in the autonomic nervous system and has been used to locate the anatomical position of synapses.   Since sympathetic and parasympathetic nerves have usually opposite effects the peripheral response is complex. Nicotine also causes the release of adrenaline from the adrenal glands and, by acting on the supra-optic nucleus, the release of antidiuretic hormone from the posterior pituitary gland.   This alkaloid causes contraction of voluntary muscle followed by paralysis. This effect is made use of in the capture of wild animals or the restraint of unbroken domestic animals.   A special dart is manufactured which injects nicotine when shot into animals.

Coniine, the active principle of hemlock, **lobeline** an alkaloid from lobelia and alkaloids in lupins have actions similar to nicotine.   Hemlock and lupins may cause poisoning in livestock.

Muscarine

This is a stable alkaloid obtained from *Amanita muscaria*, a toadstool.   It is excreted unchanged in the urine and has no therapeutic value but is considered because it has only one type of action. It stimulates post-ganglionic parasympathetic receptors and reproduces all the effects of parasympathetic stimulation. All its actions are antagonised by atropine. The responses of effector organs to autonomic nerve impulses are tabulated (Table 6.1):

Table 6.1

	Effector Organ	Adrenergic Impulse	Cholinergic Impulse
Heart	Rate	Increased	Slowed
	Stroke volume	Increased	Decreased
	Rhythm	Extra systoles and fibrillation	Bradycardia and vagal arrest
Blood vessels	Coronary	Dilated	Dilated
	Skin and mucous membranes	Constricted	Dilated
	Visceral	Constricted	Dilated
	Skeletal	Dilated	Dilated
Bronchial muscle		Relaxed	Constricted
Stomach and intestine	Motility secretions	Decreased Decreased	Increased Increased
Eye	Iris	Mydriasis	Myosis
Bladder		Sphincter contracted	Evacuated
Salivary glands		Stimulated, sparse thick juice	Stimulated profuse watery juice

Pilocarpine, arecoline, choline and *choline esters* have muscarine actions. Choline and its esters also have nicotine actions. Pilocarpine and arecoline are occasionally given by injection to stimulate intestinal movements in the horse. Arecoline is an important anthelmintic in dogs. Choline, in addition to having weak nicotinic and muscarine actions, when given by mouth prevents the accumulation of fat in the liver. Since fatty livers can be produced by feeding a choline-deficient diet it may be considered a vitamin. Various esters of choline are of therapeutic importance (Fig. 6.2).

Acetylcholine

This substance is normally present in the body and is released under the conditions already described. It is not

F

absorbed when given by mouth. and even when injected subcutaneously it produces little effect because it is destroyed very quickly by the enzyme cholinesterase. These enzymes split acetylcholine into choline and acetic acid which are

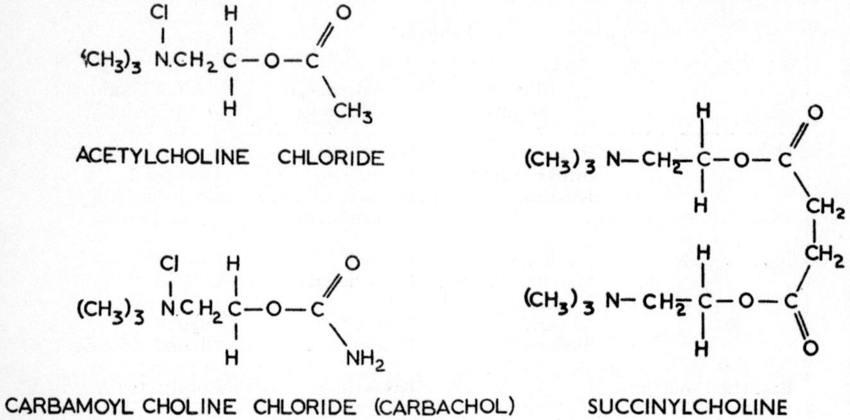

ACETYLCHOLINE CHLORIDE

CARBAMOYL CHOLINE CHLORIDE (CARBACHOL)

SUCCINYLCHOLINE

Fig. 6.2

Structure formulæ of the choline esters of veterinary importance.

Species	μ Mols acetylcholine hydrolysed/ml/hour	
	Red cells	Plasma
Horse	150 ± 6.5	98 ± 2.2
Ox	175 ± 4.5	10 ± 1.0
Sheep	83 ± 3.0	16 ± 1.2
Dog	120 ± 6.4	64 ± 6.0

Table 6.2 Cholinesterase activity in different species (courtesy P. Eyre).

substances with little pharmacological activity. The enzyme which hydrolyses acetylcholine most rapidly is true cholinesterase or acetylcholinesterase and is present in blood cells and nervous tissue; pseudocholinesterase which is present in blood plasma hydrolyses certain other choline esters more rapidly than acetylcholine. It is only when acetylcholine is given intravenously that it persists long enough for any action to be detected. Table 6.2 shows the cholinesterase activity in different species.

Acetylcholine has both muscarinic and nicotinic actions. The muscarinic effects are most marked. A fall in blood pressure is produced by an intravenous injection and this is due to a dilatation of arterioles. Larger doses inhibit the heart and produce the rest of the muscarine effects. Atropine abolishes these actions and allows some of the nicotine effects to be seen, a rise in blood pressure, for example, being produced by acetylcholine causing the release of catecholamines from the adrenal gland and sympathetic nerve endings all over the body.

Carbachol

This choline ester is as active as acetylcholine and much more stable, therefore it is active when given by subcutaneous or intramuscular injection. Although it has both nicotine and muscarine actions it is more active in stimulating contractions of the intestine and bladder than on the cardiovascular system, and is it for this reason that it is sometimes used in veterinary medicine as a hypodermic purge for large animals. The antidote to this and other choline esters is atropine. The realisation of this antagonism would probably have saved many horses from dying from inhibition of the heart when carbachol has been used to excess.

Methacholine chloride

This drug has only muscarine actions and no nicotine actions. It is stable and can be given parenterally. Its cardiovascular effects are most marked. Carbachol and methacholine resist the hydrolysing action of cholinesterase in the body.

ANTICHOLINESTERASE DRUGS

In mammals there appear to be two main cholinesterases, other phyla such as the avian, helminth or insect appear to have different cholinesterases. The two mammalian cholinesterases are called acetylcholinesterase and butyrylcholinesterase. This name is given because these two enzymes hydrolyse in the one case acetylcholine and in the other case butyrylcholine more rapidly than they do any other ester of choline. Acetylcholinesterase is known also as specific or true cholinesterase because it hydrolyses acetylcholine at con-

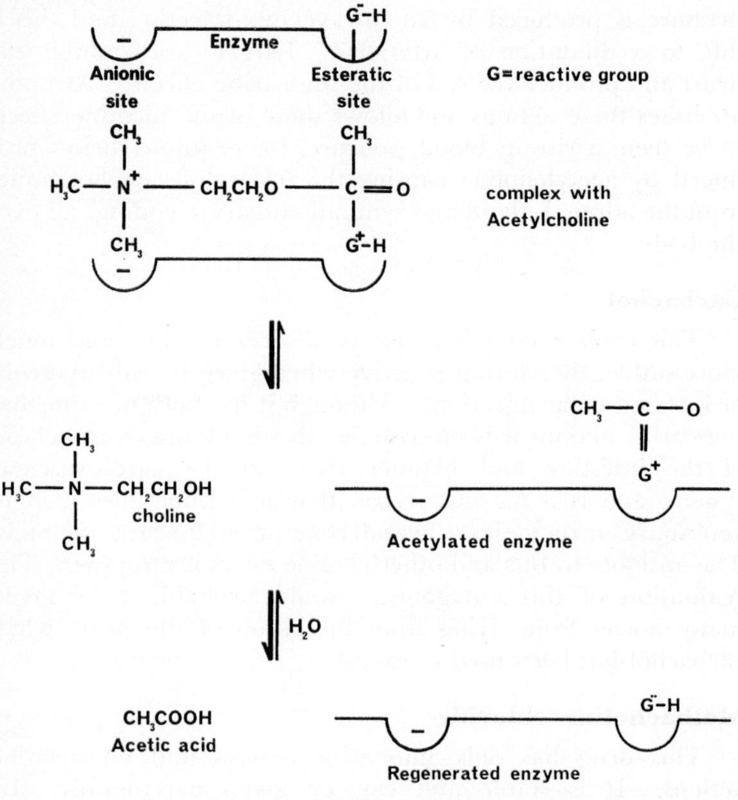

FIG. 6.3

A diagrammatic representation of the esteratic and anionic sites for binding acetylcholine on cholinesterase.

centrations which occur when this substance is released from nerves. It occurs mainly at the neuromuscular junction. The function of this enzyme is to hydrolyse the acetylcholine which is released during cholinergic nerve transmission. Butyrylcholinesterase is known also as non-specific or pseudo cholinesterase because it hydrolyses butyrylcholine faster than other choline esters. This enzyme is present in a number of cells in the nervous system, in the blood plasma and liver.

When cholinesterase is prevented from acting, acetylcholine builds up until concentrations are reached which exert the typical muscarine- and nicotine-like actions. Several drugs have the property of inhibiting cholinesterase. Drugs with this property are called anticholinesterases and fall into two categories, namely " reversible " and " non-reversible ". To explain the mode of action of anticholinesterase drugs, it is suggested that the active unit of the enzyme binds a molecule of acetylcholine at two sites, one binding with the cationic nitrogen and the other with the ester linkage (Fig. 6.3).

From the complex formed by the binding of acetylcholine to the enzyme, choline is split off leaving the acetylated esteratic site. This acetylated esteratic site reacts with water to produce acetic acid and a regenerated enzyme. The second and third steps of this process, that is the splitting off of choline and reaction of the acetylated esteratic site with water, occur very rapidly and for all practical purposes in one direction.

Eserine

This alkaloid which is also called physostigmine is obtained from the Calabar bean. It is absorbed from all sites of injection and from the gut. It is partly destroyed in the body and partly excreted in the urine.

Eserine inhibits cholinesterase by substrate competition, that is, sites on the enzyme which are naturally occupied by acetylcholine for its hydrolysis are occupied by eserine and are not available for acetylcholine, the natural substrate. It is a reversible inhibitor of acetylcholinesterase in that the part of the physostigmine molecule which occupies the esteratic site on the enzyme is very slowly hydrolysed. The rate of this hydrolysis is probably a million times slower than for the acetylated enzyme. Eserine thus increases all the muscarine actions of acetylcholine.

When eserine is given to an animal the pupil will become constricted, intestinal movements increased and the heart rate slowed. These effects are presumably due to the protection of the acetylcholine normally liberated. However, since the nicotine actions are either excitor or inhibitor these show a rather complicated picture. An amount of acetylcholine sufficient to cause a single twitch in voluntary muscle, after eserine causes a tetanic spasm. Conduction in a curarised myoneural junction may be restored by eserine, a fact used to reverse the effects of curare when this drug is employed as a relaxant during general anæsthesia. The drug is occasionally used as a hypodermic purge for horses. It may also be given in glaucoma to reduce intra-ocular pressure or to counteract the effects of atropine on the eye.

Neostigmine bromide is a synthetic analogue of eserine. Its actions are similar but more marked on the intestine than heart. It is used to increase intestinal movements and to stimulate contractions of the bladder and ureters.

Edrophonium is a competitive anticholinesterase with a short duration of action. It is probably the best antidote for overdosage with a drug acting like curare.

Several organic compounds of phosphorous inhibit cholinesterases and are important in veterinary practice because they include some important parasiticides. They are more specific in their affinity for the cholinesterases of the parasite than of the mammal, and are thus less toxic for the host than for the parasite. Most organophosphorus cholinesterase inhibitors react with the enzyme to form a very stable phosphorylated enzyme. The rate of hydrolysis of the phosphorylated enzyme depends on the particular organophosphorus compound and on the cholinesterase involved. This may vary from several hours to weeks in comparison with the fractions of a second taken for the hydrolysis of the acetylated enzyme. It will be seen from this why the organophosphorus compounds are spoken of as irreversible inhibitors of cholinesterase. As with the reversible inhibitors of the enzyme the action of the organophosphorus compound allows the normally liberated acetylcholine to accumulate and so produces an exaggerated or toxic effect. Although atropine protects against the muscarine actions of the acetylcholine produced by the inhibition of cholinesterase by drugs such as the organophosphorus compounds, atropine does not influence the inactivation of the enzyme. However, compounds have been produced, mainly various oximes and hydroximates, which will, to some extent, reactivate cholinesterase. Moreover, the best of these is only effective when given very shortly after the organo-phosphorus inhibitor. An example of one of these drugs is pyridine-2-aldoxime (2-PAM) or **Prali-doxime iodide.**

ACETYLCHOLINE ANTAGONISTS

Atropine

This alkaloid occurs in deadly nightshade (*Atropa bella-donna*) and several other plants of the potato family (*Solanaceae*) including henbane (*Hyoscyamus niger*), and thornapple (*Datura stramonium*). These plants sometimes cause poisoning in livestock. They contain in addition to atropine the related alkaloid hyoscine.

Atropine is readily absorbed from the alimentary tract or when given parenterally. Herbivores and birds are more tolerant to this drug than other species. This is due probably to the fact that they possess a specific enzyme in the liver which hydrolyses the alkaloid. Feeding *Atropa belladonna* leaves to a rabbit which possesses this enzyme does not produce signs of intoxication whereas administering an equivalent amount of atropine parenterally has a toxic effect. This is because absorption from the intestine presents the alkaloid relatively slowly directly through the portal blood to the liver where it is exposed to the atropinase. It has been possible to breed a strain of rabbits which do not possess this atropinase and hence are susceptible to poisoning by atropine when the alkaloid is given by mouth, whereas most rabbits are not susceptible to atropine given by this route. This is an example of a genetically based difference in the response to a drug of a particular breed within a species. In these and other species it is also partly oxidised in the liver and about half excreted unchanged in the urine.

Atropine antagonises all the peripheral actions of muscarine and allied drugs. The actions of most cholinergic nerves with muscarine effects are paralysed, exceptions being the vaso-dilator fibres in the *chorda tympani*, and cholinergic nerves to the bladder. Atropine does not prevent the liberation of acetyl-choline but prevents liberated acetylcholine from acting.

The central nervous system from the motor areas of the cortex to the medulla is first stimulated and then depressed. This effect is independent of the antagonism of muscarine. Impulses in post-ganglionic cholinergic nerves or the administration of muscarine-like drugs raise the tone of plain muscle. Atropine by antagonising these effects dilates the bronchi and pupil, increases the heart rate and inhibits movements of the stomach, reticulo-rumen and powerful contractions of the gut. Most of the actions of atropine are due to this antagonism of post-ganglionic cholinergic nerves. Hence it stops the secretion of tears, saliva, pancreatic juice and mucous glands in the digestive and respiratory tracts. It has no action on the secretion of milk, bile or urine.

The effect of atropine in dilating the pupil has been mentioned. It tends also to raise intra-ocular pressure and paralyse accommodation, this focuses the eye for distance. These effects on the eye are not seen in birds because the muscle of the pupil in these animals is composed of striped fibres.

In veterinary therapy the main use of atropine is in pre-anæsthetic medication when it is given to reduce the secretions of the salivary and bronchial glands. It also protects the heart from vagal inhibition which sometimes occurs during induction of anæsthesia with chloroform. Atropine is the pharmacological antidote to carbachol and similar hypodermic purges and should be used to prevent excessive action of these. This drug will also inhibit inco-ordinated contractions of smooth muscle such as produce colic. This type of pharmacological activity is known as spasmolytic or antispasmodic action. By dilation of the pupil atropine facilitates the examination of the eye. Atropine relieves the laryngeal spasm.

Homatropine

This synthetic substance is chemically allied to atropine. It is used as the hydrobromide to dilate the pupil instead of using atropine because it does not last so long and is more easily reversed with eserine.

HYOSCINE has the same peripheral actions as atropine but is purely depressant to the central nervous system. It is used in man to prevent sea-sickness and may be useful for travel sickness in dogs.

DRUGS INHIBITING SKELETAL MUSCLES AND AUTONOMIC GANGLIA

Certain drugs have the power to stop the transmission of nerve impulses at the myoneural junction and at ganglionic synapses in the autonomic nervous system. Drugs interfering with transmission at the myoneural junction produce a relaxation of skeletal muscles. This relaxation is sometimes used to facilitate surgery and it is important to realise that an animal under the influence of such a drug, although immobilised, is still capable of appreciating pain. It is essential when using muscle relaxants to ensure adequate anæsthesia.

Curare

This is the collective title for various South American arrow poisons. It is often used to refer to the purified alkaloid d-tubocurarine which was isolated from *Strychnos toxifera*.

Curare can only be given by injection because it is excreted from the body much faster than it can be absorbed from the alimentary tract. It has the inhibitor effects of nicotine without the preliminary excitement. Moreover, its paralytic action at the myoneural junction in voluntary muscle is much greater than that of nicotine. Blocking of the myoneural junction by curare was first shown by Claude Bernard, and other drugs with this property are called curare-like. Drugs acting like d-tubocurarine are also called competitive neuromuscular blocking agents because they combine with the acetylcholine receptors at the post-junctional membrane and thereby block the transmitter action of acetylcholine. Curare paralyses autonomic ganglia although the ganglion block may be preceded by brief stimulation. This action contributes to the hypotensive action of curare and in certain clinical cases makes its use undesirable. Since tubocurarine competes with acetylcholine for the acetylcholine receptors, increasing the amount of acetylcholine will swing the competition in favour of this substance and against tubocurarine. This is a matter of therapeutic significance in that neuromuscular block produced by tubocurarine can be antagonized by increasing the amount of acetylcholine present which is most readily done by administering an anticholinesterase such as neostigmine.   Some of the general systemic effects of curare such as bronchospasm and hypotension are probably due in part to curare causing the release of histamine.

Curare is sometimes used in veterinary surgery to give muscular relaxation.   When using such a substance it is essential to employ some mechanical means of maintaining respiration, although all muscles are not affected equally.   For example, the eyelids relax before the neck muscles.   The diaphragm and the respiratory muscles are the last to be affected.

Gallamine triethiodide

This is a competitive neuromuscular blocking agent which has no action on smooth muscle or the central nervous system. It does not release histamine but may cause tachycardia.   This latter effect may be due to a blocking of ganglia in the vagus. Pigs appear to be particularly resistant to muscular relaxation induced by this drug.   Since it is a competitive neuromuscular blocking agent like tubocurarine an anticholinesterase such as eserine or neostigmine is an appropriate antidote.   Gallamine has been used in darts to immobilize wild or difficult animals. It is excreted unchanged in the urine.

Decamethonium

This substance also produces muscular paralysis· Although decamethonium is no longer used in therapeutics, it is a useful drug experimentally and has also provided interesting information which is the basis for comparison of other depolarizing neuromuscular blocking agents.   Chemically it consists of two basic groups separated by ten carbon atoms. It has been suggested that the basic groups combine with the receptors on the muscle and that the space occupied by the ten carbon atoms is equal to the distance between two receptors.   Although the effect of decamethonium is similar to that of curare, it is produced in a different fashion.   Decamethonium prevents energy accumulating on the muscle surface, i.e. the development of an end-plate potential, and its main effect is, therefore, the depolarisation of the motor end-plate.   This is an important difference between decamethonium and curare, because whilst eserine antagonises

the effect of curare it increases the effect of decamethonium.
A characteristic of the neuromuscular block produced by
depolarizing agents are the (transient) muscular fasciculations

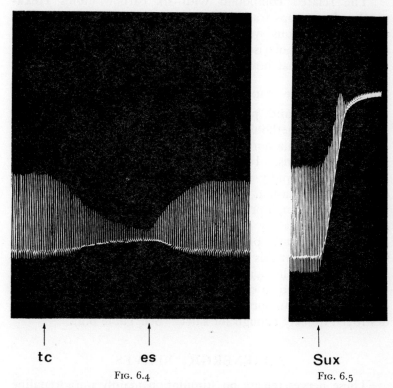

↑	↑	↑
tc	es	Sux
FIG. 6.4		FIG. 6.5

FIG. 6.4 The neuromuscular blocking effect of d. -tubocurarine and its
reversal by eserine. Biventer cervicis stimulated through the nerve at a rate of
eight impulses per minute. Concentration of tubocurarine (tc) was 20 μg/ml and
of eserine (s) was 20 μg/ml. (*Courtesy P. Eyre.*)

FIG. 6.5 The effect of a depolarising neuromuscular blocking agent suxamethonium on the chick biventer muscle. With this preparation a depolarising
agent produces a sustained contracture. The muscle was stimulated through
the nerve [eight impulses a minute]. The concentration of suxamethonium was
0/5 μg/ml. (*Courtesy P. Eyre.*)

which precede the onset of the block. Depolarizing blocking
agents are partially antagonized by d-tubocurarine. This
can be demonstrated experimentally but is of little therapeutic
moment. Avian skeletal muscle responds in a typical way
to depolarizing blocking drugs by developing a contracture

and can be used experimentally to distinguish competitive and depolarizing neuromuscular blocking agents (Figs. 6.4, 6.5).

The related compound with six carbon atoms **Hexamethonium** stops transmission at ganglionic synapses in the autonomic nervous system. Hexamethonium does not itself stimulate or depolarise the ganglion. It has little action at the neuromuscular junction.

Succinylcholine (Suxamethonium)

This compound paralyses skeletal muscle in a fashion similar to decamethonium; large doses stimulate then depress autonomic ganglia and produce cholinergic responses in plain muscle and glands. It is safer than curare or decamethonium because it is rapidly hydrolysed by the non-specific cholinesterase in the plasma. This drug has been used to cast horses prior to operation, a procedure not without risk because of the danger of respiratory paralysis. The muscular fasciculations may be particularly pronounced in the horse. It is essential to appreciate that this drug does not in any way diminish pain and proper anæsthesia must always be ensured. This technique cannot be applied to cattle because their plasma contains less cholinesterase than horses' plasma and the succinylcholine is not destroyed quickly enough for safety (See Table 6.2).

ADRENERGIC NERVES

These nerves release on stimulation mainly noradrenaline and they include the post-ganglionic fibres of the sympathetic nervous system. A convenient way of classifying the pharmacological actions of adrenaline and other sympathomimetic agents is to divide them into two categories; one group being called the alpha actions and the other beta actions. The various organs and their receptors are classified in this manner in Table 6.3. The alpha effects are mainly motor and are produced by noradrenaline. They are readily antagonised by certain drugs. The beta effects are mainly inhibitor.

Adrenaline and noradrenaline are chemically catechol amines. From a pharmacological point of view there are four important catechol amines, three of these are naturally present in the tissues, the other is synthetic. Those in the tissues are dopamine (hydroxytyramine), noradrenaline and adrenaline. The synthetic catechol amine is isoprenaline. Dopamine is about ten times less active than adrenaline. Noradrenaline has mainly motor effects on smooth muscle,

TABLE 6.3

Response to Adrenergic Impulse

Tissue	Receptor	Response
Heart		
SA node	β	rate increased
atria	β	increased contractility
ventricles	β	increased conduction rate
Blood vessels		
skin	α	constricted
muscle (skeletal)	β	dilated
visceral	α	constricted
Bronchial muscle	β	relaxed
Stomach and intestine		
motility	β	decreased
secretions	–	decreased
tone	α and β	decreased
Bladder		
sphincter	α	contracted
detrusor	β	relaxed
Eye		
iris (radial muscle)	α	contracted
Metabolism	β	increased

adrenaline produces both motor and inhibitor actions on smooth muscle whilst isoprenaline has only inhibitor actions on smooth muscle.

ADRENALINE

This is the active substance obtained from the adrenal medulla. The gland contains l-adrenaline which is much more potent than d-adrenaline. Commercial extracts usually contain both forms. Adrenaline is stable at pH 4 but alkaline or neutral solutions are quickly oxidised, forming a pink indole compound which is inactive.

Absorption of adrenaline is slow after injection excepting

intravenous injection because it produces an intense local vasoconstriction. Hence, subcutaneous injections last quite a long time.

Adrenaline increases the rate and force of the heart beat and constricts the arterioles in the viscera, skin and mucosæ.

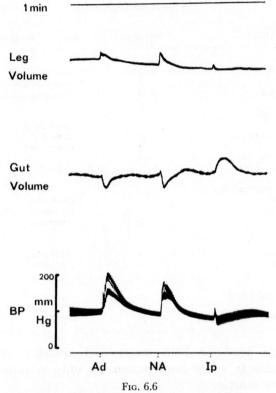

FIG. 6.6

The carotid blood pressure, gut and limb volume were recorded from a sheep given successively 2 μg/kg adrenaline, noradrenaline and isoprenaline.

The skin capillaries constrict and muscle capillaries and coronary vessels dilate. The blood in the spleen and large veins is decreased by contraction of the splenic capsule and most veins. These effects produce a rise in blood pressure and increased flow through the voluntary muscles, heart and brain. Small doses of adrenaline may only affect the muscle capillaries and so give a fall in blood pressure. Large doses may cause slowing of the heart through the carotid sinus reflex being stimulated by the rise in blood pressure.

Adrenaline dilates the pupil and contracts the nictitating membrane. It inhibits gastro-intestinal activity, dilates the

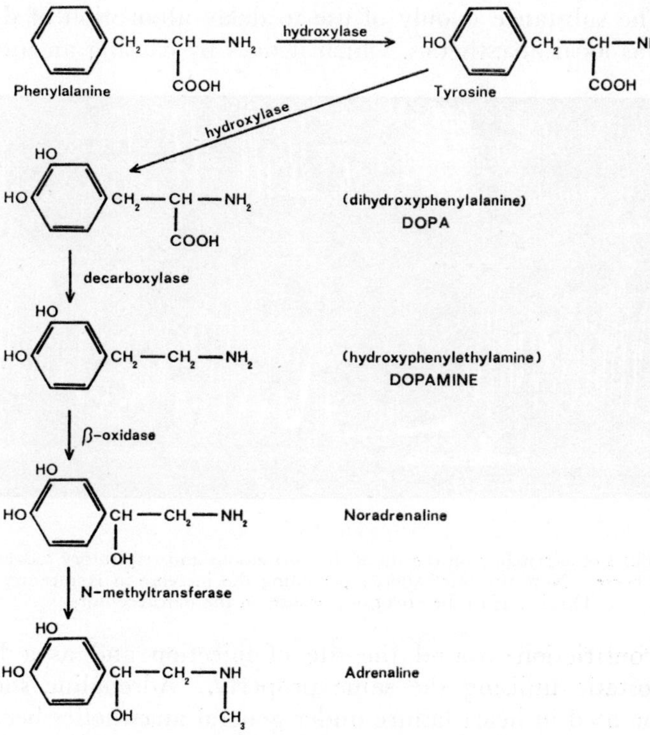

FIG. 6.7

The formation of noradrenaline and adrenaline.

bronchi, causes pilo-erection and inhibits bladder emptying. The effect on the uterus varies with the species and state of the uterus. The salivary glands produce a sparse thick juice and in the horse and cow, sweating occurs. This latter action is due to the direct action of adrenaline on the sweat glands, which in the horse at least do not appear to have a nerve supply. Metabolism is stimulated as shown by an increased oxygen consumption and a release of glycogen from the liver

and muscles, which in turn causes hyperglycæmia and glyco-
suria.   Respiration is first inhibited by stimulation of the carotid
sinus reflex resulting from the increased blood pressure.
Adrenaline improves conduction in sympathetic ganglia, the
central nervous system and fatigued nerve endings in voluntary
muscle.

The substance is only of use to delay absorption of drugs
such as local anæsthetics, which it does by causing an intense

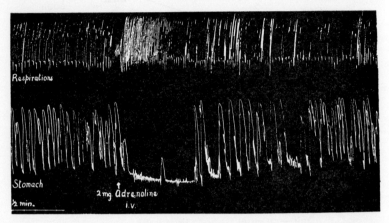

FIG. 6.8

The effects of adrenaline on the stomach contractions and respiratory movements
of the horse.   Note the brief apnœa preceding the increase in respiratory rate.
This is due to the effect of pressure on the baroreceptors.

vasoconstriction around the site of injection and as a local
hæmostatic utilising the same property.   Adrenaline should
not be used in heart failure under general anæsthetics because
of the risk of it causing ventricular fibrillation.

Noradrenaline differs chemically from adrenaline by the
lack of a methyl group (Fig. 6.7), occurs naturally as l-nor-
adrenaline and is the substance released by adrenergic nerve
stimulation.   It is a potent vasoconstrictor, so much so that
the stimulant action on the heart is obscured by the inhibitory
reflexes, which are so marked as to cause a fall in heart output.

The effects of adrenaline have been described as being
divisible into alpha and beta actions.   Noradrenaline has
strong alpha effects which include cutaneous and visceral
vasoconstriction, intestinal inhibition and contraction of

smooth muscle. This humoral agent has also weak beta effects such as dilation of capillaries in skeletal muscle and relaxation of bronchial muscle. The effects of noradrenaline

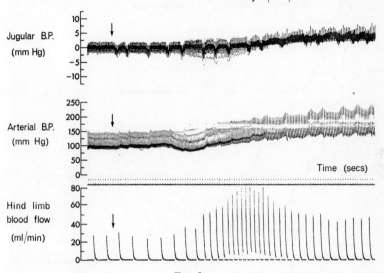

I.V. Adrenaline 1·0μg/kg/min

FIG. 6.9

The effect of adrenaline on the carotid arterial, jugular venous pressure and femoral outflow in a dog. (*Courtesy A. L. Haigh.*)

on the heart however are similar to those of adrenaline; since these actions are abolished by β blocking agents they are regarded as β effects. Noradrenaline appears to be taken up into storage sites in post-ganglionic sympathetic fibres and certain drugs such as ephedrine and amphetamine owe their activity in part to releasing noradrenaline from these storage sites. Cocaine, primarily a local anæsthetic, also has central and sympathomimetic actions. It potentiates the effects of sympathetic nerve stimulation or those of injecting noradrenaline by interfering with the uptake of noradrenaline by the sympathetic nerve fibres.

THE INACTIVATION OF CATECHOLAMINES

The action of these amines stops when their concentration falls below a certain critical level. This inactivation which

G

takes place in the tissues involves first an enzyme called
catechol ortho methyl transferase (C.O.M.T.). This
enzyme facilitates the transfer of a methyl group from adenosyl-

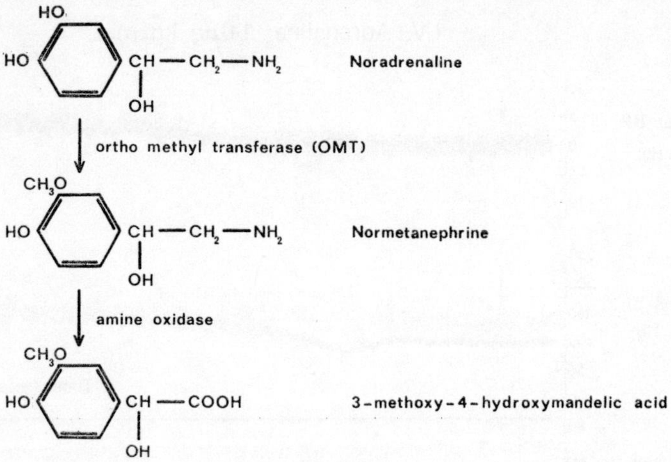

FIG. 6.10

The metabolism of noradrenaline and adrenaline.

methionine to the hydroxyl group in the meta position in
noradrenaline thus forming normetanephrine. Normetanephrine is then acted on by an enzyme called amine oxidase to
form 3-methoxy-4-hydroxymandelic acid and this is excreted
in the urine.

SYMPATHOMIMETIC AMINES

Ephedrine

This alkaloid occurs in several plants of the Ephedra
species. It is chemically similar to adrenaline but much more
stable, and this property makes it suitable to give by mouth
and to produce a more prolonged effect.

Ephedrine produces effects very similar to those of
adrenaline. However, large doses may depress the heart. It
has a stimulant action on the central nervous system.

Ephedrine, like the naturally occurring amine tyramine
and the synthetic sympathomimetic amine amphetamine, act
in part by causing noradrenaline to be released from sympathetic nerve endings. Evidence for this release of

noradrenaline by sympathomimetic amines has been obtained from experiments with an alkaloid called **reserpine**. Reserpine has the property of depleting tissues of their noradrenaline content.

Evidence for this depletion can be shown by perfusing the hind limb of an animal 24 hours after the animal has been given reserpine. Stimulation of the sympathetic nerves to such a limb does not produce vasoconstriction. However, if noradrenaline is given and the immediate vasoconstrictor action allowed to pass, stimulation of the sympathetic nerve gives the usual vasoconstrictor effect. Similarly after reserpine treatment the sympathomimetic amines such as tyramine, ephedrine and amphetamine also fail to produce their characteristic effect. Hence it follows that a large part of the effect of these amines is due to the release of stored noradrenaline since after reserpine treatment the effect can be restored by perfusing the depleted tissues with noradrenaline.

If ephedrine or amphetamine are given in excessive amounts, signs of central stimulation and pulmonary œdema are produced. Animals so affected should be kept warm and quiet, the marked excitement controlled by the intravenous injection of a short-acting barbiturate. Reduction of the blood volume by phlebotomy has been recommended for the treatment of pulmonary œdema.

Ephedrine and amphetamine are sometimes used in veterinary medicine to treat cases of anaphylaxis, depression and the prolonged recumbency associated with hypocalcæmia where there is no evidence of physical damage. They are of doubtful utility.

Amphetamine

Amphetamine is a volatile substance but forms a sulphate which is solid and so can be given by mouth in this form. About half a dose of this drug is excreted in 48 hours; the remainder is slowly destroyed in the body. In general the effects of this drug resemble those of adrenaline. It is a more powerful substance than ephedrine but, like that drug, stimulates the central nervous system and has been used to stimulate respiration and for the same purposes as ephedrine. Excessive use causes cardiovascular collapse, pulmonary œdema and convulsions.   It has been used to depress the appetite of obese dogs. Methyl amphetamine has similar actions to those of amphetamine but they are more prolonged.

Phenylephrine is a sympathomimetic amine which stimulates only alpha receptors.

Isoprenaline stimulates β receptors and is sometimes used to dilate the bronchi, (fig 5.2).

Amine Oxidase inhibitors

Some years ago it was considered that ephedrine and amphetamine owed their sympathomimetic activity to the fact that both these drugs inhibited amine oxidase which was then thought to be the major enzyme concerned in the metabolism of adrenaline and noradrenaline. However, this enzyme is only inhibited by concentrations of ephedrine and amphetamine very much higher than those necessary to produce the characteristic effects of the drugs in the animal. Hence amine oxidase inhibition does not explain their activity, whereas the concept of their causing the release of noradrenaline from its stores and also their interfering with the tissue uptake of this amine offer a more satisfactory explanation of the activity of the drugs.   However, during the past decade or so a great deal of work has been carried out on more active amine oxidase inhibitors; such drugs are of value both clinically and for investigation. Inhibiting an enzyme involved in destroying catechol amines and substances such as 5-hydroxy-tryptamine could give valuable information about these pharmacologically active amines.

One of the first amine oxidase inhibitors discovered was the hydrazine compound iproniazid. This drug had been introduced into medicine for the treatment of tuberculosis. A number of hydrazines have since been discovered which are more powerful inhibitors of amine oxidase. Other compounds such as various tryptamine derivatives have been shown to possess similar activity, α-ethyltryptamine is an example of such a compound. The amine oxidase inhibitors cause a rise in the concentration of brain amines which, in some species, is accompanied by excitement. These compounds have been used in various depressive states in man but so far have not found any therapeutic effect in veterinary medicine. They have however some interesting actions in animals. Moreover, various active amines such as tyramine are commonly present in animal foodstuffs such as silage, and it is conceivable that in the presence of an amine oxidase inhibitor these active compounds which are absorbed might reach toxic levels within the animal. This possibility is increased by the fact that the amine oxidase inhibitors produce a block which persists for an appreciable time.

Mice given hexobarbitone together with an amine oxidase inhibitor show a prolonged sleeping time which is due to the amine oxidase inhibitor interfering with the metabolism of the barbiturate by the liver microsomes. Some amine oxidase inhibitors have anti-convulsant properties in that they protect rats against convulsions produced by electrical stimulation or the injection of the analeptic drug, leptazol. Amine oxidase inhibitors can also block transmission at ganglia, although the exact mechanism whereby this is produced is unknown. Amine oxidase inhibitors have been found to interrupt pregnancy during the first half of pregnancy in rats and mice.

ADRENALINE ANTAGONISTS

Alpha adrenergic blocking agents

The pharmacological effects of adrenaline are antagonised by a number of substances. Some resemble adrenaline structurally and some do not.

The oldest antagonist is **ergotoxine,** an alkaloid present in a fungus growing on rye grains. This drug paralyses the excitor effects of adrenaline at much lower concentrations than it does the inhibitor effects. Since many of the effects of adrenaline result from a mixture of strong excitor and weak inhibitor effects, suitable doses of ergotoxine will reverse the action of adrenaline. Ergotoxine converts the typical rise in blood pressure produced by adrenaline into a fall because it blocks the vasoconstrictor receptors in the splanchnic arterioles whilst the vasodilator receptors in the muscle vessels are unaffected. Similar reversals can be shown on other tissues and adrenergic nerves are affected in the same way. Ergotamine and yohimbine have similar properties. Yohimbine in this way causes dilatation of the blood vessels of the genitalia and has been used as an aphrodisiac. Alpha blocking agents appear to act by combining with specific alpha receptors in the tissues, the beta receptors are relatively unaffected. There are many other substances with the property of antagonizing the alpha actions of adrenaline; **Dibenamine** was one of the first synthetic alpha blocking compounds and **Phenoxybenzamine** is probably the most popular. The block takes one to two hours to develop even after intravenous injection and persists for one to two days. **Tolazoline** is a drug with relatively transient alpha blocking activity. However, it has also sympathomimetic, parasympathomimetic and histamine-like activity. This drug has been used experimentally to protect dogs under cyclopropane anæsthesia against cardiac arhythmias induced by giving adrenaline.

Beta adrenergic blocking agents

An interesting development which has taken place in recent years has been the introduction of drugs with specific beta blocking activity. The first drug with this activity was dichloro-isopropylnoradrenaline. However, this drug has in addition intrinsic beta stimulating activity similar to that shown by isoprenaline. **Propranolol** is a new compound with very much greater β blocking activity than earlier drugs with this property and has little or no sympathomimetic activity. Propranolol appears to block all sympathetic activity to the heart and thus could be a very valuable drug in combating the cardiac effects of circulating adrenaline, such as make the administration of anæsthetics like chloroform and cyclopropane hazardous.

SUGGESTIONS FOR FURTHER READING

AHLQUIST, R. P. (1968). Agents which block adrenergic beta-receptors. *A. Rev. Pharmac.*, **8**, 259.
BURN, J. H. (1965). *The Autonomic Nervous system*, 2nd ed. Oxford: Blackwell.
FERRY, C. B. (1967). The autonomic nervous system. *A. Rev. Pharmac.*, **7**, 185.
KEOLLE, G. B. (1963). Cholinesterase and Anti-Cholinesterase Agents. *Handbuch der Experimentellen Pharmakologie*. Berlin: Springer.
Second Symposium on Catechol Amines (1966). *Pharmac. Rev.*, **18**.

CHAPTER VII

DEPRESSANTS OF THE CENTRAL NERVOUS SYSTEM

Narcotics, anti-convulsants, analgesics.

MANY drugs which depress the central nervous system are important in veterinary medicine because they are used to produce varying degrees of diminution of central nervous system activity varying from a mild sedation to general anæsthesia.

NARCOTICS

Hypnotics and narcotics are drugs which produce sleep and are not terms which are strictly applicable in veterinary medicine, but since many drugs so classified in human therapeutics are important veterinary drugs the terms are convenient.

Narcosis means the reversible inhibition of activity and metabolism which can be produced in almost all tissues by simple aliphatic compounds such as simple alcohols, ethers and similar compounds. The mode of action is unknown but there are some facts and several theories which help to explain.

The rapid and complete reversal of narcosis suggests that it is due to the physical rather than chemical properties of the drug. An explanation was put forward in the first decade of this century by Meyer and Overton, who, working independently, showed that there was a relationship between the ratio of narcotic's solubility in lipoids compared with its solubility in water and its narcotic potency. They suggested that because of the high lipoid content of nervous tissue it has a particular affinity for substances which have a high solubility in lipoid and low water solubility. Another suggestion is that anæsthetics act by congregating at cell surfaces like other substances which lower surface tension. Neither explanation

holds for magnesium which is insoluble in lipoids but has anæsthetic activity. A more recent attempt to explain anæsthetic
activity in terms of the physical properties of the anæsthetic
agents has drawn attention to the fact that most anæsthetics form
hydrated micro-crystals by reacting with water. It is further
suggested that the formation of such crystals in synaptic
regions of the central nervous system would impair conduction.
Although such crystals are known not to be stable at body
temperature, the theory proposes that the crystals are stabi-
lized by charged side-chains of protein. Whilst the Meyer-
Overton theory explains the distribution of many anæsthetic
agents in the body, the newer proposals in explanation of
their activity are in fact no real explanation and the matter
must remain open.

Narcotics usually depress the oxygen consumption of tissues
and the enzymes concerned in carbohydrate metabolism are
especially sensitive to narcotics.   However, since narcosis is
produced rapidly and the effect on oxygen consumption slowly
the latter is probably the result of narcosis, not its cause.
In support of a chemical explanation of narcotic activity, it
has been shown that certain barbiturates and diethyl ether
interfere with phosphorylation and since the energy-rich
phosphate bonds of adenosine triphosphate (ATP) are necessary
for the synthesis of acetylcholine, a decrease in ATP would
reduce the amount of acetylcholine available for synaptic
transmission.   Many simple aliphatic compounds have narcotic properties and are used in veterinary therapeutics.

Hypnotics usually only differ from anæsthetics in degree
and this is for the most part a matter of dosage.   Hypnotics
should produce a reliable effect without any initial excitement
and when given by mouth should be non-irritant and well
absorbed.   Clearance should be rapid to avoid cumulation and
there should be no other harmful effects such as damage to bone
marrow.   There should be a wide margin between the effective
dose and the toxic dose.   In general, although the aliphatic
hypnotics resemble the volatile anæsthetics in action they
differ in their fate in the body.   Drugs used as general
anæsthetics must be destroyed or excreted rapidly whereas
most drugs used as hypnotics are too long-acting to use as
anæsthetics.

Ethyl Alcohol (CH_3CH_2OH)

Alcohol is a narcotic, a disinfectant, a carbohydrate food and a useful solvent. It is rapidly absorbed from the gastro-intestinal tract and mostly metabolised in the body. Ethanol is metabolised by dehydrogenation ultimately to carbon dioxide and water, but forming on the way acetaldehyde and acetic acid. This oxidation is catalysed by an enzyme, ethanol dehydrogenase, and it is interesting to note that one of the richest sources of this enzyme is horse liver. It is a disinfectant acting by precipitating bacterial proteins. In veterinary practice its use is confined to disinfection of the skin.

Methyl alcohol resembles ethyl alcohol pharmacologically, the main distinction being due to the fact that in the body a large portion of the methyl alcohol is converted to formalde-hyde. Although its immediate toxic effects are less than those of ethyl alcohol it is cumulative and will produce coma lasting days accompanied by a bilateral inflammation of the optic nerve and retina resulting blindness.

Chloral Hydrate $(CCl_3CH(OH)_2)$

This white crystaline substance is used in veterinary medicine as a sedative and hypnotic for horses. It was the first synthetic hypnotic and was introduced by Liebreich in 1868. Liebreich knew that chloral hydrate in alkaline solutions liberated chloroform, and thought the same reaction would take place in the body. However, the narcotic effect is pro-duced neither by chloral hydrate itself nor chloroform but by trichlorethanol.

Chloral hydrate is readily absorbed from the gastro-intestinal tract although it is so irritant that it is necessary to give it by stomach tube well diluted. It may be given to dogs well diluted with syrup. In the body it is reduced to tri-chlorethanol which is the active substance. This is conjugated in the liver with glucuronic acid to form urochloralic acid which is excreted in the urine. The urine is then capable of reducing Fehling's solution. Some of the trichlorethanol is oxidised to trichloracetic acid. This is a strong acid which binds firmly to plasma proteins and hence persists in the blood for some days after chloral hydrate has been given.

When given by mouth to the horse or dog chloral hydrate produces its sedative effect after about 30 minutes. There is no initial excitement. It does not depress reflexes and is therefore of little use as an anticonvulsant. There is a slight fall in blood pressure due mainly to the peripheral vasodilatation. There is no good evidence of cardiac depression.

Since chloral hydrate is used occasionally in veterinary surgery as an intravenous narcotic and the margin between

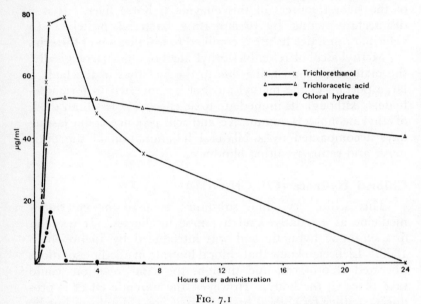

FIG. 7.1

The concentration of chloral and its metabolites in the plasma following the oral administration of 170 mg/kg to a horse.

narcotic dose and toxic dose is not great, it is important to appreciate the drug's toxic properties. In acute poisoning the blood pressure is low, temperature falls and respiration is depressed. Delayed poisoning commonly occurs after prolonged anæsthesia and is characterised by fatty changes in the liver, heart and kidneys, causing death after two or three days.

Chlorbutol is a similar hypnotic which does not irritate the gastro-intestinal tract. It is used to allay vomiting in dogs.

BARBITURATES

This important group of central depressants was discovered at the beginning of this century.   Chemically they are derived from malonic acid and urea. The thiobarbiturates have sulphur in place of oxygen in the urea portion of the molecule (Fig. 7.2). The barbiturates reversibly depress a wide range of biological functions.

There are a large number of barbiturates which differ

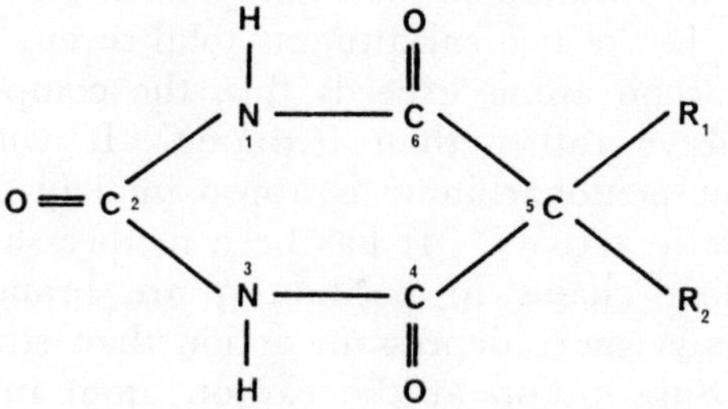

Long acting	Barbitone	Ethyl	Ethyl
	Phenobarbitone	Ethyl	Phenyl
Medium acting	Pentobarbitone	Ethyl	1−methylbutyl
	Butobarbitone	Ethyl	Butyl
Short acting	Methohexital	Allyl	1−methyl-2-pentynyl
	Thiopentone	Ethyl	1−methylbutyl
	(O at C_2 replaced by S)		

FIG. 7.2
The formulæ of certain barbiturates in common use.

from each other mainly in their duration of action which is determined by their fate in the body.   The fate in the body is affected by three factors: the solubility of the barbiturate in lipids, binding of the drug with protein and the dissociation constant of the drug.   The undissociated barbiturate has a high affinity for non-polar solvents; for example; the partition co-efficient of pentobarbitone is thirteen times that of pheno-barbitone and that of thiopentone two hundred times that of phenobarbitone. It will be seen, therefore, that the more highly lipid-soluble barbiturates are those which are short-acting with a rapid onset. They tend also to be more quickly metabolised and are almost completely re-absorbed from the renal tubule.

A great number of barbiturates have been synthesised, mainly by substitution at position 5 in the ring (Fig. 7.2). If the ring is unsubstituted at position 5 these compounds have little activity. The hypnotic activity of the barbiturate increases by substitution at position 5 until the number of carbon atoms in the two substituants total seven. When the number of carbon atoms exceeds this, the compound tends to be convulsive rather than hypnotic. It will be seen, therefore, that pentobarbitone is approximately of optimum size for hypnotic activity. It has been further shown that if the substituting chains in position 5 are branched, these compounds have more depressant action than straight chain isomerides. Substitution at the carbon atom in position 2 together with substituting one of the nitrogen atoms has given compounds with narcotic activity.

The speed at which a barbiturate acts depends on the rate at which an effective concentration penetrates into the brain, which in turn depends on the lipid solubility of the compound and on the blood supply. In the case of thiopentone, which has a high lipid solubility, it has been shown by using thiopentone labelled with radioactive carbon that those parts of the brain receiving the best blood supply are those in which the concentration of the drug is highest initially, although very soon distribution throughout the brain becomes uniform.

In the body the barbiturates are metabolised mainly by oxidation of the side-chain to form an inactive compound. This is mainly accomplished by the oxidative enzymes on the liver microsomes, which require for their activity reduced triphosphopyridine nucleotide and oxygen. This is of some practical importance as liver damage can substantially prolong the action of a barbiturate; for example, the administration (to sheep) of carbon tetrachloride which is a well known liver poison doubled the duration of action of pentobarbitone. There are some interesting and important species differences with respect to the metabolism of barbiturates. Young calves appear to be deficient in oxidative enzymes and hence even short or moderate-acting barbiturates have a prolonged action in this species. Pentobarbitone given to a calf can produce anæsthesia of twenty or more hours' duration and the animal may not recover. Sheep on the other hand appear to be well endowed with oxidative enzymes and the duration of action of pentobarbitone in sheep is not substantially longer than that of thiopentone; presumably due to the fact that the sheep can oxidize pentobarbitone as quickly as it can redistribute thiopentone. The horse appears to be similarly well sup-

TABLE 7.1

Clearance of Pentobarbitone

Species	Rate (per cent/hour)	Reference
Horse	46	Nicholson J. D. (1968) *Biochem. Pharmac.*, **17**, 1
Sheep	49	Rae, J. H. (1962) *Res. vet. Sci.* **3**, 399
Dog	15	Taylor *et al.* (1957) *Proc. Soc. exp. Biol. Med.* **95**, 462

plied with oxidative enzymes and the action of pentobarbitone in this species is little longer than that of thiopentone, whereas in the dog pentobarbitone acts four or five times as long as thiopentone. The barbiturates with the longest action are those which are mainly excreted in the urine as, for example, barbitone. Phenobarbitone, another long-acting barbiturate, is partly excreted in the urine and partly broken down in the liver. The effect of such drugs persists for more than twelve hours. Further evidence of the importance of the oxidative enzymes in the liver in influencing the duration of activity of barbiturates comes from the use of an interesting compound SKF 525A. This compound is chemically β-diethylamino-ethyl diphenyl propyl acetate; it has no apparent pharmaco-dynamic actions of its own, but appears to inhibit oxidases and esterases in the liver microsomes. If this drug is given to an experimental animal, and then followed by a barbiturate such as hexobarbitone, then the duration of action of the barbiturate is substantially prolonged. Phenobarbitone has an interesting property independent of its narcotic activity in that it appears to stimulate liver enzyme systems and can in the case of barbiturates cause tolerance to develop by increasing the activity of the oxidative enzymes of the liver.

Barbiturates whose effect is of six to eight hours' duration include Amylobarbitone, Pentobarbitone and Butobarbitone. These substances are largely broken down in the liver.

The short-acting barbiturates given intravenously last about fifteen minutes and include Thiopentone and Hexobarbitone. A more recently introduced barbiturate is *methohexitone*. This is a rapidly-acting oxy-barbiturate, which although it is an oxy-barbiturate has a very high solubility in fat, and is rapidly detoxicated. The high solubility in lipids of the unionised moiety of the short-acting barbiturates, which when carried to the brain in high concentrations allows similarly high concentrations to be taken up by that tissue, is the main reason for the rapid onset of action. The short duration of action is due to a redistribution of the drug and not to rapid metabolism. As thiopentone is taken up by tissues with a slower rate of perfusion the plasma concentration falls and the drug diffuses out of the brain. The fat depots also become sites where thiopentone is concentrated because of its high solubility in lipids. After the initial redistribution, the fall in plasma concentration is due to the increasing uptake by the fat depots and metabolism. When this drug is slowly released from the fat, it is metabolised in the liver. Most of the information about short-acting barbiturates has been obtained from work on thiopentone, which is still one of the most useful and widely used of this group of drugs. The fact that substantial amounts of the drug remain in the body after the action appears to have passed accounts for the fact that repeated doses are cumulative.

The duration of action is potentiated by the intravenous administration of glucose or intermediaries in its metabolism, such as lactate, pyruvate and glutamate. This should be kept in mind when using parenteral fluid replacement after a barbiturate anæsthesia.

All the barbiturates depress the central nervous system.

They differ only in degree and are not analgesic unless consciousness is affected. They are particularly depressant to the
motor areas of the cortex and are therefore useful in controlling convulsions of cortical origin. Depression of the sensory

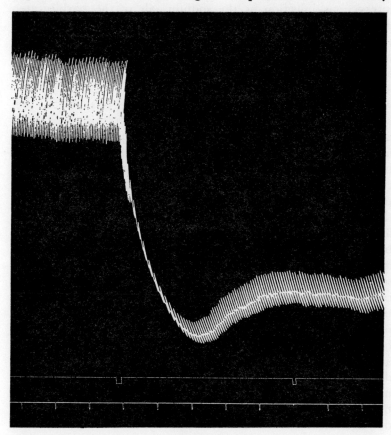

FIG. 7.3

The effect of pentobarbitone (10 mg/kg i.v.) on the respirations of a rabbit. The
height of the tracing above the base line shows the volume of air breathed. Time
interval 10 secs.

areas requires larger doses. There are two theories which
attempt to explain the action of the barbiturates—one suggests
they act by depressing the utilisation of oxygen by the brain
and the second that they prevent the synthesis of acetylcholine in the brain by blocking the conversion of pyruvate to

acetate. However, since the function of acetylcholine in the brain is still obscure the matter remains open.

In veterinary surgery Thiopentone and Pentobarbitone are widely used to produce anæsthesia. They are given by intravenous injection as the sodium salt of the barbiturate. The intravenous route is chosen because it allows the dose to be adjusted most readily to the animal's requirements. Moreover, these sodium salts form solutions which are markedly alkaline and are therefore irritant; the intravenous route avoids this irritation.

The barbiturates are particularly depressant to the respiratory centre and overdosage causes death from respiratory failure; pulmonary œdema is occasionally produced. Three factors are involved in the respiratory depression produced by barbiturates; firstly neurogenic factors involving the respiratory centres, secondly the carbon dioxide concentration in, and the pH of, arterial blood, and thirdly hypoxic factors involving the chemoreceptors of the carotid body and the aorta. The first of these factors is affected most by barbiturates, followed by the second and third. The sensitivity to carbon dioxide is actually abolished during barbiturate anæsthesia. This has some practical importance in that attempts to stimulate respiration, which has been unduly inhibited by too much barbiturate, by increasing the carbon dioxide content of the inspired air are unlikely to succeed. Therapeutic doses of barbiturates have little effect on the cardio-vascular system, although larger doses depress the vasomotor centre and may dilate and injure the capillaries, thus producing shock. They have little effect on the digestive tract or on renal function. The barbiturates reduce the basal metabolic rate but do not damage the liver. The motor activity of the uterus is un-affected, but respiration is depressed in the newborn because the barbiturates pass across the placenta. This is an important factor in choosing an anæsthetic for a Cæsarian section. The cerebrospinal fluid pressure is unaffected.

Barbiturates produce death either by direct paralysis of respiration or by causing a prolonged coma which may lead to a broncho-pneumonia. In treating barbiturate overdosage during anæsthesia artificial respiration is invaluable.

Bemegride is probably the best antidote but either

Bemegride or Picrotoxin may be used; they should be injected slowly intravenously until muscular twitching is produced. The long-acting barbiturates are liable to cause cumulation, and when used over a period the dose should be reduced accordingly.

The barbiturates can give any degree of central depression required depending on the compound chosen and on the dose and rate of administration. The short and medium-acting barbiturates are given intravenously to produce anæsthesia. The longer-acting compounds are used in small animal practice as anti-convulsants.

ANTI-CONVULSANT DRUGS

Phenytoin Sodium is an anti-convulsant drug chemically similar to the barbiturates, excepting that the barbituric acid ring is replaced by the 5 membered hydantoin ring (Fig. 7,4.) It is well absorbed from the gut and destroyed in the body, less than 0·1 per cent appearing in the urine. A single dose of this compound may persist in the cat's body for several days, because the cat is deficient in enzymes which metabolise the drug; hence this drug in the cat is cumulative. Experimentally this compound was found to prevent convulsions produced in the cat by electrical stimulation of the brain. Clinically it will suppress epileptic convulsions, and although it is not a general anti-convulsant like phenobarbitone, it has little hypnotic action.

Trimethadione is a drug which prevents Leptazol-induced convulsions and is also useful in controlling epileptic convulsions. It has been found to damage the bone marrow.

Mephenesin is a drug which depresses selectively subcortical and spinal poly-synaptic pathways. It is thus a centrally acting relaxant of voluntary muscle producing relaxation without loss of consciousness and not affecting myoneural transmission. Absorption takes place rapidly from all routes but it is quickly cleared, the effect of a single dose lasting less than one hour. This rapid clearance is a marked defect as it would otherwise be a very useful antagonist to strychnine for use in cases of poisoning. Concentrated solutions of mephenesin given intravenously have produced

H

hæmoglobinurea and even anuria by causing hæmatin crystals to precipitate in the kidney.

Primidone is a powerful anti-convulsant, said to be

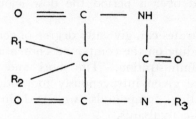

BARBITURATE NUCLEUS

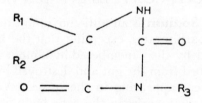

HYDANTOIN NUCLEUS

FIG. 7.4
The barbiturate and hydantoin nucleus.

better than the barbiturates and hydantoins and less hypnotic. It is used in dogs to control epileptiform convulsions and hysteria and to control convulsions in the foal.

Prolonged treatment may cause inco-ordination.

PHENOTHIAZINE ATARACTICS

An ataractic may be defined as a drug which produces in an animal a state of indifference to its surroundings. A number of derivatives of phenothiazine have been produced which possess this property. Several of these drugs have proved very useful in veterinary practice, both to facilitate handling of difficult animals of all species and, in particular, to pre-medicate animals prior to general anæsthesia. When used in this latter way ataractics not only make the induction of anæsthesia easier but reduce the amount of anæsthetic required and hence the liklihood of toxic sequelae.

Chlorpromazine inhibits a large number of enzymes and in consequence produces a wide range of pharmacological effects, the most conspicuous being due to depression of various functions of the central nervous system. Chlorpromazine inhibits the hypothalamus, the reticular formation and the chemoreceptor trigger zone. This latter property is utilized

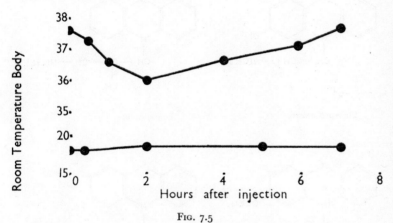

FIG. 7.5

The hypothermic action of chlorpromazine (1.5 mg/kg) in the horse.

when the drug is given to prevent vomiting, but it should be realised that chlorpromazine does not inhibit vomiting arising from stimuli from the gastro-intestinal tract or vestibular apparatus. Chlorpromazine has weak antihistamine, anticholinergic, antispasmodic and hypotensive actions. The hypotension may be due to its strong anti-adrenaline activity.

The animal given chlorpromazine remains conscious but is ataxic, refuses food, and shows some muscular relaxation, the head and tail drooping. The animal appears sedated but will react to stimuli. The effect of anæsthetics and hypnotics is enhanced. Body temperature falls and the production of hypothermia facilitated. The uptake of oxygen by the tissues is reduced. Chlorpromazine is antagonistic to central stimulants and large doses may produce respiratory failure.

The drug is well absorbed from the gut and destroyed in

the body.   The phenothiazine ataractics have a complex metabolism and in the dog less than 3 per cent of a single dose of chlorpromazine has been recovered from the urine unchanged. Many oxidation products are produced and in the dog tens of metabolites have been identified.   Chlorpromazine is even more persistent in the cat than in the dog and it is important that this long persistence of the phenothiazines is appreciated. In veterinary practice, administration by the intramuscular

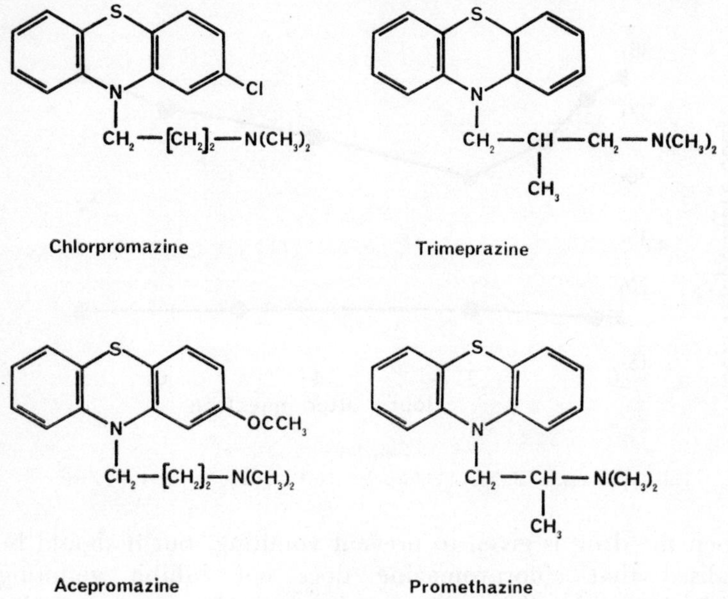

Chlorpromazine   Trimeprazine

Acepromazine   Promethazine

FIG. 7.6
Four phenothiazine derivatives.

route is usually preferred, the drug being used to render animals more tractable or as pre-anæsthetic medication.

Promazine has properties very similar to those of chlorpromazine but is much weaker.   It has proved popular in veterinary therapeutics.

Trimeprazine is similar to chlorpromazine in its activity but has stronger antihistaminic actions.   It is used both as an ataractic and as an antipruritic.   It is claimed that the ataractic action of trimeprazine is more reliable than that of chlorpromazine in the case of cats and horses.

Acepromazine has a potency similar to or even greater than chlorpromazine and it is alleged that acepromazine is less erratic in its ataractic activity, especially in the horse. It has been a popular drug for use in this species.

Promethazine is a phenothiazine used mainly as an antihistamine but has ataractic properties.

Miscellaneous Hypnotics

Phenycyclidine hydrochloride is a drug with both ataractic and narcotic action. Sometimes drugs with actions like this are called neuroleptics. Phenycyclidine does not appear to have any appreciable action on either the respiratory or circulatory systems and it does not affect muscle tone. However, it causes some stimulation of salivation. It is quickly absorbed and excreted. The main use of this drug is in the control of primates other than man and is no longer recommended for use in other species. It is a drug which has been used in the capture of wild animals; for this purpose it is administered by means of a dart. In primates catalepsy is produced. This is a state in which the body remains passively in any position it has been placed. In equines this drug produces an alarming excitement.

Dehydrobenzperidol is a neuroleptic agent which can be given by intramuscular injection and has proved useful in the sedation of the pig.

Cannabis Indica is obtained from a resin occurring in the leaves and stem of the hemp plant. It is a habit-forming drug in man and therefore scheduled under the Dangerous Drugs Act. It is probably the oldest drug of addiction and was used by the Assassins to prepare themselves for carrying out political murders. Man is first depressed then excited and the sense of space and time distorted. Fantastic dreams are experienced and pain is decreased.

This drug was used as a hypnotic in horses but was erratic in action. Newer synthetic substances of similar structure have been prepared and may be more reliable.

Bromides are occasionally used to produce a mild degree of sedation. They produce this effect because the bromide ions replace chloride without affecting any tissue except brain.

They have little effect on the sensory areas and are not analgesic. Large doses depress reflexes and motor activity and also produce " Bromism ". This condition is characterised by dullness, inco-ordination and skin eruptions. It is treated by increasing the chloride intake : since the kidney is unable to distinguish chloride from bromide, if it is excreting a lot of chloride it must at the same time excrete a lot of bromide. Conversely, restricting the chloride intake prolongs the effect of bromide.

Bromides are readily absorbed from the small intestine, distributed throughout the extracellular fluid and excreted in the urine.

ANALGESICS

Analgesia means the relief of pain. Simple depressants of the central nervous system, such as chloral hydrate, will dull pain, but do not produce relief until the animal is nearly comatose. A true analgesic such as morphine will relieve pain in certain species without producing any other marked effect.

The relief of pain is one of the most important responsibilities of a veterinary surgeon. It is essential, therefore, that he is fully acquainted with drugs which have this effect. Pain can be relieved by local anæsthetics, by counter-irritants, by certain drugs acting centrally such as morphine and by a number of antipyretics.

Analgesics should not be given to an animal if there is any risk of obscuring the diagnosis as pain is often an important clinical feature of a disease. Analgesics do not take the place of specific treatment if such is available. Tests of analgesic activity depend on the response of an experimental animal to a noxious stimulus; this response involves movement on the part of the animal. Common tests of this type are such as involve the measurement of the duration of the exposure of a rat's tail to radiant heat before the tail twitches, or the strength of the electrical stimulus which is required to make a mouse squeak when the underskin of the tail is stimulated. Tests such as these involve what are termed superficial nociceptors. Nociceptors are defined as those sensory nerves which respond to noxious stimuli. Other tests have been devised which involve the stimulation of so-called deep nociceptors. Examples of these are the writhing movements produced in mice by the intraperitoneal injection of substances such as acetic acid or bradykinin. Analgesics are tested by seeing whether these various responses can be reduced or abolished by an appropriate dose. However, it is realised in human medicine that the results of such experiments with analgesics in animals give not only inconsistent results, but results which are not always applicable when applied to the analgesia of pain arising from disease or trauma. The study of analgesics in natural pain occurring in domesticated animals is even more difficult.

Analgesics are conventionally divided into two groups, the so-called narcotic analgesics and a second group, the analgesic-antipyretics. The oldest and best-known member of the first group is the alkaloid morphine, but this group contains not only drugs chemically related to morphine but a number of synthetic compounds of quite different structure.

Opium is the name given to the dried exudate obtained when the unripe fruit of the Oriental poppy is incised. It is one of the oldest analgesics known and owes its activity to the alkaloid morphine which it contains together with numerous other alkaloids, the more important being narcotine, papaverine, codeine and thebaine.

Morphine

This is one of the most important drugs for treating intractable pain in man; in veterinary medicine its use is restricted to the dog. Morphine depresses the higher functions of the brain, stimulates then depresses the medullary centres and stimulates spinal reflexes. In the dog, rabbit and bird it is purely depressant, producing analgesia, sleep and, in large doses, coma. In the cat it causes delirium, and in the horse, ox and pig the effect is unreliable, sometimes producing narcosis and sometimes excitement. Morphine and its derivatives are probably the best analgesics for the dog and in this species, like man, it may produce a pin-point pupil by exciting the oculo-motor nerve nucleus. In other species the pupil is dilated because of the excitement caused by this drug.

The vagal centre is stimulated, slowing the pulse and increasing gastro-intestinal activity. In species with a developed vomiting centre the drug first stimulates and then depresses vomiting. Bronchial secretion is similarly stimulated then depressed. Cutaneous vaso-dilatation is produced with a consequent heat loss. The respiratory centre is depressed, respirations becoming slow and deep then intermittent. Large doses kill from depression of the respiratory centre. The cough centre is also depressed.

Morphine affects the alimentary tract, first, by increasing movements through the stimulation of the vagal centre and, secondly, through the contraction of the plain muscle of the gut impeding passage of digesta and thus leading to constipation. This is accentuated by the reduction in secretion of the intestinal glands and depression of the defæcation reflexes. Morphine produces the retention of urine by contracting the sphincters of the bladder and so making emptying difficult.

The drug is readily absorbed from the gut or after injection. In the body some is conjugated and excreted in the urine but more is destroyed by the liver. About 30 per cent is excreted in the fæces. Tolerance is quickly acquired to this drug.

The main use of morphine in veterinary practice is to pre-medicate the dog prior to anæsthesia with ether or similar anæsthetic. It is also used as an analgesic and to depress the cough centre and so relieve troublesome coughing. There is, however, a danger of depressing the respiratory as well as the cough centre. Crude preparations of opium are sometimes used to relieve diarrhœa.

The other opium alkaloids fall into two chemically distinct groups. Morphine, codeine and thebaine are phenanthrene derivatives; narcotine and papaverine are isoquinoline derivatives. Their pharmacological effect on plain muscle gives a similar grouping. Morphine, codeine and thebaine stimulate plain muscle wheras narcotine and papaverine inhibit it.

The opium alkaloids vary considerably in their effect on the central nervous system. As their narcotic action decreases the stimulant action on the spinal cord and medulla increases. Arranged in descending order of narcosis they are morphine, codeine, narcotine, papaverine and thebaine, the last substance producing strychnine-like convuslions.

Codeine resembles morphine in its activity but is less potent. It is mostly excreted unchanged in the urine and is used to relieve coughing, being given to dogs by mouth as codeine phosphate or syrup of codeine phosphate.

Papaverine has only slight narcotic activity but is a powerful inhibitor of plain muscle. It has been used to relieve colic but is of doubtful value.

Diamorphine or heroin is made by acetylating morphine and is a much more active drug but is more liable to produce a rapid deterioration in morals and health of addicts. It is absorbed from all routes of administration, including the nasal mucosa. In the U.S.A. manufacture is prohibited.

Apomorphine is prepared by treating morphine with mineral acids to remove a molecule of water from a morphine molecule. This greatly reduces the narcotic activity but increases the stimulant effects; in particular stimulation of the vomiting centre through its action on the chemoreceptor trigger zone. It produces vomiting when given by injection and is used for this purpose in dogs. Drugs with this property are called central emetics.

Methadone is a synthetic substance with many of the properties of morphine. It produces analgesia to about the same extent but is also depressant to respiration, and produces vomiting and addiction in man. This drug is well absorbed by most routes of administration and is mainly metabolised in the body, 20 to 30 per cent being excreted in the urine.

Pethidine hydrochloride has about one-tenth the analgesic power of morphine. When first introduced pethidine was claimed to have antispasmodic activity; however, recent experiments have shown that whilst pethidine is not as spasmogenic as morphine, it cannot be claimed to be an anti-spasmodic.

Respiration is rarely depressed but nausea and vomiting are produced and in man euphoria leading to addiction. The drug can be given orally or by intramuscular injection. Although pethidine is metabolised at a rate of about 17 per cent of the dose per hour in man, in the dog the rate of metabolism is 70 to 90 per cent of a given dose per hour; hence to be effective in this species the drug would have to be given frequently to produce an effect lasting more than 30 minutes.

Diethylthiambutene is used as the hydrochloride in

dogs to produce analgesia and narcosis. It is similar to morphine and is used for the same reasons. It is much less likely to produce vomiting but, like morphine, causes respiratory depression, which is more persistent than with morphine, and defæcation. In cats it produces excitement. When given by subcutaneous injection, diethylthiambutene is

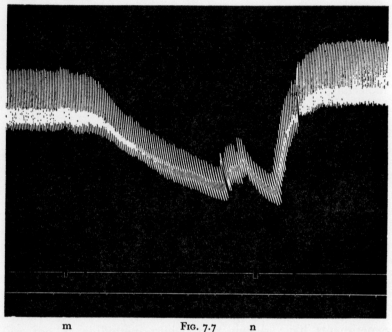

m   FIG. 7.7   n

The effect of morphine m(2·5 mg/kg) on the respirations of a rabbit and the antagonistic action of nalorphine n(2·5 mg/kg). The height of the tracing above the base line shows the volume of air breathed. Time interval 10 secs.

more rapidly absorbed than is morphine, but it is poorly absorbed from the gut.

Etorphine is a recently produced very potent derivative of morphine. This compound apparently is effective in a dose of about half a milligram per thousand pounds body weight. So far its use has been confined to the narcotization of wild game and occasionally to facilitate the handling of difficult horses and cattle. The advantage of this compound as an agent to immobilize wild game is that it can be injected by a dart and a very small volume of solution is required to contain an effective dose.

Dextromethorphan is the d-isomer of the codeine analogue of levorphanol.   This drug apparently has no analgesic or addictive properties, is devoid of narcotic activity and exerts no action on the gut.   However, it raises the threshold for stimuli to coughing and has been used thera-

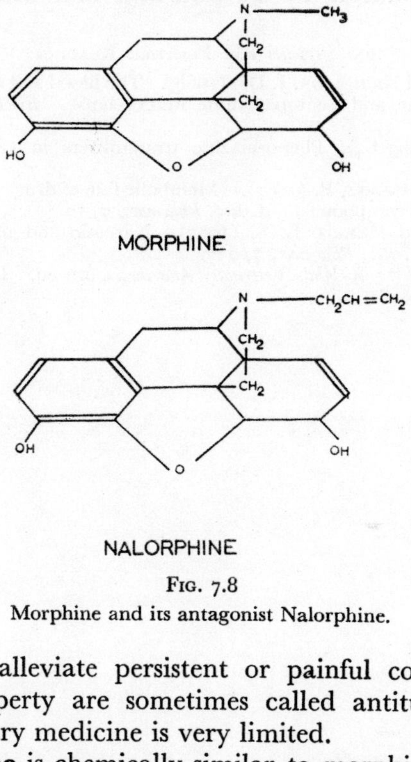

MORPHINE

NALORPHINE

Fig. 7.8

Morphine and its antagonist Nalorphine.

peutically to alleviate persistent or painful coughs.   Drugs with this property are sometimes called antitussives;   their use in veterinary medicine is very limited.

Nalorphine is chemically similar to morphine (Fig. 7.8), but pharmacologically acts as a competitive antagonist to morphine and morphine substitutes such as methadone and pethidine.   The degree of antagonism depends on the dose of nalorphine, large doses of morphine requiring large doses of nalorphine (see fig. 7.7).

When given to a normal animal nalorphine is depressant to the central nervous system, especially to respiration.   It reduces the tone of plain muscle and increases intestinal activity.   The main use is in the dog to terminate the effects of morphine or morphine substitute.   Since the effects of nalorphine are less persistent than those of morphine, animals so treated must be kept under observation for twelve hours after treatment.

Cats after nalorphine do not show excitement and mydriasis when given morphine.   Nalorphine does not reverse the central depression produced by barbiturates and other anæsthetic agents.

SUGGESTIONS FOR FURTHER READING

ALEXANDER, F. and NICHOLSON, J. D.   (1968).   The blood and saliva clearances of phenobarbitone and pentobarbitone in the horse.   *Biochem. Pharmac.*, **17**. 203.

BOYES, G. R.   (1963–64).   Phenothiazine tranquilizers in veterinary practice, *Vet. A.*, **5**, 32.

BUSH, M. T. and SANDERS, E.   (1967).   Metabolic fate of drugs: barbiturates and closely related compounds.   *A. Rev. Pharmac.*, **7**, 57.

FRASER, H. F. and HARRIS, L. S.   (1967).   Narcotic and narcotic antagonist analgesics.   *A. Rev. Pharmac.*, **7**, 277.

HALL, L. W.   (1966).   *Wright's Veterinary Anæsthesia*, 6th ed.   London: Bailliere, Tindall & Cassell.

CHAPTER VIII

DEPRESSANTS OF THE CENTRAL NERVOUS SYSTEM

General Anæsthetics

ANÆSTHETICS AND ANÆSTHESIA

Historical

ALCOHOL, opium and substances containing hyoscine were used from earliest times to dull the pain of surgical procedures. Surgical anæsthesia was introduced with almost explosive rapidity in the early years of the nineteenth century. Humphry Davy showed the possibilities of nitrous oxide anæsthesia in 1798, and in 1842 Crawford Long used ether as an anæsthetic for minor procedures but did not publish his results until after Morton produced surgical anæsthesia with ether in 1846. Surgical anæsthesia with chloroform was first demonstrated by Simpson in Edinburgh in 1847. In September 1846 the possibility of surgical anæsthesia was not generally recognised; by November 1847 ether and chloroform were in widespread use and the possibilities of nitrous oxide and ethyl chloride anæsthesia recognised.

The discovery of the anæsthetic properties of nitrous oxide is especially interesting. Sir Humphry Davy studied the pharmacological properties of this gas between 1798 and 1800. He anæsthetised himself on several occasions and showed the necessity of administering oxygen together with the nitrous oxide. His suggested use of this gas in surgery was neglected for forty years whereas the ludicrous effects of "laughing gas" were exploited in side-shows.

Wells, an American dentist, extracted a tooth under nitrous oxide anæsthesia in 1844, but his demonstration at the Massachusetts General Hospital failed and not until 1870 was nitrous oxide used generally. Ether was one of the earliest synthetic organic drugs, and its powers of intoxication were well known. Jackson and Morton witnessed the failure of

Wells to anæsthetise with nitrous oxide, and two years later in 1846 Morton used ether for the painless extraction of teeth. On 16th October 1846 he demonstrated its use in public as a general anæsthetic for major surgery. On 19th December 1846 ether was used in London by Liston and thereafter its use became widespread.

The third outstanding discovery was that of chloroform by Sir James Y. Simpson as an anæsthetic in human obstetrics. Simpson had investigated the possibilities of several volatile substances for this purpose and the use of chloroform was suggested by a chemist named Waldie. Fortunately for chloroform the patient on whom the first operation under chloroform was to be performed died before the drug arrived and so the drug escaped blame for killing the patient. Both ether and chloroform were soon in wide use and controversy about their respective merits arose. However, when the facts were assembled it became clear that chloroform was responsible for a number of fatalities and that ether was the safer drug. Nevertheless, in veterinary surgery chloroform is still a valuable anæsthetic under certain circumstances. Following the discovery of chloroform there was no major advance in general anæsthesia until the second decade of the twentieth century when ethylene and later cyclopropane were introduced.

FATE OF VOLATILE ANÆSTHETICS

Volatile drugs given by inhalation are quickly absorbed and rapidly excreted, hence the depth of anæsthesia can be altered quickly during the administration, and when administration stops recovery soon follows. The uptake and distribution are largely dependent on the solubility of anæsthetic in blood and tissues. At the beginning of anæsthesia the concentration of anæsthetic in arterial blood is much greater than in venous blood. However, as the anæsthesia progresses the concentration in venous blood rises as the tissues, especially those rich in fat, acquire a higher concentration of anæsthetic. The concentration of anæsthetic in both arterial and venous blood gradually rises and the difference between them falls. Absorption from the alveoli falls until the concentration of anæsthetic in the blood and alveoli is in equilibrium.

The uptake, distribution and excretion of volatile anæsthetics is governed by the concentration of anæsthetic inspired, the alveolar ventilation, the partition coefficient of the anæsthetic and the blood supply of the tissue. The boiling point, saturated vapour pressure, maximum concentration and partition coefficient between blood and gas, and fat and blood, for the various anæsthetic agents is shown in Table 8·1. Induction of anæsthesia is slower with the more blood-soluble anæsthetic agents such as ether, than with the less soluble agents like halothane. This is because the solubility in blood represents a large reservoir for soluble agents which continue to enter it for an appreciable time before it is filled, whereas the reservoir for insoluble gases is smaller and can be filled more quickly, hence they can more quickly pass from blood to brain. Similarly a soluble drug such as ether takes longer to be eliminated than a less soluble agent such as cyclopropane, because more is held in solution in the blood, which has a potentially larger capacity for ether than for the less soluble cyclopropane. Although the more soluble ether is rapidly taken up from the alveoli by the blood, an effective concentration does not arise in the brain very quickly as a substantial amount of the ether, because of its solubility, is retained in the blood. These facts explain why it is necessary to induce anæsthesia with a high concentration of anæsthetic and maintain it with a lower concentration. In fact the art of the administration of volatile anæsthetics is that of adjusting the concentration of volatile anæsthetic needed to produce and maintain surgical anæsthesia. Both absorption and excretion are exponential; the latter is particularly important in ensuring quick excretion of most of the dose. It is not necessary to saturate the body with anæsthetic as brain cells on which it acts are especially sensitive to it. Moreover, the brain has a better blood supply than most tissues which ensures a better supply of the anæsthetic.

ADMINISTRATION OF VOLATILE ANÆSTHETICS

The rate at which volatile liquids vaporize depends upon their physical characteristics such as boiling point, saturated vapour pressure etc. which are shown in Table 8.1.

In anæsthetic apparatus other factors such as the surface

TABLE 8.1

Anaesthetic	B.P. (°C.)	Saturated Vapour Pressure at 20°C. (mm. Hg)	Maximum Concentration obtainable at 20°C.	Partition coefficient		
				Blood/Gas	Brain/Blood	Fat/Blood
Ether	35	442	58%	12	1·1	5
Halothane	50	243	32%	2·3	2·6	60
Chloroform	61	160	21%	10	1·2	26
Trichloroethylene	87	59	8%	9	—	106
Methoxyflurane	105	25	3%	13	—	63
Cyclopropane	−33	—	100%	0·5	—	20
Nitrous oxide	−88	—	100%	0·5	1·0	3

The physical characteristics of some volatile and gaseous anaesthetics.

area of anæsthetic presented, which depends on the diameter of the bottle, influence the rate of vaporisation. It is affected by whether air or oxygen is bubbled through the liquid or

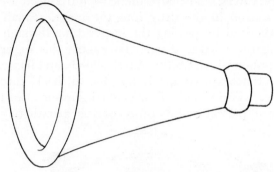

FIG. 8.1
Conical rubber mask suitable for dogs and other small animals.

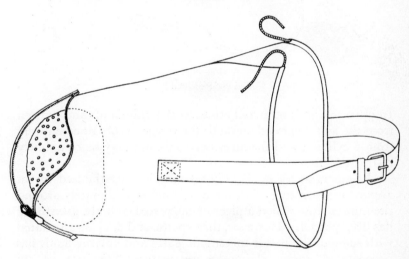

FIG. 8.2
Canvas mask for the administration of volatile liquid anæsthetics to the horse. The anæsthetic liquid is applied to the sponge.

over the surface of the liquid Gauze pads or wicks, soaked in anæsthetic, are sometimes used to facilitate vaporization. The liquid anæsthetic is sometimes contained in a water-jacketed bottle so it can be volatilised more readily by warming.

I

Horses and cattle under the conditions of general practice may be given volatile anæsthetics by means of a mask fitting the muzzle fairly closely and usually having inspiratory and expiratory valves. The anæsthetic is introduced by placing a gauze soaked in the drug into the mask. Small animals are anæsthetized by passing the inspired air through a bottle containing the volatile drug. To enable this to be done a mask is applied which fits the muzzle closely and has expiratory valves so that expired air is not blown back through the anæsthetic. These methods are called semi-open in that they allow for a partial re-breathing of the anæsthetic mixture.

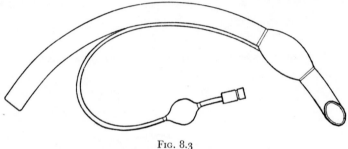

FIG. 8.3
Cuffed endotracheal tube.

In open methods of anæsthetisation the animal obtains oxygen from the air; in closed methods the oxygen is obtained entirely from a cylinder and the anæsthetic mixture may be completely re-breathed.

In emergencies small animals may be anæsthetised by an apparatus consisting of a tin can, fitting approximately around the muzzle, into which a piece of gauze soaked in the anæsthetic has been placed. However, the expense and dangers associated with some of the newer anæsthetic gases and volatile fluids has necessitated more elaborate apparatus. The use of an anæsthetic machine not only allows a more accurate control of the concentration of anæsthetic, but also enables the degree of oxygenation to be more safely regulated. In such an apparatus the anæsthetic gas is delivered from a cylinder through a flow meter, mixed with oxygen similarly delivered and enters the animal's lungs either through the animal's nostrils or through an endotracheal tube. The former method involves the use of a tightly fitted mask, whilst passing an endotracheal tube necessitates premedication with a suitable hypnotic. The

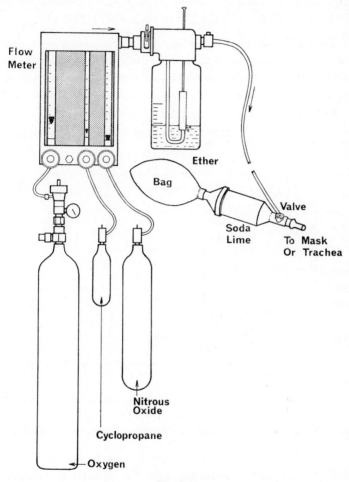

Flow
Meter

Ether

Bag

Valve

Soda
Lime

To Mask
Or Trachea

Nitrous
Oxide

Cyclopropane

Oxygen

FIG. 8.4

Diagram of a simple anæsthetic machine for the administration of gaseous and volatile liquid anæsthetics..

carbon dioxide is removed from the system by soda lime contained in a suitable cannister.

With all anæsthetic apparatus it is essential to keep the dead space to a minimum and to have tubes of sufficient diameter so as to reduce the resistance to gas flow and so interfere with respiration as little as possible.

THE STAGES OF ANÆSTHESIA

To facilitate understanding and comparison of general anæsthetics it is convenient to describe four stages of anæsthesia. The first stage is that of analgesia, the second of excitement, the

Guedel's Classification.			Reflexes etc. Present					
			Respiration	Pulse	Swallowing	Corneal	Eyeball Movements	Temperature
Stage 1.		Analgesia.	Rapid & irregular	Rapid	+	+		Normal
Stage 11.		Delirium.	Very irregular	Rapid	+	+	+++++	Slight increase
Stage 111. Surgical Anaesthesia	Plane 1.	Sleep.	Slow regular	Normal	-	+	+++++ ++++ +++ +,+	Gradual fall
	Plane 2	Sensory loss	Slow regular	Normal	-	+ to - - - - -		↓
	Plane 3.	Loss of muscle tone	Thoracic abdominal	Rapid & fall in B.P.	-	-		↓
	Plane 4	Intercostal Paralysis	Shallow abdominal	Rapid & weak	-	-		
Stage 1V.		Medullary Paralysis			-	-		

FIG. 8.5

Stages and plans of general anæsthesia. These are best shown in the dog under ether.

third of surgical anæsthesia and the fourth of medullary paralysis. Surgical anæsthesia is divided into four planes. These are represented diagrammatically in Fig. 8·5.

Stage I—Analgesia

In this stage sensitivity to pain is diminished and there is a slight increase in pulse rate but not respiratory rate. It is important for smooth induction of anæsthesia not to disturb the respiratory rhythm.   The end of this stage is marked by unconsciousness.

Stage II—Delirium

The animal is unconscious at the onset of this stage and the influence of the higher centres is abolished, which results in struggling and attempts to remove the mask.   These efforts are often followed by a period of deep breathing and care is required to avoid the onset of cardiac or respiratory failure. It is advisable to stop administration of anæsthetic during the deep breathing and only resume once normal respiration is re-established.   The swallowing and vomiting reflexes may be active and the latter especially should be anticipated.   It is important to pass through this stage as quickly as is consistent with safety; premedication with suitable sedatives facilitates this progress.

Stage III—Surgical Anaesthesia

The first plane of surgical anæsthesia is considered to begin with the onset of regular automatic breathing.   The rate and depth of respiration is increased and there is marked movement of the eyeballs.

The second plane should follow the first plane smoothly with the rate and volume of respirations increased.   The tone of voluntary muscle is lost and the *recti abdominis* muscles relax. This plane is usually sufficient for most surgical operations on domestic animals.

The third plane is required very occasionally.   It is marked by paralysis of the intercostal muscles and quietening of respiratory movements.   Respiration becomes entirely dependent on the diaphragm.

The fourth plane is marked by the rapid irregular respirations and small pulse.   The respirations tend to stop.

Stage IV—Medullary Paralysis

In the last stage the animal is markedly cyanosed, the pupils dilated and the eyeballs glazed and staring.   Death very quickly supervenes.

In veterinary anæsthesia the most reliable indications of

progress are the various changes in respiration. The ocular reflexes whilst useful are less consistent than respiration.

Whilst the Guedel classification of the stages of anæsthesia is very convenient for studying the process, it is essential to realise that all the various stages and planes are unlikely to be shown during an individual anæsthesia, and that the classification was developed from a study of ether. This classification, for example, tends to overemphasise the effects of the anæsthetic on respiration and minimize circulatory effects. Whilst this is correct in the case of ether, it does not give sufficient weight, for example, to the hypotension produced by halothane.

The stages of anæsthesia are greatly modified by preanæsthetic medication. Ruminants under general anæsthesia usually show a rise in body temperature instead of the more usual fall. This is because in the ruminant heat is continuously produced by the fermentation of digesta in the rumen, yet under anæsthesia, both the heat regulating centre and respiratory centre are depressed so that the heat of fermentation is less readily dissipated.

Pre-anaesthetic Medication

The induction of general anæsthesia is greatly facilitated and and many of the complications of anæsthesia avoided by the use of other drugs in addition to the anæsthetic agent. The phenothiazine ataractics are used in all species to facilitate the induction of anæsthesia. These agents also reduce the amount of anæsthetic required by the animal. Chloral hydrate, given by mouth, is sometimes used for the same purpose in horses. Atropine is often given to reduce salivary and bronchial secretions.

Induction of Anæsthesia

Anæsthesia in all the domesticated species is often induced by the intravenous injection of a short-acting barbiturate such as thiopentone. This procedure facilitates the introduction of an endotracheal tube and the use of inhalation anæsthetics like cyclopropane or it may precede the administration of an irritant anæsthetic of relatively low potency such as ether. It is sometimes possible to induce anæsthesia by using halothane in a mask and then transferring the animal to a different volatile agent. The intravenous injection of a drug such as thiopentone has many advantages in veterinary surgery, for example, the stage of excitement can be very nearly abolished by regulating the rate at which the injection is made. The risks of physical injury to the animal are reduced because induction by an intravenous agent is much more rapid than by inhalation. It is, however, not always possible to adopt this technique and under some circumstances it is even possible to induce anæsthesia by cyclopropane given by a mask.

Ether

Di-ethyl ether, discovered in 1546 by Valerius Cordus, is a volatile liquid boiling at $35°$ C, highly inflammable and explosive when mixed with air. When exposed to light and air ether forms various peroxides which are more irritant than ether and so tend to make it more toxic. Copper helps to prevent this oxidation, hence copper tubes are often used in anæsthetic bottles containing ether.

Ether is a weaker anæsthetic than chloroform since it requires four times the concentration to produce anæsthesia. Induction is slow and difficult with ether, and although it is less irritant than chloroform in equal concentrations, since four times as much is required, the total irritant effect is greater. Cold ether vapour is very irritant, and it is good practice to use a warming device. Ether stimulates the sympathetic centres, increasing blood pressure, pulse rate and blood sugar. It has a direct depressant action on the myocardium; this is countered to some extent by increased sympathetic activity which produces a high cardiac output. This drug does not sensitise the heart to catechol amines. The secretions of the bronchial and salivary glands are increased and may interfere mechanically with respiration. Premedication with atropine reduces these secretions. Ether produces a neuromuscular block, which potentiates the action of drugs with curare-like activity, but not depolarising neuromuscular blocking agents. Although most of the ether administered is excreted in the expired air, some is metabolised to ethanol and acetaldehyde.

Chloroform

This volatile liquid is readily oxidised by light or oxygen to phosgene. It is advisable to buy it in small containers and not keep the residue of a bottle. It is a very powerful anæsthetic which makes it easy to administer but increases the danger. All statistics agree that chloroform is more dangerous than any of the other anæsthetics in common use. Nevertheless, in certain circumstances in veterinary practice the advantages outweigh the dangers.

Chloroform reduces the oxygen-carrying capacity of the blood, and by depressing the vasomotor centre produces a fall in blood pressure. The respiratory centre is also depressed so that respirations may cease suddenly whilst the blood pressure is still high. It is essential when using this drug to ensure an adequate oxygenation of the tissues.

Since situations arise in veterinary practice in which the surgeon has no alternative to chloroform anæsthesia, it is essential to recognise the risks associated with this drug. Death may occur either during induction, in the course of a prolonged anæsthesia or two or three days after the anæsthesia. The last type of death is termed delayed chloroform poisoning. When death occurs during the induction the heart stops suddenly, due to ventricular fibrillation. This can be produced experimentally by stimulating the vagus nerve or giving adrenaline to an animal under chloroform. Obviously adrenaline should never be given to an animal under chloroform. Pre-medication with atropine helps to prevent the effects of vagal stimulation.

The cat is particularly liable to develop ventricular fibrillation under chloroform. However, cardiac irregularities occur with many anæsthetics in addition to chloroform; cyclopropane and halothane, for example, are anæsthetics which may give rise to this condition. These cardiac arrhythmias are more common in conditions of inadequate carbon dioxide excretion. Arrhythmias produced by the action of released adrenaline on the heart can best be prevented by the use of a beta blocking agent such as propranolol.

Deaths which occur during a prolonged anæsthesia are usually due to the depressant effect of chloroform on the myocardium. This effect is distinct from the ventricular fibrillation produced during induction. Chloroform also predisposes to shock, which is an important consideration in some operations. Respirations may stop suddenly during prolonged anæsthesia.

Delayed chloroform poisoning usually occurs twenty-four hours after the anæsthesia. This complication is more likely to occur when the liver has been deprived of glycogen and if anoxia is allowed to develop during anæsthesia. In man and dog the clinical signs resemble those of acidosis such as vomiting, acetonuria, followed by coma and death. The horse shows complete loss of appetite, jaundice, constipation and later coma and death.

Chloroform produces fatty changes in the liver, kidney and heart. Even a brief administration of chloroform can produce liver damage, and this drug should only be used when no safer agent is available.

Halothane (Fluothane), a recently introduced volatile anæsthetic, is slightly more potent than chloroform. This anæsthetic is non-explosive and non-inflammable. It is very expensive and is commonly administered by a closed circuit apparatus in which there is re-breathing of the expired gases. For operations of short duration such as castration of the cat, it can be given by means of a mask. Halothane is not potent a analgesic. Induction with halothane is smooth and relatively fast because the drug is non-irritant and being poorly soluble in blood it is quickly taken up by the brain.

However, muscular relaxation is not as good as with chloroform or ether at comparable levels of anæsthesia. Moreover, muscle relaxants such as d-tubocurarine are contra-indicated because they produce a fall in blood pressure which may be dangerous. The hypotension produced by halothane was considered to be due to a ganglion blocking action of the drug. However, this is a minor component, the circulatory depression being due mainly to a direct action of the drug on the myocardium and blood vessels. There is also a reduced sympathetic outflow and increased parasympathetic action, due to the action of halothane on the central nervous system. Vascular tone is also reduced causing vasodilatation. Cardiac irregularities sometimes occur under halothane; these are

usually associated with hypercapnia. Lowering the carbon
dioxide concentration usually restores normal cardiac ryhthm,
although halothane also sensitises the heart to catechol
amines. Halothane has some depressant action on respiration;
it reduces the reflex response to an increased carbon dioxide
concentration. Recovery from this anæsthetic is usually
rapid and quiet. It is, however, by no means completely
excreted through the lungs. By using halothane labelled
with radio-active chlorine and rats as experimental animals,
it has been shown that only 60 per cent of a given amount of
halothane was excreted in the first thirty hours after administration. Moreover, these animals were found to continue
excreting radio-active chlorine in the urine for two weeks
after the drug had been administrated. This shows that a
proportion of the halothane administered is metabolised in
the body. The slow clearance of halothane may be due in
part to the uptake of this drug by the fat. The fat : blood
partition coefficient of halothane is 60, whereas the same figure
for ether is 5. Halothane inhibits the tone and motility of
the gastrointestinal tract and uterus. There have been few
reports of liver damage being caused by this drug, but this
seems to be more likely when oxygenation has been inadequate.

Methoxyflurane is a non-explosive, non-inflammable
liquid which has been used to anæsthetise the dog and cat.
Although methoxyflurane is a more potent anæsthetic than
halothane, induction and recovery are more prolonged. This
is because methoxyflurane has a boiling point of 105° C.
at room temperature, the partial pressure of the vapour
produces an inspired concentration of only 3 per cent of the
anæsthetic gas. Moreover, this drug has a high solubility
in blood, which tends to hold the drug in appreciable quantities
in the blood rather than allowing an anæsthetic level to be
attained quickly in the brain. Given by either open or closed
methods it produces a good degree of analgesia. It has some
neuromuscular blocking activity. It produces a progressive
degree of hypotension and is very depressant to the respiratory
reflexes. If the carbon dioxide concentration is greatly
increased, methoxyflurane may cause liver damage. The
prolonged recovery makes this drug unsuited for large animals.

Cyclopropane is a colourless gas forming an explosive

mixture with air. The anæsthetic properties of this drug were discovered in 1929. It is similar in potency to ether but is non-irritant. Cyclopropane must be given in a closed circuit apparatus. The inspired concentration of cyclopropane for anæsthesia should be 30 per cent of the gas in oxygen.

It is expensive and gives poor muscular relaxation. Respiration is depressed and blood pressure rises. Cardiac irregularities may occur as a result of catechol amines being released by carbon dioxide retention. Despite a normal systemic blood pressure being maintained, cyclopropane causes capillary constriction and thus may impair the tissue perfusion. The depression of ventilation is produced by a central action and a rise in the carbon dioxide concentration does not cause reflex stimulation. In addition, since the anæsthetic is given with high concentrations of oxygen, this removes any stimulation of respiration arising from hypoxia. It is essential therefore, when using this anæsthetic, to maintain the ventilation rate, if necessary, by artificial means. It is used in some veterinary hospitals and for experimental surgery on farm animals.

Trichloroethylene resembles chloroform but is less potent. In veterinary practice, it is used for anæsthesia of dogs, cats and pigs. It is frequently supplemented by nitrous oxide. It does not irritate the bronchi and is less toxic to the liver. Full relaxation cannot be obtained with this drug, and it probably has the same cardiac effects as chloroform. Trichloroethylene differs from the other inhalation anæsthetics in its effect on respiration. At deep planes of surgical anæsthesia tachypnoea develops, which is in contrast to the more usual depression of respiration produced by other anæsthetics. Trichloroethylene must never be used in a closed circuit apparatus because it forms a toxic compound with soda lime.

Ethyl chloride is a powerful anæsthetic but maintenance is difficult. It has similar dangers to chloroform. This drug when sprayed on the skin gives a transient local anæsthesia.

Nitrous oxide is used in conjunction with other inhalation drugs for the induction of anæsthesia and during the maintenance of anæsthesia as a supplement to drugs such as ether, methoxyflurane and trichloroethylene. When using nitrous oxide, it is important to realise that the oxygen concentration of the anæsthetic gas mixture must be at least 20 per cent O_2.

Carbon dioxide can be compressed to form a solid known as " dry ice ". Pigs are sometimes exposed to the vapour from dry ice to produce anæsthesia as a prelude to slaughter. Guinea-pigs may also be anæsthetized by exposure in this fashion to carbon dioxide.

CHOICE OF ANÆSTHETIC

This varies with the circumstances. If the resources of a veterinary hospital are not available then methods requiring bulky cylinders of gas and elaborate flow meters cannot be considered. This eliminates the possibility of using agents such as cyclopropane. On the other hand, since many operations on the horse are of short duration, chloroform despite its dangers may be the drug of choice, having regard to its potency and simplicity of administration, the brevity of the operation reducing the risks of pulmonary complications and liver damage.

The ruminant is a particularly poor subject for general anæsthesia. This is because of the high risk of the development of pneumonia and/or ruminal tympany. The risk of pneumonia is accentuated by the continuous salivation shown by these animals which increases the risk of inhaling saliva. There is also a possibility of regurgitated rumen contents being inhaled. General anæsthesia inhibits ruminal movements and the eructation mechanism and, since fermentation in the rumen continues, gas is produced which cannot escape. This gives rise to tympany which by increasing intra-abdominal pressure may reduce the animal's tidal volume and, by compressing the large veins, reduce the venous return to the heart. Most surgeons prefer to use epidural or paravertebral nerve blocking with local anæsthetic in the bovine. Sheep can be anæsthetised with an intravenous barbiturate or, if facilities exist, with cyclopropane. Anæsthesia in calves can be induced and maintained with halothane. This avoids the problem presented by this species in their inability to metabolise barbiturates. Although the administration by intravenous injection of drugs, such as chloral hydrate in the larger animals and pentobarbitone in small animals, has practical advantages, these drugs are eliminated much more slowly than the volatile anæsthetics and overdosage is less readily corrected. Recovery from these agents may be prolonged and fatalities are more likely to occur. In large animals recumbency may be protracted and undue excitement be shown during recovery The introduction of potent ataractics has extended the surgery which can be performed using these drugs to maintain unconsciousness, whilst analgesia is attained by the use of appropriate local analgesic techniques. Although the agents available for pre-anæsthetic medication and for general anæsthesia have increased in number, which has given the anæsthetist a wider choice of anæsthetic, this has resulted in a wider margin of safety in general anæsthesia but has placed greater demands on the anæsthetist's skill and knowledge. Within the past decade anæsthesia has become a speciality in the veterinary profession and, although such a specialist requires to have considerable experience, his knowledge must be based on a thorough understanding of the pharmacological properties of the drugs used. Nevertheless, with all anæsthetics, the skill of the anæsthetist is a very important factor and familiarity with the agent chosen is essential.

SUGGESTIONS FOR FURTHER READING

EVANS, F. T. and GRAY, T. C. (1965). *General Anæsthesia*, 2nd ed. London: Butterworths.

FEATHERSTONE, R. M. and MUEHLBAECHER, C. A. (1963). The current role of inert gases in the search for anæsthesia mechanisms. *Pharmac. Rev.*, **15**, 97.

HALL, L. W. (1966). *Wright's Veterinary Anæsthesia*, 6th ed. London: Bailliere, Tindall & Cassell.

MITCHELL, B. (1966). Anæsthesia in small animal practice. *Vet. Rec.*, Clin. Suppl. 3.

Symposium on Inhalation Anaesthetics (1965). *Br. J. Anaesth.*, **37**, 644.

WEAVER, A. B. (1966). Recent developments in anæsthesia of large animals. *Vet. Rec.*, Clin. Suppl. 3.

WESTHUES, M. and FRITSCH, R. (1965). *Animal Anæsthesia*, Vol. II. Edinburgh: Oliver & Boyd.

VANDAM, L. D. (1966). Anæsthesia. *A. Rev. Pharmac.*, **6**, 379.

CHAPTER IX

DEPRESSANTS OF THE CENTRAL NERVOUS SYSTEM

ANTIPYRETICS AND ANTI-INFLAMMATORY AGENTS

ANTIPYRETICS are drugs which lower the body temperature by acting on the heat regulating centre. Since this property is often combined with that of producing a mild analgesia, it is convenient to consider them alongside the more powerful analgesics. These drugs may be called analgesic-antipyretics, and are usually classified into three categories according to their chemical structure. On this basis the three groups are the salicylates, the para aminophenol derivatives, such as phenacetin, and the pyrazolon derivatives, for example, phenylbutazone. Unlike the narcotic analgesics the antipyretic analgesics are inactive when tested by a number of anti-nociceptive tests such as those already described. However, acetylsalicylate is particularly effective in the mouse peritoneal test where the deep nociceptors are stimulated. There is some evidence which suggests that the analgesic antipyretics act peripherally. This may be because certain of them such as the salicylates have anti-inflammatory activity which will be discussed later.

With the advent of specific drugs to combat infections, antipyretics are not often used in the treatment of fever but are used mainly for their analgesic properties.

One of the oldest antipyretics is quinine, the alkaloid obtained from the bark of the Cinchona tree. However, the most important action of this drug is on the schizonts of the malaria parasite which is not of veterinary importance. It acts as a bitter when in the mouth, is absorbed readily from the gut, about half being excreted in the urine and half being destroyed in the body. After absorption, quinine lowers the body temperature by increasing heat lost through vasodilation and decreasing heat production by depressing metabolism. It is a mild analgesic. The cinchona alkaloids have an important action on heart muscle; they increase the refractory period, and this property is utilised in the treatment

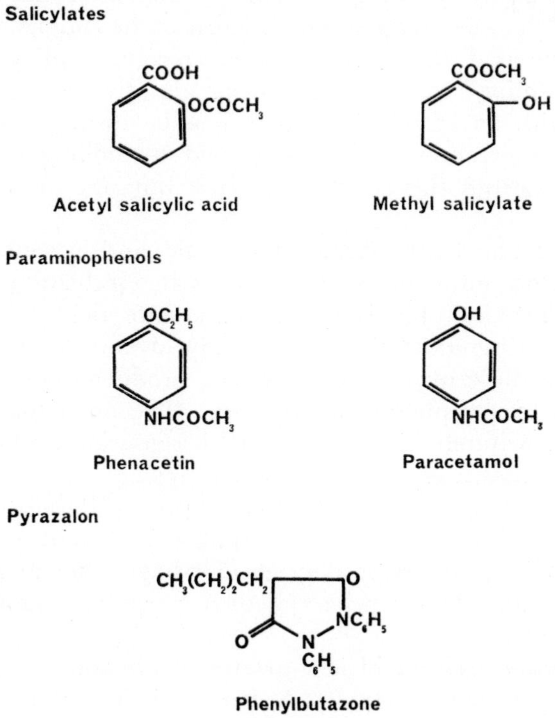
Salicylates
COOH
OCOCH3
COOCH3
OH
Acetyl salicylic acid
Methyl salicylate
Paraminophenols
OC2H5
NHCOCH3
OH
NHCOCH3
Phenacetin
Paracetamol
Pyrazalon
CH3(CH2)2CH2
O
NC6H5
N
O
C6H5
Phenylbutazone

FIG. 9.1
The formulæ of some antipyretic analgesics.

of certain arrhythmias of the heart. Voluntary muscle is affected in the same way, but this is not an effect of therapeutic importance.

Salicylic acid was first used in the form of bark from the Willow tree which contains a glycoside salicin. This glycoside yields salicylic acid on hydrolysis. It is now used in the form of white crystals of sodium salicylate which are very soluble in water.

Salicylates are quickly absorbed from the gut and excreted in all secretions. However, the greater portion is excreted in the urine partly unchanged, partly oxidised and partly combined with glucuronic acid. Since the cat lacks a glucuronide-forming enzyme, salicylates are potentially particularly dangerous in this species and toxic levels may be reached if large or continuous dosage is used. A single dose may take one to two days to be excreted, and because of the conjugation with glucuronic acid, the urine of animals receiving salicylates will reduce Fehling's solution; such urine also gives a red or violet colour with ferric chloride which can be distinguished from the colour given by aceto-acetic acid by boiling the urine. Boiling destroys the aceto-acetic acid but not the salicylate conjugate.

Salicylic acid is weakly bacteriostatic, and in concentrated solutions or ointments destroys the skin epithelium without pain. This kind of activity is called keratolytic.

The antipyretic action is seen only in animals with fever. It acts on the central nervous system, producing an increased heat loss by peripheral vasodilation. The analgesic effect is produced without the loss of other sensations. The drug increases the urinary excretion of uric acid.

Salicylates are not devoid of toxic actions. Large doses may cause vomiting in the dog, dyspnœa and skin eruptions. Repeated large doses produce hæmorrhages due to a fall in prothrombin. This can be remedied by giving vitamin K or an analogue.

Acetylsalicylic acid is a palatable substitute for salicylic acid, usually given in tablets because it is insoluble, unstable and incompatible with most drugs. Its use is confined to the dog and cat to produce analgesia. It is partly hydrolysed in the intestine, but some is absorbed unchanged. The actions of this drug differ from those of salicylic acid in several respects. Some individuals show an allergic response, and it causes hypoprothrombinæmia more easily than salicylic acid.

Phenylbutazone is a pyrazole derivative related to amidopyrine, used to relieve painful conditions affecting muscles and skeletal structures. It has also an antipyretic action. These, however, are not its sole properties as it influences the tissue reactions involved in inflammation and pain.

The tubular re-absorption of sodium and chloride ions is increased by this drug, and may lead to œdema. Phenyl-butazone should not be used where there is evidence of disease of the heart, liver or kidney. Moreover, it is advisable to reduce the salt intake of animals receiving phenyl-butazone.

The use of this drug is confined to the dog and horse. It is given by mouth, absorption from the gut being rapid, a peak concentration in plasma being reached in about two hours. Intramuscular injections give a peak plasma concentration in six to ten hours because the drug is fixed to muscle protein and absorption delayed.

Phenylbutazone disappears from the body of the horse or dog within a few hours after absorption, but in man it is meta-bolised at the rate of about 10–15 per cent per day, hence there is a much greater risk of chronic poisoning from this drug in man than in the horse or dog, and these are the species most likely to be given the drug in veterinary medicine.

The main toxic effects in the dog are nausea and œdema of the limbs, but in man there are many others, including skin sensitisation and damage to hæmopoetic tissues.

Methylsalicylate or oil of wintergreen is a colourless liquid with a characteristic taste and smell. The main use of this oil is as a counter-irritant applied locally to the skin. However, it is readily absorbed from the skin and after absorption has an action like sodium salicylate.

Phenylsalicylate or Salol is insoluble in water and passes unchanged through the stomach. In the small intestine it is hydrolysed to phenol and salicylic acid. The only use of this drug is as a coating to pills to enable them to pass unchanged through the stomach.

Aniline and p. aminophenol have antipyretic activity but are rather toxic. However, both acetanilide and phenacetin have been used as anti-pyretics but are now frequently replaced by **paracetamol**. When phenacetin is given to the dog it is deacetylated because the appropriate enzyme is present in the dog. This gives rise to the free amine. Since an acetylating enzyme is lacking in the dog, the free amine persists and this can give rise to toxic effects by the formation of methæmoglobin. The replacement of phenacetin by paracetamol in man was due to the paracetamol being a major metabolite to which phenacetin owed its activity.

ANTI-INFLAMMATORY AGENTS

Since many analgesic-antipyretic agents are used in the treatment of disease arising from inflammation of connective tissue, it is convenient at this stage to consider collectively drugs used for their anti-inflammatory properties. The four cardinal signs of inflammation are heat, pain, redness and swelling. To these a fifth may be added, namely loss of function. Three of these signs, pain, redness and swelling were collected under a common heading by the distinguished pathologist of the last century, Cohnheim, who described " increased vascular permeability " as an important feature of inflammation. Cohnheim's concept of increased vascular permeability consequent to local injury as an important factor in inflammatory change has been strengthened considerably in recent years by the discovery of a number of chemical compounds or their precursors normally present in the tissues, which are or may be liberated at the site of injury and have the pharmacological property of causing small blood vessels to leak. Amongst the substances with these properties are histamine, 5-hydroxytryptamine and bradykinin.

Although it is generally considered that the vascular change affects mainly the capillary vessels which show an increased permeability, there is some evidence that the principal vessels involved may be the small venules. In addition to the increased vascular permeability, there are various changes in the biochemical environment around the inflamed area which may contribute to increasing the resistance of the region to infection by bacteria. Another important feature involved in the inflammatory change is the migration of polymorphonucleoleucocytes to the site of tissue injury. Where the tissue injury is caused by bacteria, the rate and efficiency of ingestion of the invading micro-organisms by polymorphonucleoleucocytes and the fate of these bacteria within the blood cells are important features which determine the development of the lesion.

Chronic inflammatory change and the repair of injured tissues is characterised by the proliferation of capillary blood vessels, the laying down of fibroblasts and an increase in the deposition of collagen. Since the signs of inflammation which appear after tissue injury are the same regardless of the cause of the injury, it was attractive to many people to consider these signs as being mediated by a single chemical substance. The similarity between these signs and the actions of histamine caused Lewis and his collaborators to consider the possibility that the inflammatory response was due largely to the release of histamine. Unfortunately there are a number of facts which do not support this hypothesis. The reaction of blood vessels during injury differs from their reaction to local injections of histamine, and drugs which antagonise the effects of histamine have no influence against many of the reactions produced in inflammation. Later workers thought that 5-hydroxytryptamine might be an important mediator of the inflammatory response. This amine is present in the mast cells of rodents and certainly appears to play a part in certain of the inflammatory responses occurring in rats and mice.

In addition to the possible involvement of substances of small molecular weight like histamine and 5-hydroxytryptamine there has been a considerable opinion that certain products of protein decomposition might be involved in producing the local and general effects of both inflammation and shock. Preparations have been made from the exudate produced during inflammation, which have the property of increasing the permeability of capillaries, and these preparations also cause the accumulation of leucocytes. The name leucotaxin has been given to such preparations. Early preparations undoubtedly contained a number of active substances such as, for example, the polypeptide bradykinin. It is, however, probable that a peptide is produced during tissue injury which is not bradykinin, and which has the properties already mentioned as being attributable to leucotaxin.

Independent of the work on leucotaxin an important plasma-kinin forming system has been discovered. Plasma kinins are derived from plasma globulins and are polypeptides with the property of causing dilatation of blood vessels and contraction of smooth muscle. Bradykinin is an important member of this group of substances.

Bradykinin

It has been known for more than forty years that urine contains a substance which on injection causes a fall in blood pressure. This substance can be obtained in substantial quantities from the pancreas. Later work showed that substances with similar activity could be isolated from both saliva and plasma, and it was discovered that these substances which were originally called Kallikreins had an indirect action. They behaved as though they were enzymes splitting off a pharmacologically active substance from an inactive precursor present in the blood. It was shown later that certain snake venoms as well as the enzyme trypsin act on plasma globulin to produce a substance which lowers the blood pressure and causes a slow contraction of intestinal muscle. A pure substance with these properties has been isolated and synthesised and is a nonapeptide called Bradykinin. There are undoubtedly other plasma kinins with similar pharmacological properties. In very low doses these substances cause vasodilatation, increased capillary permeability and œdema. They also evoke pain by acting on sensory nerve endings. They act on a variety of smooth muscles sometimes causing contraction, sometimes causing relaxation. These kinins appear to be involved in the inflammatory response. Fortunately, as a safeguard against the excessive formation of these pharmacologically active peptides, an enzyme called kininase is present in the blood which rapidly destroys plasma kinin, and once a specific inhibitor for this enzyme can be discovered, work on plasma kinins will proceed very rapidly.

PHARMACOLOGICALLY ACTIVE SUBSTANCES AND INFLAMMATION

If lymph is collected from a dog's leg after the limb has been subject to mechanical injury, such as by pressure or burning, it can be shown that the concentration of plasma kinin in the lymph is increased and, moreover, the flow of lymph is greater after the injury. Some histamine also appears in the lymph after injury and histamine itself can cause an increase in the plasma kinin-forming activity of the lymph as well as increasing the lymph flow.

Injecting turpentine into the intra-pleural space of rats causes a pleurisy. The inflammatory exudate produced by the pleurisy is not only rich in protein but within the first thirty minutes after the turpentine injection contains substantial quantities of histamine and 5-hydroxytryptamine. However, an hour after the injection these substances are no longer detectable. This experiment has been used to support the idea that the role of histamine in the inflammatory response is to initiate the vascular reaction. This concept is supported by the fact that the administration of an antihistamine in doses small enough to specifically inhibit histamine will cause a marked delay in the appearance of the turpentine exudate. However, by two to four hours after the injection, the volume of exudate is the same as in rats not treated with an antihistamine. A similar result has been obtained after rats have been depleted of histamine by means of injections of the histamine-releasing substance compound 48/80. Animals treated with 48/80 show a delay in the appearance of full volumes of exudate which is greater even than the delay shown by animals given antihistamine treatment. Thus it appears that histamine is probably involved in initiating the inflammatory response but not in sustaining the response.

Pleural exudates produced in the manner described also contain a substance which is very similar if not identical with Bradykinin. Although a great deal has been learned about inflammation by the use of pharmacological techniques which are necessary to study active substances such as histamine, 5-hydroxytryptamine and bradykinin, a great deal more is required before the inflammatory response can be fully understood and, by implication, properly treated. However, it has been known for a considerable time that certain drugs have value in alleviating the effects of inflammatory change in certain tissues, and some of these such as certain antipyretic analgesics have already been discussed. However, various drugs derived from the adrenocortical hormones have proved even more potent in affecting the inflammatory change, and it is proposed to discuss these.

THE ADRENOCORTICOTROPHIC HORMONE AND THE ADRENOCORTICAL STEROIDS

It has been known for several decades that many of the body's responses to harmful stimuli depend on the integrity of the adenohypophyseal-adrenocortical system. An interesting theory was put forward by Selye, in which he suggested that certain diseases of so-called " adaptation " are the result of complex responses of susceptible tissues to the adrenocortical hormones and nearly twenty years ago it was shown that the corticosteroids alleviated the inflammatory changes in mesenchymal tissues.

Corticotrophin

The pharmacological effects of the corticosteroids may be produced by administering corticotrophin. This hormone of the anterior pituitary gland stimulates the adrenal cortex to release the corticosteroids, mainly cortisone and cortisol. Corticotrophin is rapidly destroyed in the body and if it is used in treatment, it is necessary to give either frequent intramuscular injections or to use a long-acting preparation. Since the discovery of potent synthetic substitutes for the corticosteroids, there is less need to use corticotrophin, and it is now usual to use one of these potent synthetic analogues.

Cortisone and Cortisol

These hormones are synthesised by the adrenal cortex from cholesterol. The adrenocortical hormones used for their anti-inflammatory properties are the glucocorticoids. These substances are called glucocorticoids because they raise the concentration of glucose in the blood. They are gluconeogenic because they convert amino acids to glucose and decrease utilisation of glucose by the tissues. The conversion of amino acids to glucose by these compounds reduces the amount of amino acids which is available for conversion into protein. This leads to the defective repair of tissues and in young animals growth may be retarded by the prolonged treatment of an animal with glucocorticoids. The lack of amino acids may lead also to spontaneous fractures of bones because the bones are weakened by this lack, which is often combined with an inhibition of osteoblast activity producing a condition called osteoporosis.

The classification of adrenocortical hormones into glucocorticoids and mineralocorticoids is not absolute and most of the hormones of the adrenal cortex have some of either activity; hence the glucocorticoids may cause sodium retention and loss of potassium in the urine. The glucocorticoids appear to be involved in the promotion of glomerular filtration and the maintenance of urine flow. It is, however, in alleviating inflammatory change that they find their main therapeutic employment.

The presence of the glucocorticoids appears to increase the power of the body to withstand various stresses, such as those of trauma, infection or cold. It is, however, important to realise that a situation which may be stressful to one species of animal is not necessarily stressful to another. A simple test of the release of glucocorticoids can be carried out by counting the circulating eosinophils. In man and the laboratory rat, excitement or the injection of adrenaline will cause the number of circulating eosinophils to fall by more than 50 per cent. However, neither the injection of adrenaline nor excitement appear to have any effect on the circulating eosinophils of the domesticated ungulates. This is not because these species are insensitive to corticotrophin or the glucocorticoids, but apparently because excitement and adrenaline injections are not stressful to these species. The eosinopenia and lymphocytopenia produced by the glucocorticoids may be secondary to their action on the vascular system and it is the effect on the blood vessels which seems to govern their anti-inflammatory action.

When administered in large amounts cortisone and cortisol suppress the inflammatory response. Apparently this effect is produced by the hormones decreasing the permeability of capillaries, but they may also reduce the blood flow to the inflamed area by vasoconstriction. The anti-inflammatory effect produced by cortisol is much greater than that of cortisone. This is because cortisone is active only after conversion in the liver to cortisol; hence cortisol is the more suitable preparation for local application to suppress the inflammatory response in tissues such as the conjunctiva.

Since the glucocorticoids suppress the inflammatory response and fever many of the objective clinical signs of infection may pass unnoticed, and it is essential that a diagnosis should be reached before these drugs are administered. When the glucocorticoids are used therapeutically, especially in infective conditions, it is essential to give large doses of appropriate antibiotics simultaneously, both to control and prevent infection because the suppression of the inflammatory response greatly favours the spread of infection. The administration of these drugs may disturb the healing of surgical wounds; although this is a serious potential hazard, it has not so far proved an important contra-indication to the use of these drugs. It is important to realise that the continued administration of glucocorticoids suppresses the normal secretion of corticotrophin, and when the administration of the glucocorticoid stops, there may be signs of corticotrophin lack produced by this feedback mechanism. The signs of a too rapid withdrawal of glucocorticoid therapy are the same as those of acute adrenal insufficiency (see p. 19).

The importance of the anti-inflammatory action of the glucocorticoids led to the introduction of methods of testing anti-inflammatory activity, as it is only by the development of adequate assay techniques that better anti-inflammatory drugs can be produced. There are four main types of test. One type measures the effect of a drug on the erythema or pyrexia produced in inflammation. A second type measures the effect of a drug on tissue permeability. This is usually done by measuring the passage of a dye attached to plasma protein through a membrane such as the synovial membrane or into a tissue such as the skin. The dye Evans blue, used in measuring plasma volume, is commonly employed. A third type of test is based on changes in the volume of an organ such as the rat's foot. The injection of an irritant into such a structure increases exudation and hence volume. Formalin, dextran and egg albumin have been used as irritants. More severe inflammatory reactions leading to exudation, granulation and even necrosis have been used. In these tests an irritant such as croton oil or a non-absorbable foreign body such as cotton wool are introduced under the skin or into a pouch in the cheek of certain animals. These substances give rise to the formation of a granuloma; this can be cut out and weighed The greater the inflammatory action, the greater the size of the granuloma and the anti-inflammatory agent can be tested by comparing the effects of a similar irritant with and without the anti-inflammatory drug.

THE RELATION BETWEEN STRUCTURE AND ACTION OF THE CORTICOSTEROIDS

On studying the relationship between the activity of various corticosteroids and their chemical structure, it was found that certain features in the molecule were important in conferring anti-inflammatory activity. The conventional labelling and numbering of the steroid molecule is shown in Fig. 9·2. The anti-inflammatory properties of cortisone appear to depend on the ketone group on carbon 3, carbons 4 and 5 unsaturated, oxygen at carbon 11 and dihydroxyacetone chain at carbon 17. The introduction of a double bond between carbons 6 and 7 produced a loss in anti-inflammatory potency, whereas a double bond between carbons 1 and 2 increased anti-inflammatory activity without affecting mineralocorticoid activity.

Prednisone and Prednisolone

These are synthetic analogues of cortisone and cortisol respectively. They have four to five times the anti-inflammatory activity of the naturally occurring glucocorticoids and therefore have the advantage of requiring a smaller dose to produce the same effect. This reduces the risk of salt and water retention. As with cortisone and cortisol, Prednisolone is the main anti-inflammatory compound as prednisone is only active after conversion into prednisolone. These synthetic glucocorticoids are used as anti-inflammatory agents in the treatment of certain skin and orthopedic conditions. In the latter it is sometimes necessary to give them by intra-articular or peri-articular injection. Prednisone and Prednisolone are powerful suppressors of the secretion of corticotrophin. Like cortisone and cortisol they are used for their gluconeogenic action in the treatment of ketosis in dairy cows. This is a disease of post-parturient cows, which has a misleading title, because ketosis is a clinical feature which

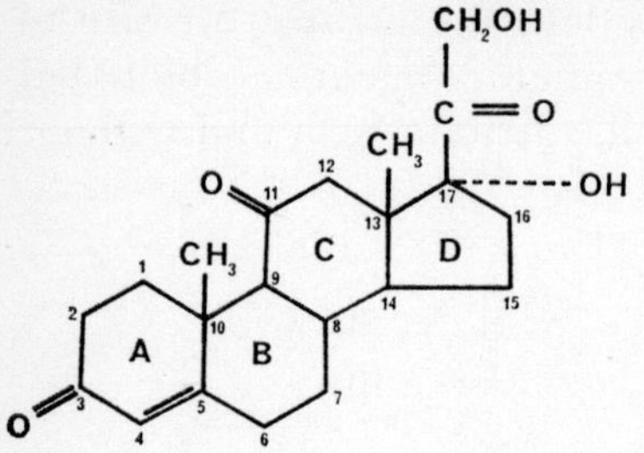

Cortisone

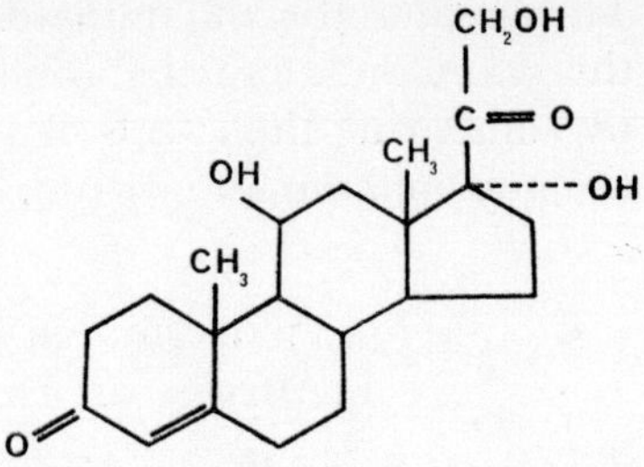

Cortisol

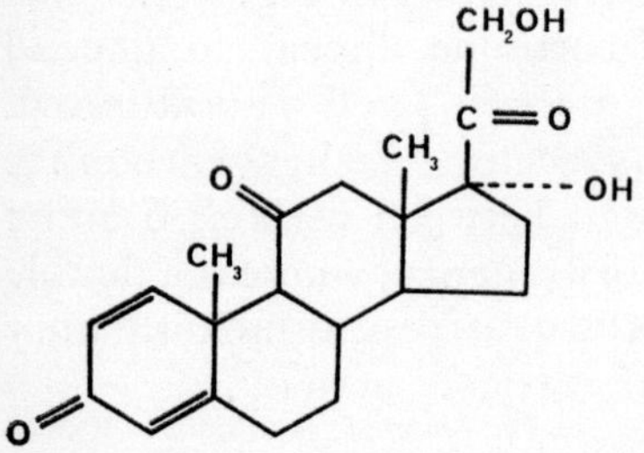

Prednisone

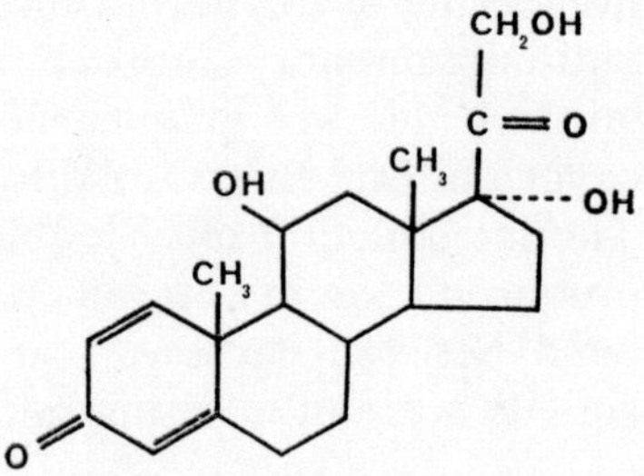

Prednisolone

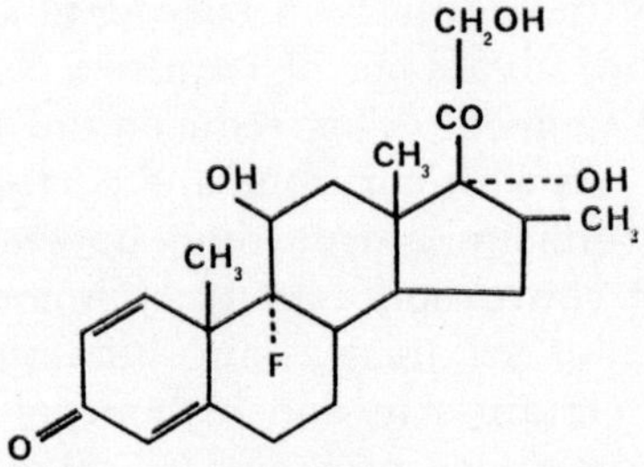

Betamethasone

FIG. 9.2
The formulæ of some adrenocorticosteroids.

occurs in several other disorders. Prednisone and Prednisolone are given by intramuscular injection in the treatment
of ketosis. When these drugs are given to dogs and cats to
alleviate a chronic inflammatory condition, they are given
in tablet form. There is no evidence that the synthetic
corticosteroids have any advantage over the naturally occurring
compounds when they are used as local applications in
the treatment of inflammatory conditions of the skin or eye.

Betamethasone and Dexamethasone

Glucocorticoid activity is greatly increased when a
fluorine atom is introduced into the 9 alpha position of the
corticosteroids. Two such compounds are available for
therapeutic use, they are the isomers Betamethasone and
Dexamethasone. The anti-inflammatory activity of these
substances is about five times as great as that of Prednisone,
and they are virtually devoid of mineralocorticoid activity.
However, they may produce a negative calcium balance
because they increase the loss of this element in the faeces.
They are used for the same purposes as the other corticosteroids.

When glucocorticoids are given to cattle in large doses
they are liable to suppress, but not prevent, the tuberculin
reaction. Their use therefore may, on occasion, confuse the
results of tuberculin testing.

The adrenocorticosteroids are present in the plasma bound
to the alpha globulin fraction. The half clearance time of
cortisone from the body is approximately thirty minutes,
whereas for Prednisolone it is about twenty minutes. The
corticosteroids are not stored in the tissues, but their metabolism
may be delayed in liver disease, pregnancy and starvation.

PYRETICS

The body temperature may be raised by a variety of
methods such as exposure to heat, injury to the corpus striatum
which increases carbohydrate metabolism without compen-
satory heat loss, by bacterial toxins and by pyrogenic drugs.
Fever is usually due to infection with living organisms but
can be reproduced by injecting killed bacteria or toxins.

The only therapeutic importance of pyrogenic substances lies in the fact that the distillled water used for intravenous injections may contain them. Such pyrogens are formed by non-pathogenic bacteria growing in distilled water. Water intended for injection should be sterilised as as soon it is distilled, and thereafter kept under aseptic conditions.

SUGGESTIONS FOR FURTHER READING

EISENSTEIN, A. B. ed. (1967). *The Adrenal Cortex*. London: Churchill.
KUZELL, W. C. (1968). Non-steroid anti-inflammatory agents. *A. Rev. Pharmac.*, **8**, 357.
SMITH, M. J. H. and SMITH, P. K. (1966). *The Salicylates*. New York: Interscience Publishers.
SPECTOR, W. G. and WILLOUGHBY, D.A. (1968). *The Pharmacology of Inflammation*. London: English Universities.

CHAPTER X

STIMULANTS OF THE CENTRAL NERVOUS SYSTEM

Caffeine, strychnine, leptazol, bemegride

MEDULLARY STIMULANTS

THE regulation of the body's vital functions is carried out by special nerve cells situated in the medulla. They are usually called the vital or medullary centres and include the respiratory centres, the vasomotor centre, the vomiting and vagal centres. These centres are affected by a number of drugs, some of which cause stimulation, some depression and some a mixture of stimulation and depression. Drugs of the stimulating category are called **analeptics** or "arousing" agents.

In veterinary therapeutics the medullary stimulants are of most value as stimulants of the respiratory centres. They are used mainly to stimulate respiration in animals which have stopped breathing during anæsthesia. It is usual nowadays to resuscitate such animals by means of artificial respiration and the medullary stimulants are a group of drugs which are of declining therapeutic importance. Two of the oldest stimulants of the central nervous system are caffeine and strychnine. They are no longer used to any great extent in therapy, but the latter is of toxicological importance.

Caffeine

This alkaloid occurs in tea and coffee and chemically is derived from purine. Theobromine and theophylline are also purine derivatives with similar actions to caffeine. Caffeine is readily absorbed from the gut. In the body it is partly oxidised and partly demethylated. The purines are excreted in the urine as methyluric acids or methylxanthines, about 10 per cent of the parent drug being excreted unchanged.

The central nervous system is stimulated from the cortex downwards and there is no subsequent depression. Caffeine increases the motor effects of conditioned reflexes and, by acting on the motor area of the brain, decreases fatigue, thus increasing the work which a group of muscles can do. The respiratory, vasomotor and vagal centres are stimulated, and caffeine is sometimes used to stimulate respiration. Very large doses produce convulsions similar to strychnine convulsions.

Caffeine increases the blood flow through the brain and kidney, causing the latter organ to produce more urine. This increased blood flow is produced by the drug acting on the heart and blood vessels both directly and through the medullary centres. Its restriction to the brain and kidneys is due to these organs being poorly supplied with vasoconstrictor nerves. Caffeine acts directly on the heart muscle to increase the rate and force of contraction; at the same time the heart is slowed from stimulation of the vagal centre. Although the vasomotor centre is stimulated, the vasoconstrictor effect is counteracted by the drug dilating the vessels directly. The diuresis produced by caffeine is partly due to the effects on circulation and partly due to the drug decreasing tubular reabsorption of water.

The formation of prothrombin by the liver is increased by caffeine which by this action resembles vitamin K. The drug is used mainly as a diuretic, but occasionally to counteract centrally depressant drugs. It is usually given as the double salt caffeine and sodium benzoate because this is more soluble.

Theophylline has actions similar to caffeine but is a more powerful diuretic. Theobromine has no action on the central nervous system and is used only for its diuretic properties.

Strychnine

This alkaloid occurs together with the chemically and pharmacologically similar Brucine in the Nux Vomica bean. Strychnine is more active and is absorbed quickly from the gut. It is rapidly fixed by the tissues amd mostly destroyed in the liver by enzymes on the microsomes of hepatic cells.

About 20 per cent is excreted unchanged in the urine; this takes about twelve hours and it is, therefore, somewhat cumulative. Many proprietary "tonics" contain small amounts of strychnine and their use by animal owners has given rise to cases of poisoning. Although strychnine is a particularly painful poison, it can still be legally employed to destroy moles and seals. It is surely time that a relatively painless poison was employed to kill these unfortunate creatures. An appreciation of the actions of strychnine is important to the veterinarian to enable him to take appropriate counter-action in cases of poisoning.

Strychnine has a bitter taste which in the mouth stimulates the taste buds, and in debilitated animals may cause a reflex stimulation of gastric secretion. However, the drug's most important action is on the central nervous system. Reflexes are first stimulated and then depressed; the motor effects of spinal reflexes are increased and the latent period diminished. Nerve impulses in the spinal cord are restricted to their appropriate path by inhibitory neurones. Strychnine produces its characteristic pharmacological effects by inhibiting these inhibitory neurones, thus producing an exaggeration of the reflex effects of sensory stimuli and a general enhancement of neuronal activity. Although it antagonises the respiratory depression produced by morphine, the excitatory effects of morphine on the central nervous system are additive with those of strychnine. The blocking by strychnine of many postsynaptic inhibitory processes and consequent facilitation gives rise to increased irradiation, so that the nerve impulses are more widely spread within the spinal cord and the response to a nerve impulse involves more muscles than would normally be the case. Large doses exaggerate these effects, so that any small sensory disturbance sends all the voluntary muscles into violent convulsions which are extremely painful. These are followed by depression of the central nervous system and relaxation of the muscles. In a strychnine convulsion the limbs and trunk are extended, because in domestic animals the extensor muscles are usually stronger than the flexors, the position being termed opisthotonus.

The lethal properties of strychnine have led to its use for the destruction of dogs and cats. Such a procedure is quite unjustified because of the intense pain produced by the convulsions. Strychnine should never be employed for this purpose.

Strychnine exerts its main effect on the spinal cord, and,

although the sensitivity to stimuli of the medullary centres is increased, drugs are available which exert a greater effect on the centres than the cord and are to be preferred. Strychnine is used as a bitter in the form of prepared Nux Vomica, which is the powdered bean standardised to contain 1·2 per cent strychnine.

In strychnine poisoning the animal is restless; sensory stimuli, such as noise, cause jerking of the limbs and even convulsions. The convulsions are characteristic, the animal adopting a position of opisthotonus. Respiration usually fails after five or six convulsions. The treatment consists of controlling the convulsions by means of a barbiturate such as sodium pentobarbitone given intravenously, the animal being placed in a dark loose box or kennel and every effort made not to disturb the animal. Mephenesin, a drug acting on the inter-neurones of the spinal cord, has been suggested as a specific antidote to strychnine. Unfortunately, it is cleared relatively quickly and the dose has to be repeated almost hourly. In veterinary practice this is rarely possible. Atar-actics are also useful in the treatment of strychnine poisoning.

Picrotoxin

This is a non-nitrogenous white crystalline substance prepared from seeds which come from an East Indian plant *Cocculus anamirta*. It is absorbed from all routes of administration, but since it is only used in emergency to stimulate respiration the intravenous route is the best. Since this drug leaves the circulation rapidly and is quickly destroyed, the dose can be repeated after a very short interval. It is a powerful stimulant of the central nervous system, the effect on the mid-brain and medulla being most marked. The cortex is also stimulated and may lead to convulsions. Stimulation of the central nervous system eventually leads to depression.

Picrotoxin is an effective antagonist to the central depression produced by the barbiturates and this is its only therapeutic indication. It is too toxic to use in unanæsthetised animals and is of no value in morphine poisoning.

When using picrotoxin in barbiturate overdosage the solution should be injected slowly intravenously until tremors of the voluntary muscles are observed; to give more than is necessary to produce this effect is harmful. Certain plants poisonous to livestock contain active principles pharmacologically similar to picrotoxin. The best antidote to these poisons as to picrotoxin is a barbiturate given intravenously.

Leptazol

Leptazol is a white crystalline substance, very soluble in water, and sterilisable by boiling. It is rapidly absorbed and quickly destroyed in the body so that half a convulsive dose can be repeated after an interval of two hours.

Leptazol is a powerful cerebral and medullary stimulant. It is probably the best analeptic or " arousing " drug available, and counteracts the depression produced by hypnotics such as the barbiturates. The drug, however, has no value as a circulatory stimulant.

Nikethamide is available as a synthetic water-soluble oil which is slowly absorbed from the gut or subcutaneous injection and is best given intravenously. It stimulates respiration in doses which do not produce any other effect. However, as an analeptic it is less potent than leptazol.

Bemegride

This powerful stimulant of the central nervous system is used to antagonise the medullary depression produced by barbiturates. Because Bemegride is chemically similar to the barbiturates, it was thought to be a specific competitive antagonist. However, its antagonism is probably due entirely to its analeptic properties. It will usually arouse dogs, sheep and rabbits from barbiturate-produced anæsthesia; cats are not awakened although the anæsthesia is lightened.

Bemegride is given in solution by intravenous injection. If this is not possible, the intraperitoneal route may be employed. The dose should be repeated at ten-minute intervals until muscular tremors are seen. Bemegride's action lasts for only half an hour, and cases treated should be kept under observation in case a relapse occurs.

SUGGESTIONS FOR FURTHER READING

HAHN, F. (1960). Analeptics. *Pharmac. Rev.*, **12**, 447.

L

CHAPTER XI

LOCAL ANALGESIC AGENTS

THE effects of drugs on the various functions of the central and autonomic nervous systems have been considered. It remains to discuss substances which act directly on nerve fibres and nerve endings, by far the most important being the local analgesics which are drugs with the property of reversibly impairing conduction in nerve fibres and paralysing nerve endings. Sensory fibres are blocked more easily than others because they are the fine unmyelinated C fibres, which are easily penetrated by the drug.

Local anæsthetics act at the cell membrane where they interfere with the transient increase in the permeability of the membrane to sodium ions which is produced by depolarisation of the membrane and is an essential part of both the generation and conduction of the nerve impulse. Local analgesics block conduction without depolarising the nerve because these drugs stabilise the cell membrane. It has been suggested that the action of local analgesics in stabilising the membrane potential of nerve fibres may be brought about by their causing an increase in the surface pressure of the lipid layer, which forms the nerve membrane, thus closing the pores through which the sodium and potassium ions pass. Although it is in the form of the free base that the tissues are penetrated and local analgesia produced, the free base of the various local analgesic drugs is only slightly water-soluble and usually is unstable. Local analgesics are usually used in the form of a water-soluble salt which forms a slightly acid solution. However, these salts must be neutralised in the tissues, the free base liberated and the tissues penetrated before local analgesia is produced.

Local analgesics are used in a variety of ways to produce the effect desired. They may be applied directly to a mucous membrane to prevent pain arising from irritation or manipulation of the membrane. Most commonly they are injected subcutaneously or around nerve trunks; analgesia of a greater area of the body may be produced by injecting a local analgesic epidurally and paralysing a number of spinal nerve roots. A sub-arachnoid injection, or true spinal analgesic, has a similar effect but is less commonly used in veterinary surgery.

A local analgesic must produce analgesia without damage to nervous structures and must be non-irritant. After absorption a local analgesic should have a low toxicity and should be effective in low concentrations. The analgesia produced should persist long enough for the surgical interference to take place, and should be produced quickly. The drug should act after injection and when applied locally to mucous membranes. However, few substances have all these properties, and amongst the defects which might be present in a local analgesic are the following: stimulation of sensory nerves may occur before analgesia; there may be local or general toxic effects; the drug may not penetrate mucosæ and may be unstable in solution or insoluble in water.

Spinal anaesthesia may be produced by the injection of local analgesic solutions sub-durally; on occasion, in small animals, the needle punctures between the lumbar vertebræ or the lumbar sacral space piercing the dura and arachnoid. In this case the injection is made into the cerebro-spinal fluid and the specific gravity of the injected solution can influence its distribution and, hence, the zone of analgesia. In human surgery the extent to which the nerve roots are blocked can be varied by altering the specific gravity of the injection fluid; in veterinary surgery the volume of solution determines the extent of spread of the anæsthetic and hence the zone of anæsthesia produced. Spinal anæsthesia is not without risk, although epidural injections as commonly used in the cow are reasonably safe. There is a risk of paralysing the intercostal nerves or even the phrenic nerves if too large a volume is used. The blood pressure may fall partly because of blocking the splanchnic nerves and partly because the reduced respiratory movements may impede the return of the blood to the right heart.

GENERAL PROPERTIES OF LOCAL ANALGESICS

Local analgesics affect the central nervous system, autonomic ganglia, the myoneural junction and muscle fibres, in addition to their inhibitory effect on conduction in nerve axons. On the central nervous system they cause stimulation followed by depression and may give rise to death from respiratory failure. Medullary stimulants are ineffective in the treatment of this type of respiratory failure because the local analgesics themselves are central stimulants and the depression is characteristic of excessive stimulation, probably resulting from exhaustion of the mechanism. It has been suggested that as in the case of strychnine the stimulation produced by local analgesics is due to a selective depression of inhibitory neurones.

Cocaine is the oldest local analgesic and is obtained from the leaves of the South American plant *Erythroxylon coca*. It is destroyed by prolonged boiling. Absorption takes place from mucous membranes but not from intact skin, and after absorption it is partly destroyed by the liver and partly excreted in the urine. Cocaine is a very effective local analgesic paralysing sensory nerve trunks and endings without initial stimulation. It potentiates the action of adrenaline and therefore has a vasoconstrictor effect. Cocaine dilates the pupil but the light reflex remains, unlike the mydriasis by atropine. However, it has dangerous central actions which may be shown by doses lower than those required for local analgesia.

This drug produces a stimulation of the central nervous system which is followed by depression and starts at the highest centres. Large doses cause convulsions and small doses slow the heart by stimulating the vagal centre. Moderate doses increase the heart rate by central and peripheral sympathetic stimulation. It is scheduled under the Dangerous Drugs Act. Cocaine is too toxic to use if a substitute can be found and neither cocaine nor butocaine should be injected.

In an attempt to find a less toxic substitute for Cocaine **Procaine** was synthesised in 1905 and is still widely used. It has only one-quarter the toxicity of cocaine, forms a stable solution in water and does not lead to addiction. However, it has poor powers of penetration and is therefore no good for the anæsthetisation of mucosæ, being used mainly as an injection. Chemically most local analgesics are esters and are metabolised by hydrolysis. This takes place in both the liver and blood plasma, and it is probable that the enzyme responsible for the plasma hydrolysis is plasma cholinesterase. The fact that plasma cholinesterase may be responsible for much of the metabolism of certain local analgesics is of particular importance in the veterinary field when one considers the difference in the amount of plasma cholinesterase in different species. Local anæsthetics are often mixed with adrenaline, which limits absorption and acts as a local hæmostatic, although this latter effect is not always advantageous as it may conceal hæmorrhage which should have been dealt with by ligation of the bleeding points. The pH of concentrated solutions of drugs such as procaine may cause irritation by their acidity.

Many compounds have since been tested and several have come into general use. **Butocaine** is a good anæsthetic for mucous membranes but is too toxic to inject. **Amethocaine** is suitable for injection and anæsthetising mucous membranes. **Orthocaine** and **Benzocaine** are insoluble local anæsthetic powders used only as dressings for painful superficial lesions. **Cinchocaine** is much more effective than procaine but is also more toxic. It is suitable for surface anæsthesia and produces a prolonged effect. However, Cinchocaine may cause an inflammatory reaction at the site of injection. A more recent local anæsthetic is **Lidocaine** which gives anæsthesia both on injection and after local application. When used as a 1 to 2 per cent solution it acts quickly and has about the same toxicity as procaine. It is also called **Lignocaine.** Lidocaine is non-esteric and is metabolised in the liver and not by cholinesterase. This may explain in part the longer action of Lidocaine.

Sometimes local anæsthetic solutions have the enzyme *hyaluronidase* added to them. This enzyme splits the hyaluronides, which form an important part of connective tissue, and thus facilitates spread and penetration of the anæsthetic after injections.

SUGGESTIONS FOR FURTHER READING

HALL, L. W. (1966). *Wright's Veterinary Anæsthesia*, 6th ed.   London: Balliere, Tindall & Cassell.

RITCHIE, J. M. and GREENGARD, P. (1966).   On the mode of action of local anæsthetics.   *A. Rev. Pharmac.*, **6**, 405.

WESTHUES, M. and FRITSCH, R. (1964).   *Animal Anaesthesia*. Vol. I., Local anæsthesia.   Edinburgh: Oliver & Boyd.

CHAPTER XII

DRUGS ACTING ON THE ALIMENTARY SYSTEM

Antacids, carminatives, emetics

THE pharmacology of the digestive tract of the domestic animals is complicated by the diversity of form and by the fact that an important part of the digestive process is carried on by micro-organisms in the tract. These micro-organisms may be deliberately or inadvertently affected by drugs.

Salivary secretion in man and dogs can be stimulated by the

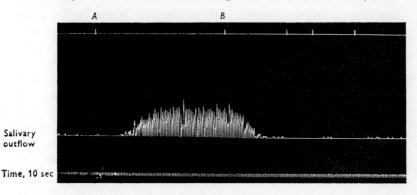

FIG. 12.1

The effect on parotid salivation in the horse of pilocarpine (0·3 mg/kg) (A) and atropine (0·2 mg/kg) (B) (Adapted from Alexander, 1966, *J. Physiol.*, **184,** 646).

sight or smell of food. This is called the psychic secretion and is not marked in the other domestic animals. Stimulation of the taste buds in the mouth causes an increase in secretion, and, in ruminants, eating and rumination has a similar effect. Salivation in the horse occurs as a consequence of mastication. A copious secretion is produced by pilocarpine, physostigmine and other parasympathomimetic drugs; inhibitors of the parasympathetics such as atropine also inhibit salivation. This

fact is made use of in pre-medication before a general anæsthetic, although in ruminants atropine only decreases the
salivary flow and does not stop it completely.

The saliva of ruminants does not contain digestive enzymes
but functions mainly as a buffer to neutralise the fatty acids
formed during fermentative digestion in the rumen and is
secreted continuously. Ruminant saliva also contains a
substance which decreases the surface tension of the rumen
liquor and this may be a factor in producing bloat. Horse
saliva resembles that of the dog more closely than ruminant
in composition, a point of difference being the relatively high
calcium content of horse saliva.

BITTERS

Reflexes from the taste buds when stimulated cause an
increased secretion of saliva and gastric juice in the dog. The
response to these reflexes is stimulated by bitter-tasting substances acting on the taste buds. These substances which are
called *Bitters* have no effect when given by stomach tube and
work best in debilitated dogs. There seems little purpose in
giving bitters to ruminants as these animals secrete an acid
juice continuously from the abomasum. The continuance of
this secretion depends on the passage of digesta through the
abomasum and is independent of vagal innervation. The other
parts of the ruminant stomach are non-secretory.

Bitters are classified into three groups, aromatic, simple
and compound. Aromatic bitters include compound tincture
of Gentian, extract of Orange Peel, and Gentian powder.
Simple bitters, so called because they do not contain tannic
acid and are therefore compatible with iron and alkaloids,
include Quassia; compound bitters such as compound tincture
of Gentian are incompatible. Many alkaloids have a bitter
taste hence Quinine and Strychnine are used as bitters.

ANTACIDS

There are few indications for the use of antacids in
veterinary practice. In certain cases of disturbed ruminal
function alkalies may be given to counteract excess acidity,

and some inflammatory conditions of the dog's stomach may benefit from an antacid.

Sodium bicarbonate is the commonest antacid, acting quickly with the release of CO_2. When bicarbonates are given to ruminants, the CO_2 is removed by eructation after being formed in the rumen. The usual reason for giving bicarbonate to ruminants is when some indiscretion of diet has given rise to the production of large quantities of lactic acid in the rumen instead of the normal volatile fatty acids. This lactic acid can readily give rise to acidosis and a recognisable clinical syndrome. The sodium bicarbonate not only neutralises the lactic acid formed during fermentation in the rumen but may also be absorbed into the body where it assists to rectify the acidosis. The administration of sodium bicarbonate in excess to all species can give rise to an alkalosis.

Magnesium carbonate acts similarly to sodium bicarbonate; **magnesium oxide** does not release CO_2 but has the possible drawback of causing purgation. Frequent dosing with carbonates or bicarbonates may produce alkalosis causing vomiting and tetany in dogs. **Magnesium trisilicate** is an insoluble powder reacting slowly with acids to form magnesium chloride and colloidal silica. It acts as an absorbent and antacid and cannot cause alkalosis. Calcium carbonate is also an effective antacid but also has a constipating action which may sometimes be disadvantageous. Several salts of bismuth have been used as antacids. However, these compounds do not neutralise the gastric juice and are potentially toxic, hence there is no justification for their further employment.

DRUGS ACTING ON STOMACH MOVEMENTS AND SECRETIONS

Drugs can affect stomach movements by acting on the gastric muscles, reflexly by stimulating nerve endings in the gastric mucosa or through the autonomic nervous system. Parasympathomimetic drugs increase and sympathomimetic drugs inhibit stomach movements. Gastric activity is inhibited also by atropine, and stomach emptying is delayed by the spasm of the pylorus produced by morphine.

Gastric secretion is stimulated by excitation of the psychic reflex in some species, by drugs with muscarine actions and by drugs such as alcohol, histamine and insulin. In ruminants insulin reduces abomasal secretion. The secretion of gastric

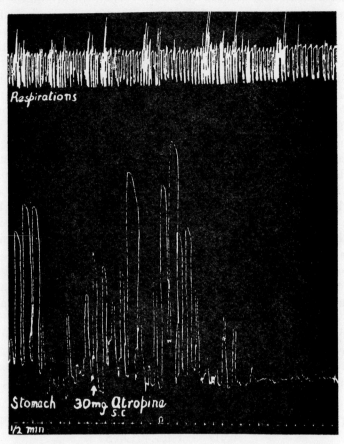

Fig. 12.2

The inhibition by atropine of the stomach contractions of the horse. (Adapted from Alexander, F., 1951, *Q. Jl. exp. Physiol.*, **36**, 139.)

juice is inhibited by atropine, irritant drugs producing gastritis and by the direct action on the pylorus and duodenum of fats, cold and acids stronger than 0·2 per cent.

As the structural differences might suggest, there are differences in the way in which the stomachs of the different species respond to drugs. Stomach movements in the horse stop when food is withheld for more than twenty-four hours. They are also inhibited by atropine and adrenaline but are not affected by carbachol or histamine. The reflex closure of the œsophageal groove in ruminants enables fluids to enter the omasum and abomasum directly. This reflex is stimulated by the presence in the mouth of a 1 per cent solution of copper sulphate or a 10 per cent solution of sodium bicarbonate. The reflex in sheep responds better to copper sulphate and in cows to sodium bicarbonate. The œsophageal groove reflex is inhibited by atropine and during general anæsthesia. The solutions which stimulate the reflex are useful adjuncts to give prior to the administration of other drugs which are required to act in the abomasum such as certain anthelmintics.

Carminatives are substances which facilitate the expulsion of gas from the stomach. They are of particular value in ruminants because these animals produce large quantities of gas in the rumen during the fermentation of carbohydrates. This gas is normally removed by belching but if this mechanism is disordered, carminatives may assist the removal of the gas. The carminatives commonly used in veterinary practice are the volatile oils such as oil of turpentine and volatile drugs such as ether, alcohol and preparations of ammonia.

Antizymotics are drugs which kill or inhibit the rumen bacteria thus stopping fermentation and consequently gas production. Formalin and the volatile oils are used for this purpose. Certain antibiotics such as the tetracyclines and streptomycin may be used as antizymotics. The protozoa which are normally present in large numbers in the rumen and are probably an important factor in rumen digestion can be killed by very low doses of copper sulphate.

Anti-frothing agents are substances which are given to ruminants to raise the surface tension of the rumen liquor and thus allow gas bubbles to rise to the dorsal sac of the rumen. When gas bubbles are trapped in the rumen contents, as in the clinical condition of " frothy bloat ", the gas formed during fermentation cannot be removed by belching; it accumulates with fatal consequences unless appropriate remedies are applied. The remedies include the administration of an anti-frothing agent to allow the gas to separate and rise into the dorsal sac.   The accumulated gas is then released by stomach tube or by trocar and cannula.   The drugs used as anti-frothing agents include **oil of turpentine,** polymerised **methyl silicone** and **polyricinate**   These drugs are either given by mouth or injected directly into the rumen.   The treatment of this type of bloat may also include the spraying of the pastures on which it occurs with anti-frothing agents such as arachis oil and mineral oil.

In recent years a polymer of *polyoxyethylene* and *polyoxypropylene* has proved an effective prophylactic in bloat.   This substance acts on the surface tension of the rumen liquor. Penicillin and other antibiotics have also been used with some success in the prevention and treatment of bloat.

VOMITING

The vomiting reflex is controlled by a centre in the medulla which is situated near the cough and vagal centres.   This centre is poorly developed in the horse and ruminant.   These animals do not vomit in the true sense, although in certain pathological conditions stomach contents are ejected through the nasal passages.   The vomiting centre can be stimulated directly or by peripheral stimuli.   These stimuli include disturbances of the labyrinth, the stimulation of vagal nerve endings in the pharynx, stomach and duodenum and the stimulation of sensory nerves to the heart and viscera.   Situated in the area postrema of the medulla is the chemoreceptor trigger zone (**CTZ**).   This zone can be stimulated by certain drugs such as morphine and some of its derivatives such as apomorphine to produce vomiting.   Destruction of the CTZ still allows the vomiting centre to respond to peripheral stimuli. Certain drugs which have anti-emetic properties such as the phenothiazine tranquilisers exert their effect on the CTZ and hence are more likely to be of value in preventing vomiting arising from the administration of drugs acting on the CTZ than vomiting brought about by stimuli from nerve endings in the alimentary tract or from the labyrinth.

Local or **reflex emetics** are drugs which stimulate sensory nerve endings in the stomach and duodenum.   They

include solutions of the salts of certain heavy metals and
vegetable drugs such as Ipecacuanha.

Copper or **zinc sulphate** in 1 per cent solution given
by mouth to dogs produce emesis within a few minutes.   This
prompt action prevents damage to the gastric mucosa, and since
these metals are absorbed very slowly there is little risk of
poisoning.   There is no nausea after the emesis or purgation;
in fact small doses of these salts are astringent to the intestine.
A crystal of washing soda given by mouth to a dog is also an
effective means of inducing vomiting.

Ipecacuanha contains the alkaloids *emetine* and *cephaline*
to which it owes its emetic properties.   These alkaloids irritate
all mucous membranes causing lachrymation, conjunctivitis
and increased bronchial secretion.   Emetine by mouth produces vomiting in thirty minutes.   When this drug is given
parenterally, much bigger doses are required.   A probable
explanation of this difference is that emetine has to be excreted
into the alimentary tract and perform its irritating action there.
The slow action of Ipecacuanha makes it a much less suitable
emetic to use to empty the stomach in cases of poisoning.   In
sub-emetic doses it increases bronchial secretions and sweating
and is used as an expectorant.

Tartar emetic produces vomiting but is too toxic to use for
this purpose.   However, it has been given by intravenous
injection in certain protozoal diseases.

Central emetics are drugs which stimulate the vomiting
centre through their action on the CTZ.   They are effective
in a smaller dose when given by injection than when the drug
is given by mouth.

Apomorphine is the most important central emetic and
acts selectively on the chemoreceptor trigger zone producing
vomiting within ten minutes after a subcutaneous injection.
When given by mouth, twice the dose is required and the
effect is not produced for thirty minutes.   Dogs whose CTZ
has been destroyed no longer respond to the injection of
apomorphine, although copper sulphate given by mouth still
produces vomiting.   This is part of the evidence for the
existence of a CTZ separate from the actual vomiting centre.
Therapeutic and large doses of apomorphine are depressant.
Birds and pigs are said to be insusceptible to apomorphine

emesis. Morphine also stimulates the CTZ in the dog as do the medullary stimulants. However, these drugs are never used for this purpose.

MOTION SICKNESS

Travel sickness can be a problem in transporting dogs and cats and certain drugs are useful in the prevention of this condition. Motion sickness is a problem in human medicine and considerable effort has been applied to the study of drugs which are capable of preventing this condition. Dogs have been used as experimental animals for the study of motion sickness remedies, but unfortunately drugs which have been found effective in the dog have been less effective in man and vice versa.

In man the drugs of value in the prevention of motion sickness fall into two groups: the anti-acetylcholine drugs of which the most effective is the alkaloid hyoscine and a second group, the antihistamines, i.e., promethazine, diphenhydramine and various piperazine antihistamines such as cyclizine and meclizine. The piperazine derivatives are equally effective as anti-motion sickness remedies as the other antihistamines and have fewer side actions and hence are the antihistamines of choice in this particular purpose, but in dogs and cats the central depression of the other antihistamines has advantages. Vomiting induced experimentally in dogs by putting them in a swing is not alleviated by the anti-acetylcholine type of drug but is, to some extent, prevented by the antihistamine type of agent. Barbiturates, whilst ineffective as anti-motion sickness agents in man, were shown to have an appreciable action when tested experimentally in the dog.

Vomiting arising from drugs acting on the CTZ or as a result of a disease process in which a so-called toxin acts on the CTZ is best prevented by drugs of the phenothiazine type of antihistamine. Vomiting is often part of a clinical syndrome and occurs, for example, in intestinal obstruction and uræmia. Vomiting of this kind is treated by treating the cause. An undesirable feature of certain drugs is that they cause vomiting, and drugs such as sodium salicylate or digitalis given by mouth may have this disadvantage. Giving the drug in dilute solution may avoid this difficulty.

SUGGESTIONS FOR FURTHER READING

BRAND, J. J. and PERRY, W. L. M. (1966). Drugs used in motion sickness. *Pharmac. Rev.*, **18**, 895.

JOHNS, A. T. and McDOWALL, F. H. (1962). Bloat in cattle. *N. Z. Jl Agric. Res.*, **5**, 1.

WANG, S. C. (1965). Emetic and antiemetic drugs. *Physiol. Pharmac.*, **2**, 256.

CHAPTER XIII

DRUGS ACTING ON THE ALIMENTARY SYSTEM

Reticulo-rumen, purges, astringents

THE EFFECT OF DRUGS ON RETICULO-RUMENAL MOVEMENTS

THE reticulo-rumen shows a basic sequence of contractions which does not vary appreciably. The reticulum makes a double contraction at regular intervals of about one minute. This contraction forces the liquid digesta into the rumen and probably some digesta passes into the omasum with each reticular contraction. Digesta appears to pass continuously from reticulum to omasum and also to flow continuously from the abomasum. The movements of the reticulo-rumen depend upon the integrity of the vagi and there are various areas in the medulla which produce reticular contractions when stimulated. Rumination and the œsophageal groove reflex also depend on an intact vagal innervation. Carbachol and similar parasympathomimetic agents usually increase the amplitude of the reticular contractions but not the frequency, and this increase is followed by inhibition. Acetylcholine and histamine inhibit the activity of both rumen and reticulum. It has been suggested that the inhibitory action of acetylcholine is due to the adrenaline which it releases from the adrenal gland. In support of this suggestion it has been shown that carbachol, in doses inhibitory to rumenal movement, also produced a rise in blood sugar. Carbachol is known to have strong nicotinic actions which would give rise to the release of adrenaline from the adrenal medulla, which in turn would produce the rise in blood sugar concentration. However, since both histamine and acetylcholine have marked effects on the cardiovascular system the inhibition of reticular rumenal movements by these drugs could be due to their interference with the flow of blood to these organs. Moreover, although adrenaline normally inhibits reticulorumenal movements, if the reticulum is quiescent, an injection

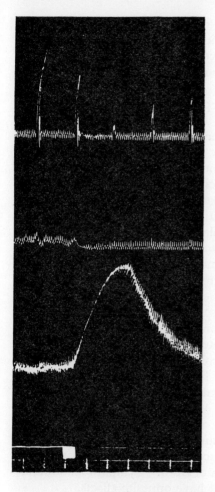

Fig. 13.1

The inhibition of reticular contractions in sheep by adrenaline (3 mg). Records from above down: Biphasic reticular contractions; Abomasal pressure, Arterial blood-pressure. (Adapted from Brunaud, M., & Navarro J., 1953, *Bull. Acad. vet Fr.,* **26,** 597.)

of adrenaline or splanchnic stimulation produces a contraction. Atropine inhibits movement of the rumen and reticulum.

A mixture of alkaloids collectively known as **veratrine** are obtained from plants of the *Veratrum* species. They have been used in man as hypotensive agents, and are of veterinary interest because when injected into ruminants they produce a phenomenon which is very similar to vomiting. It has been suggested that **veratrine** may be of use in the treatment of a certain type of bloat; at present the status of this agent is uncertain.

Very little absorption of drugs or products of digestion takes place in the stomach of simple-stomached animals. This is because most drugs are given as salts which ionize in the stomach and it is only the non-ionized moiety which passes through the gastric mucosa. The movement of uncharged molecules across the gastric epithelium is governed by their lipid solubility; for example, three barbiturates with similar pKa are absorbed at rates proportional to their lipid/water partition coefficients. Acidic drugs such as acetylsalicylic acid are readily absorbed through the gastric mucosa. However, in ruminants an appreciable absorption of both drugs and products of digestion takes place in the reticulo-rumen. Drugs such as pilocarpine, atropine, phenothiazine, cyanide and metabolites as, for example, ammonia and fatty acids, are absorbed through the rumen wall. The vital ions sodium and potassium pass through the rumen wall, the passage of potassium being passive but that of sodium is selective, and can take place against a concentration gradient. Water is absorbed along with sodium. Inorganic phosphate is both absorbed from the rumen and diffuses into the rumen.

Bile is continuously excreted by the liver and, in animals possessing a gall-bladder, is collected there and concentrated with the addition of mucin. Emptying of the gall-bladder is controlled in part by the vagal reflex and partly by humoral agents.

Cholagogues are drugs which stimulate the liver to excrete bile. It is doubtful if any drug has this property. Vagal stimulation or drugs with muscarine actions contract the gall-bladder and relax the sphincter of Oddi. Sympathetic stimulation and drugs which mimic it have opposite effects.

The hormone cholecystokinin which contracts the gall-bladder is released by the presence of fat in the duodenum. This contraction throws bile salts into the duodenum causing the liberation of secretin, which in turn stimulates pancreatic secretion and the secretion of bile by the liver thus refilling the gall-bladder. Hypertonic solutions of magnesium sulphate in the duodenum cause contraction of the gall-bladder as does the injection of secretin. Bile salts themselves are used sometimes as cholagogues, being available as *Dehydrocholic acid*.

Certain drugs such as phenolphthalein are excreted in the bile, and this property is utilised in the X-ray examination of the biliary system. An iodine-containing derivative of phenolphthalein, *Iodophthalein* or sodium tetra-iodo-phenol phthalein, is sometimes given to dogs by mouth and outlines the gall-bladder in about ten hours. **Iodipamide methylglucamine** may be used for the same purpose. **Iodophendylate** is a radio-opaque substance which can be injected into the subarachnoid space where it is immiscible with the cerebro-spinal fluid and is used for diagnostic purposes; both the latter diagnostic agents are given by injection.

DRUGS ACTING ON THE MOVEMENTS OF THE INTESTINES

The intestines under normal conditions are constantly active, the purpose of their activity being to mix the digesta with the secretions of the intestines and associated glands and to expose this mixture to the intestinal mucous membrane. There are two basic types of activity: namely, mixing movements and propulsive movements, the latter moving the digesta along the tract from duodenum to anus. The division into these types of activity is not rigid. The mixing movements tend to move digesta aborally and the propulsive movements tend to mix the digesta. The aboral progression of digesta by mixing movements is brought about by the spontaneous activity of the plain muscle of the intestine which shows a gradient from duodenum to rectum. The rhythmic contractions decrease in rate from duodenum aborally. The propulsion of digesta is brought about mainly by the intrinsic nerve plexi and involves a co-ordinated contraction of the gut preceded by relaxation aborally.

Intestinal movements are influenced by the autonomic nervous system, vagal stimulation increasing and splanchnic stimulation decreasing the movements. Similarly, drugs with muscarine actions increase intestinal motility, and this effect is antagonised by atropine. Atropine also diminishes the

propulsive movements of the intestine.   The intestines are also
influenced by painful stimuli or irritation of the peritoneum
which reflexly produce splanchnic inhibition.   The response
of the pyloric and ileocæcal sphincters to both nerve stimulation
and adrenaline is opposite to that of the rest of the intestinal
muscle.

The rate of passage of digesta along the alimentary tract
varies in the different species and may affect the fate of drugs
given by mouth.   In carnivores a large part of digestion takes
place in the stomach, and thereafter the food residue passes
through the small intestine as a soup-like chyme, becoming
firmer in consistency in the colon due to the re-absorption of
water.   The passage from mouth to anus takes less than
twenty-four hours.   Herbivores having a more complex gut
take rather longer over this process, but in the horse not as long
as might be expected.   Food residues first appear in horse
fæces about twenty-two hours after feeding and are not completely excreted until after forty-eight hours.   In foals the over-
all rate of passage is similar to that in the adult, but the time
spent in the stomach is much longer in the suckling foal than
after weaning.   The digesta in weaned foals passes quickly
through the stomach but remains longer in the large colon.
In ruminants the rate of passage is much slower; about 80 per
cent of food residue is excreted in from seventy to ninety hours
after ingestion.

Drugs may influence intestinal movements by acting on
the intrinsic or extrinsic nerves of the bowel or by direct action
on the plain muscle.   The sympathomimetic and parasympathomimetic drugs and their antagonists affect gut movement
as discussed (p. 69, 81) earlier. Histamine, barium, salts of lead,
nitrates and the opium alkaloids act directly on the intestinal
muscle.

Pituitary extract stimulates the plain muscle of the gut,
and in dogs this empties the colon and rectum.   In the horse,
however, the capillary contraction produced by this drug
renders the bowel anoxic, this inhibits movements and so
masks any direct stimulation of the bowel muscle this drug
might exhibit. Carbachol and physostigmine are used clinically
to stimulate bowel movements especially in the horse. Atropine
inhibits violent contractions of the gut and is useful in treating

some types of colic. It is, of course, the antidote to carbachol and physostigmine and should be used if these drugs produce any untoward effects. Barium salts produce a violent contraction of intestinal muscle and profuse diarrhœa. Barium chloride was used in earlier times as a purge for the horse but this proved a dangerous practice.

PURGATIVES

It is sometimes therapeutically desirable to hasten the rate of passage of digesta along the tract. This is accomplished by the use of a purgative. Purgatives act either by increasing the bulk of non-absorbable contents in the bowel or by irritation or stimulation of the nerves or muscle of the gut.

Purgatives which increase bulk include Agar Agar, a Japanese sea-weed, liquid paraffin and the saline purges. **Agar Agar** in the presence of water swells to form a gel which is not absorbed. It is suitable for use in the dog and cat only as it is a carbohydrate and would be fermented in the alimentary tract of herbivores. **Liquid paraffin** is a mixture of aliphatic hydrocarbons. It is non-irritant and non-absorbable. It acts in part by softening the fæcal mass and lubricating the rectum and by virtue of its bulk. A practical objection, especially in household pets, is its tendency to leak through the anal sphincter. It also interferes with absorption of fat-soluble vitamins.

The **saline purges** all act in a similar fashion and depend on the fact that certain anions and cations are only slowly absorbed from the gut. These ions include magnesium, sulphate, phosphate, tartrate and citrate which, in the form of salts, remain in the gut, water passing through the intestinal wall until the cathartic salt is in isotonic solution with the tissues. This solution distends the gut and reflexly increases peristalsis, thus hastening the passage of contents along the small intestine, an increased volume of fluid enters the colon, which responds in a similar fashion to the small intestine, thus producing defæcation. If a saline purge is required to act quickly, it must be given in isotonic solution so that time is not taken for water to pass from the tissues into the gut or vice versa to make the saline solution isotonic.

Magnesium sulphate is a powerful saline purge typical of the class. It is not used for horses and if purgation is delayed there is a very slight risk of absorption of magnesium ions and depression of the central nervous system. *Magnesium oxide* and *carbonate* are primarily antacids with slight cathartic properties. The latter salt is used sometimes as magnesium limestone to dress pastures on which hypomagnesæmia occurs.

Sodium sulphate is the saline purge of choice for horses and cattle. It is the cheapest and most effective saline cathartic which is best given by stomach tube because it has an unpleasant taste and the dose is rather copious. Sodium chloride is sometimes given to horses by stomach tube, in which species it acts to some extent as a saline purge.

Irritant purges increase intestinal movements by stimulating nerve endings in the intestine. Such drugs should not irritate the stomach or cause vomiting, and the irritation must be very slight, never producing inflammatory changes in the intestine. Drugs acting in this manner include sulphur, the anthracene purges and phenolphthalein, the mercurial purges and the drastic purges.

Sulphur is an inert powder which acts as a purge because it is converted in the intestine into hydrogen sulphide or other sulphides which are irritant. These sulphides are partially absorbed and excreted as sulphates in the urine. Sulphur is no longer used in veterinary practice but is sometimes given to dogs and cats by their owners.

Castor oil is a bland non-irritant oil which is sometimes used externally as a protective dressing. It has no action on the stomach, but in the intestine it is hydrolysed by lipase to liberate ricinoleic acid, which by irritating both the large and small intestine stimulates peristalsis and evacuation of the contents. The hydrolysis of castor oil depends on the presence of bile and lipase so the drug will not act in conditions where bile is absent. It is not used in adult horses or ruminants but is the purge of choice in foals and calves in which the large colon and rumen respectively have not fully developed.

The **anthracene purges** owe their activity to active principles derived from anthracene. Most of these drugs contain *emodin* (tri-hydroxymethylanthraquinone) and several contain *chrysophanic acid* (di-hydroxymethylanthraquinone).

In such drugs such as aloes, senna, cascara sagrada and rhubarb these active principles are combined with sugars to form glycosides which require hydrolysis before the active principle is free to act.

The glycosides are absorbed from the small intestine, hydrolysed in the body to liberate emodin or chrysophanic acid which then act on the large intestine. This takes several hours whereas emodin given parenterally or placed in the jejunum of cats acts in about half an hour. Moreover, emodin or extracts of senna placed in the jejunum are effective even after the large and small intestines have been separated surgically. This evidence shows that the long latent period of the naturally occurring anthracene purges is due to the time taken for their hydrolysis in the body and not the time for them to pass down the gut to the colon. These purgatives cause contraction of the colon and uterus and should never be given to pregnant animals because of the risk of producing abortion. There is some evidence that the anthracene purges interfere with the reabsorption of sodium from the gut. This may contribute to their purgative action. Emodin is converted in the body to chrysophanic acid which is excreted in the milk and urine. The chrysophanic acid acts as an indicator, turning red with alkalis.

Aloes, the traditional purge for horses, has been replaced by the synthetic **Danthron** compound [*dihydroxyanthra-quinone*] which has the advantage of being suitable to give mixed with the food. When given in this way *dihydroxyanthra-quinone* takes about twenty-four hours to act; given as a suspension in water it acts more quickly. It is suitable for all the domestic animals when given in an appropriate dose.

Cascara sagrada is an anthracene purge used only in the dog and cat. It is the mildest anthracene purge and the gut does not become tolerant. It is given as either a dry or liquid extract.

Rhubarb, in addition to the anthracene active principles, contains a tannin and is therefore liable to produce constipation after purging because of the astringent action of the tannin on the bowel mucosa. To overcome this disadvantage it is combined with a saline purge. For example, Gregory's powder consists of powdered rhubarb and magnesium salts. Rhubarb as the powder or in the form of Gregory's powder (Pulv. Rhei Co.) is given to foals, calves and dogs to produce purgation.

Phenolphthalein is similar to the anthracene purges in the way it acts and in chemical structure. It is given by mouth to dogs and cats, dissolves in the alkaline contents of the small intestine and is partly absorbed. The absorbed portion is partly excreted in the bile and partly in the urine. The excretion in the bile allows some of the dose to be re-absorbed repeatedly and thus prolongs the effect of the drug. Excessive prolongation of action may lead to irritation of the kidneys.

The sub-chloride of mercury, **calomel,** is an insoluble compound which is slowly converted into a more soluble form in the gut. It is usually a powerful purge, but should it not act, a saline purge must be given immediately to limit the absorption of mercury and consequent toxic effects. Calomel is rarely used now as safer means exist of producing a similar effect. Metallic mercury may be used as a purge when it is ground into very fine droplets with chalk as in Grey Powder. Occasionally Grey Powder is used for foals, calves, dogs and cats. It has been suggested that the mercurial purges act in a similar fashion to mercurial diuretics and by inhibiting enzymes with sulphydryl groups interfere with water absorption in the colon. The inhibition of water absorption distends the colon and so causes evacuation.

Dioctyl sodium sulphosuccinate is an anionic-active agent which has a detergent-like effect on the contents of the intestine. It causes the production of softer fæces and appears to have a laxative action. A 1 per cent solution may be used as an enema in cases of fæcal impaction. This anionic detergent is used occasionally to facilitate the disintegration of tablets.

Enemata are usually solutions of sodium chloride or soap injected into the rectum to stimulate defæcation. An infusion of *Quassia* is occasionally used as an enema to remove *Oxyuris equi*. An enema of glycerine is sometimes used to treat constipation in dogs and cats. Enemata should be warmed before administration and injected by gravity not a pump. A suppository is occasionally inserted into the rectum of a dog or cat to stimulate defæcation.

The drastic purges colocynth, jalap and croton oil have no place in veterinary therapeutics.

Adsorbents are preparations used to remove undesirable substances, gases or poisons from the intestine. Substances are said to be adsorbed when they stick on the surface of a solid. Hence the greater the surface area of the solid the better adsorbent it is likely to be.

Kaolin, a naturally occurring aluminium silicate, is the commonest adsorbent used in veterinary medicine. It is practically insoluble, and when given by mouth forms a protective coating on the bowel wall. However, the main value lies in its adsorption of toxins in certain entero-toxæmias. Magnesium trisilicate acts both as an antacid and adsorbent. *Prepared chalk* is used also in veterinary medicine as an adsorbent but is less effective than kaolin.

Preparations of Belladonna are used to relieve spasm of the intestinal muscle and are termed **Antispasmodics**.

Astringents are drugs which precipitate proteins and so form an insoluble layer of precipitated protein on the skin or mucous membrane. This layer protects the underlying tissue from further irritation and also inhibits exudation, secretion and small hæmorrhages. When given by mouth astringents tend to stop diarrhœa but are not as good as kaolin.

There are two classes of astringent, metallic astringents and vegetable astringents. The former includes salts of lead, zinc and aluminium which are used on the skin, and salts of iron and copper which are occasionally used as intestinal astringents. The vegetable astringents act by liberating tannic acid which precipitates protein. *Tannic acid* is not used as it irritates the stomach, damages the liver on absorption and precipitates food protein. The vegetable astringents liberate tannic acid slowly as they pass along the gut. *Catechu* is the main vegetable astringent used in veterinary medicine. Tannic acid should never be used to treat burn injuries because of the risk of damaging the liver with tannic acid absorbed from the burned surface.

Diarrhœa is a common symptom in all the domesticated species. When it is produced by a specific agent the correct treatment is to eliminate the causal agent; various antibiotics have a useful function in this type of treatment where the cause is a specific organism. Occasionally diarrhœa can occur in which there is no obvious causal agent, and it has to be treated symptomatically. Astringents and adsorbents can be useful drugs in controlling this condition and it is important to remember that water and electrolytes can be lost in substantial amounts during diarrhœa and restorative treatment may be essential. Use can also be made in the treatment of diarrhœa of the spasmogenic action of morphine. This alkaloid increases the tone of the intestinal muscle and so delays the movement of digesta along the alimentary tract. It is usual in treating diarrhœa with morphine to use a preparation containing crude opium such as tincture of opium, or powdered opium.

SUGGESTIONS FOR FURTHER READING

ALEXANDER, F. (1963). *Digestion in the Horse*. Contribution to the Rowett Research Institute, Collected Papers for 50th Anniversary. Edinburgh: Oliver & Boyd.

DOUGHERTY, R. W., ALLEN, R. S., BURROUGHS, W., JACOBSON, N. L. and McGILLIARD. A. D. (1964). Physiology of Digestion in the Ruminant. *Second International Symposium*, Ames, Iowa.

FARRAR, J. T. and ZFASS, A. M. (1967). Small intestinal motility. *Gastroenterology*, **52**, 1019.

MENGUY, R. (1964). Motorfunctions of the Alimentary Tract. *A. Rev. Physiol.*, **26**, 227.

TEXTER, E. C. (1964). The control of gastro-intestinal motor activity. *Am. J. dig. Dis.*, **9**, 585.

TRUELOVE, S. C. (1966). Movements of the large intestine. *Physiol. Rev.*, **46**, 457.

CHAPTER XIV

DRUGS ACTING ON THE CIRCULATORY SYSTEM

Cardiac glycosides, vasodilators, antihistamines, shock

THE HEART AND BLOOD VESSELS

THE circulatory system can be influenced by drugs acting either directly on the heart or blood vessels or indirectly through the nerves supplying these structures. The heart is the most important muscle in the body and its efficiency as a pump is its most essential function. Contraction of this muscle in health takes place in an organised fashion. The wave of excitation begins at the sino-auricular node, passing over the auricles to the atrio-ventricular node and so over the ventricles. This contraction gives rise to changes in electrical potential which can be recorded by an electro-cardiograph and these records are sometimes of great diagnostic value. The wave of excitement which spreads through the bundle of His and Purkinje fibres appears to be checked at the atrio-ventricular node. This delay allows the ventricles to fill. The work done by the heart is regulated by the initial pressure which controls the rate of filling.

The activity of the heart is dependent on the coronary circulation maintaining an adequate supply of oxygen and nutrients. The heart is always under some degree of control through the vagus nerve, although this control is greater in the horse and dog than in sheep and oxen. There is intermittent control through the sympathetics and further reflex control from the pressor receptors in the aortic arch and carotid sinus.

Heart failure may be caused by a variety of circumstances, for example, in shock, the vaso-motor mechanism fails. Injury to the heart valves impairs the pumping efficiency and leads to heart failure. Poisoning of the heart muscle impairs its efficiency and so gives rise to failure as do the various arrhythmias. Alterations of the refractory period, the excitability and rate of propagation of the cardiac excitatory waves may make them self perpetuating. If this alteration is well organised a very rapid atrial rate of four or five times the

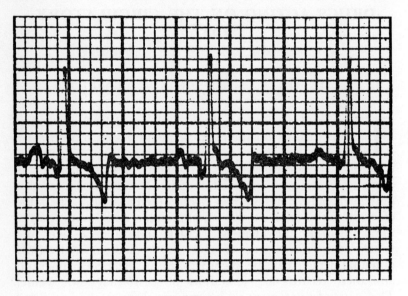

FIG. 14.1

An electrocardiograph showing atrial fibrillation in the dog.
(*Courtesy G. F. Boddie.*)

normal may occur. This condition is called atrial flutter. When these alterations are disorganised causing a random ineffective activity of the atria, the condition is called atrial fibrillation. Some of these conditions can be alleviated by drugs, such as the cardiac glycosides and quinidine.

THE CARDIAC GLYCOSIDES

The common foxglove, *Digitalis purpurea*, is the source of some important *cardiac glycosides* and was introduced into orthodox medicine from folk-lore by William Withering in the eighteenth century. Its leaves contain the glycosides **digitoxin,** gitoxin and gitalin. The Balkan woolly foxglove,

Digitalis lanata, contains **digoxin**. Digitoxin is the principal glycoside of *Digitalis purpurea* and like digoxin is a crystalline substance. However, commercial samples of digitoxin vary slightly, but digoxin is a well-defined substance of constant chemical composition. The cardiac glycosides comprise a combination of genin or aglycone with sugar. The aglycones resemble in chemical structure the sterols (see Fig. 16.6). The effect on the heart of the aglycones is similar to that produced by the corresponding glycosides but they are less firmly fixed to the cardiac tissue and are more easily washed out. It is generally considered preferable to use digoxin, which is a definite chemical entity, than the various galenical preparations of digitalis which vary in composition.

Digitalis and the other cardiac glycosides act directly on the heart and also through the vagus. They increase the force of contraction and excitability of heart muscle, increasing heart output so that the heart does the same work at a smaller volume. This effect is best shown in a failing heart. The increased cardiac output improves the circulation, relieving œdema due to venous congestion and improving the oxygenation of the tissues. There is a transient rise in arterial pressure and a fall in venous pressure.

The rate of conduction of the impulse from auricles to ventricles is decreased and the refractory period increased. Large doses eventually cause heart block. Acting through the vagus nerve these drugs slow the heart rate and block conduction from the sinus node to the ventricle. These vagal effects are antagonised by atropine and a partial heart block produced by overdosage with a cardiac glycoside may be relieved by treatment with atropine. When the vagi are blocked with atropine, digitalis prolongs the refractory period of the atrial muscle, but when the vagi are intact the refractory period is shortened. The vagal effects produced by digitalis are not uniform, so that in some regions of the heart the refractory period of the cardiac muscle is greatly reduced and not in others. Thus digitalis causes atrial flutter to be converted into atrial fibrillation. This effect of digitalis in converting atrial flutter to fibrillation is usually regarded as clinically desirable because it is generally easier to control the ventricular rate in fibrillation than in flutter.

The excitation-contraction response of the heart muscle is probably mediated by the transport of ions across the cell membrane. The entry of sodium ions into the cell is probably controlled by the enzyme ATPase. When sodium enters the cell calcium ions are released and thus become available for the contractile proteins. It has been shown that the cardiac glycosides inhibit the active transport of sodium and potassium by antagonising ATPase and it has also been shown that low concentrations of glycoside potentiate ATPase. These observations have led to the suggestion that the cardiac tonic effects of the glycoside are due to potentiation of the enzyme and the toxic effects due to inhibition. Digitalis often causes vomiting, probably by acting on the vomiting centre, but it may be through gastric irritation or by its action on the heart. Cats are especially liable to vomit if treated with this drug.

The cardiac glycosides are of value in stimulating a failing heart and in the treatment of auricular fibrillation. In this latter condition these drugs slow conduction in the bundle of His and so allow the ventricles time to empty before the next impulse arrives. They have a diuretic effect in œdema of cardiac origin, but this is due to the improvement in the renal circulation allowing the formation and excretion of more urine.

The glycosides of digitalis are quickly absorbed from the gut but are destroyed in the rumen. Digoxin is sufficiently water-soluble for it to be given by injection. The glycosides are quickly fixed by the tissues, particularly by the heart and voluntary muscle. They are mostly destroyed in the body and only traces appear in the urine.

Digitoxin becomes so firmly fixed to heart muscle that the effect of a series of doses persists long after administration has stopped. It is therefore cumulative. Gitoxin and gitalin are more water-soluble than digitoxin so act more rapidly and are more easily washed out. Digitalis is usually given by mouth as the tincture; digoxin is available as tablets or for injection. The use of preparations of digoxin is confined almost entirely to the dog and cat. There are several reports of the successful treatment of atrial fibrillation in the dog and horse. Sometimes digitalis has been used to control fibrillation as a preliminary to subsequent treatment with quinidine, and, on occasion, even in the case in which digitalis alone has been used, the heart has reverted to a normal sinus rhythm on withdrawal of the drug.

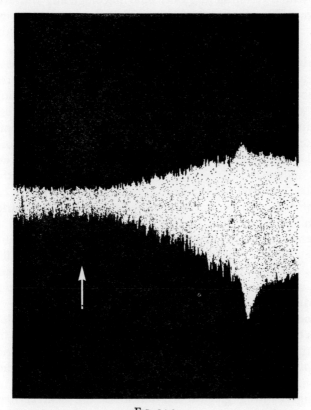

FIG. 14.2

The effect of ouabain on the contractions of the isolated guinea pig auricles.

Strophanthus has similar actions to digitalis but is less effective because it is partly destroyed by the intestinal enzymes. It was first used by African natives as an arrow poison. The active principle Strophanthin G or Ouabain is a pure crystalline substance which may be injected intravenously to produce a rapid effect. It is destroyed in the body much more quickly than digitalis and is preferred for use in cats or where digitalis causes vomiting.   Crystalline Ouabain or Tincture of Strophanthus are available.

The bulb of **Squill** contains the glycosides Scillaren A and B which resemble digitalis pharmacologically but are less effective.   The tincture or syrup of Squill is used as an expectorant.   Red squills is a rat poison, but this action is not due to the cardiac glycosides.

Quinidine, the dextro-rotary isomer of quinine, is used specifically to treat auricular fibrillation.   It actually cures the condition, unlike digitalis which only reduces the harmful effects of the fibrillation.   It is a myocardial depressant. Quinidine slows conduction in the bundle of His and depresses the excitability of heart muscle.   The frequency of the auricular contractions is reduced and the length of the refractory period increased.   It is rapidly excreted, hence maximum doses are required all the time.   Sometimes quinidine causes sudden death, because the sudden alteration of auricular rhythm dislodges clots in the auricular appendix and these form emboli which block the coronary vessels.   Quinidine has been successfully used in the treatment of atrial fibrillation in both the dog and horse.   It is regarded as usually desirable to use quinidine in this condition after prior digitalisation as this reduces the hazards of quinidine.

Procainamide is a drug with similar pharmacological actions to procaine, but with more marked effects on the heart, It is, moreover, less readily hydrolysed by plasma esterases than procaine.   The cardiac actions of procainamide are very similar to those of quinidine.

Drugs causing general excitation of the central nervous system usually stimulate the vagal centre more strongly than the sympathetic, hence strychnine causes slowing of the heart. Parasympathomimetic drugs such as physostigmine decrease the heart rate; atropine and like substances increase heart rate by abolishing vagal control.   Adrenaline increases the heart rate and output, which is due largely to an increased mobilisation of blood which increases the venous return.   The rise in blood pressure also contributes.   However, if the rise is great, stimulation of pressor receptors causes reflex vagal slowing of the heart.

DRUGS ACTING ON BLOOD VESSELS

Many drugs act on plain muscle, and since this includes the plain muscle of the blood vessels they also affect the circulation. The nitrites, papaverine and certain xanthine derivatives act on plain muscle to produce vasodilation. Papaverine and the xanthines have been discussed earlier. The nitrites, whilst of little therapeutic importance in veterinary medicine, merit mention because in certain circumstances nitrite poisoning may occur in ruminants.

All the nitrites act in a similar fashion, differing mainly in the rate and duration of action. Inorganic nitrates have no such action except in ruminants, in which species they are reduced to nitrites by the rumen bacteria, the nitrite is absorbed and causes methæmoglobinæmia. The nitrites cause relaxation of plain muscle, that of the arterioles being particularly affected, producing a vasodilatation and fall in blood pressure.

Histamine is a substance with very marked pharmacological activity. It causes dilatation and increased permeability of the capillaries. Although it is usual to speak of the increased permeability being shown by the capillary blood vessels, it is probably the very small venules which show this phenomenon. The effect of histamine on the arterioles varies with the species; in rodents the arterioles contract, in cats the contraction is only slight and in the dog there is dilation of the arterioles. Big doses of histamine cause blood to collect in the capillaries and the plasma to be filtered off; this results in hæmal concentration and produces a clinical condition which is called shock. In cats this effect predominates. In man the effect on capillaries is shown in the triple response which occurs after histamine has been scratched into the skin. The response shows as local redness, local arterial dilatation from an axon reflex and local œdema.

Histamine causes contraction of nearly all smooth muscle. However, different species vary in their response to histamine, the guinea-pig is very sensitive and histamine causes death in this animal by producing a marked broncho-constriction. The rabbit is much less sensitive. Death in this species is caused by histamine constricting the pulmonary vessels, and in the dog death is said to be produced by constriction of the hepatic

N

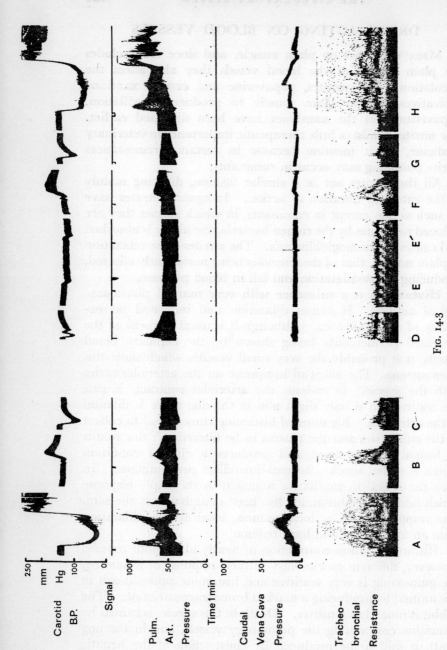

FIG. 14.3

The effect of histamine, 5HT, bradykinin, mepyramine and egg-albumin on a sheep previously sensitised to egg-albumin. At A, 0·5 µg/kg histamine; at B, 10 µg/kg 5HT; at C, bradykinin 1 µg/kg at D; mepyramine 2 mg/kg at E; 0·5 µg/kg histamine; at G, 10 µg/kg 5HT, at H; 1 µg/kg bradykinin; at I, 1 g albumin. The veins. In ruminants and the pig, histamine also produces hypotension although these species are not particularly sensitive. The hypotension in ruminants and the pig is due to histamine constricting the pulmonary vessels which decreases the return of blood to the heart, reducing the heart output and thus the blood pressure.

When histamine is slowly absorbed it greatly increases gastric secretion. Atropine reduces but does not abolish this effect, and it is not prevented by antihistamines. This stimulation if repeated sufficiently will produce gastric ulceration. Histamine also increases the secretion of the salivary, lacrimal, bronchial and intestinal glands. The effect on these glands, particularly on the salivary gland, is antagonised by antihistamine drugs.

Histamine is formed by the decarboxylation of histidine, a change which can be brought about chemically or by bacteria. It is stable, soluble in water and in alcohol. Histamine is present in the body in high concentrations in the skin, intestinal epithelium and lungs. It is stored in the mast cells where it exists as granules bound to heparin. The histamine in the skin and intestine, however, does not all exist in the mast cells because these cells are very few in number in these tissues; in non-mast cell sites, histamine can be quickly made from histidine by a specific decarboxylase. This manufactured histamine is not stored and hence these tissues are able to produce substantial quantities of histamine very quickly.

During anaphylaxis or after the administration of certain drugs the tissue histamine is released into the circulation when it produces a variety of effects, such as a fall in blood pressure, œdema, bronchospasm and itching. If histamine is applied to the superficial layers of the skin it produces itching, application to the deeper layers causes pain. The reaction between an antigen and its appropriate cell-fixed antibody, as occurs in anaphylaxis, causes the release of histamine and, in some species such as the dog, this released histamine is responsible for most of the phenomena observed during anaphylaxis. However, released histamine is not responsible for all features of the various hypersensitivity reactions and other substances are involved such as 5-hydroxytryptamine, heparin, plasma kinins and slow-reacting substance (SRS). In ruminants histamine and 5-HT do not appear to be involved to an appreciable extent in the anaphylactic response. There is some evidence that bradykinin may be released in these animals. Chemically plasma kinins are polypeptides and SRS is probably an unsaturated fatty acid.

Tissue injury may release not only histamine but can increase the activity of the enzyme histidine decarboxylase, which increases the amount of histamine formed. This release of histamine as a consequence of increased histidine decarboxylase activity may account for the delayed vaso-dilatation which occurs in inflammation. Amongst the drugs which release histamine are curare, strychnine and morphine, the chemo-therapeutic agents quinapyramine, the diamidines and organic arsenicals, proteolytic enzymes, bacterial toxins and snake venoms. A powerful and specific releaser, known as 48/80, is composed of simple polymers of N. methyl methoxy-phenylethylamine mixed with formaldehyde. Some drugs liberate heparin, bradykinin and hydroxytryptamine as well as histamine.

Histamine is well absorbed from all parenteral sites of administration, but only a little is absorbed after oral administration. This is because histamine, given by mouth or produced in the gut by the activity of bacterial decarboxylating enzymes, is rapidly metabolised by intestinal bacteria and by enzymes in the intestinal mucous membrane. However, a little may gain entry to the body, and this is metabolised partly by methylation to produce methyl-histamine and partly by oxidation to imidazole acetic acid. In sheep the major route of inactivation of histamine appears to be by oxidative deamination and no inactivation by methylation occurs in this species, whereas in the dog and cat methylation predominates. The oxidation of histamine is catalysed by an enzyme histaminase. In mice less than 1 per cent of an injected dose of histamine appears in the urine as the free compound. Herbivorous animals excrete in the urine a substantial quantity of acetyl histamine which is pharmacologically inactive. It arises mainly as a result of the acetylation of histamine by intestinal bacteria. Most of the information about histamine has been obtained by using a method of estimation, which consists of measuring the effect of a specially prepared extract of tissue on the isolated guinea-pig ileum and comparing it with the effect of a known amount of histamine. When other biological preparations such as the cat's blood pressure and the guinea-pig uterus are used and give the same answer, the probability of the active substance in the extract being histamine is increased. This evidence may be supported by using specific antagonists. This is another example of a parallel quantitative assay (see p. 64).

HISTAMINE ANTAGONISTS

Under circumstances such as those described above, histamine may be released from the tissues and cause harm. Drugs to counteract these harmful effects are, therefore, of importance. This antagonism to histamine may be classified into physiological, competitive or destructive antagonism (non-competitive).

Physiological antagonists are substances, such as adrenaline and other sympathomimetic amines, which have actions opposite to those of histamine and are therefore antagonistic to it.

Competitive antagonists probably act by competing for the same receptors in the tissue. Some, but by no means all, competitive antagonists have a molecular structure similar to that of the agonist. They are usually compared and tested by measuring their power to protect guinea-pigs against death from histamine poisoning or in preventing the contraction of an isolated piece of smooth muscle treated with histamine.

A number of histamine antagonists have been synthesised. They include **Diphenhydramine** (Benadryl), one of the oldest antihistamines; **Mepyramine** (Neoantargan); **Tripelennamine** (Vetibenzamine); **Dimenhydrinate** (Dramamine); **Promethazine** (Phenergan); and **Trimeprazine** (Vallergan).

Mepyramine is a typical antihistamine. It is specific and very active, protecting guinea-pigs against 80 times a lethal dose of histamine. It antagonises the actions of histamine on the blood vessels, bronchi and intestines, but not on gastric secretion. Mepyramine has a powerful local anæsthetic effect and a quinidine-like action on the heart.   It has little atropine-like effect whereas the other antihistamines have atropine-like actions and are less specific. The antihistamines protect against the effects of histamine released either in anaphylaxis or by drugs, they do not prevent the release of histamine in these circumstances. The degree of protection to anaphylactic shock by antihistamines varies with the species, for example, they give no protection against anaphylaxis in mice, little in ruminants, an appreciable amount in the dog and complete protection in the guinea-pig. Whether or not an anti-histamine protects against anaphylaxis depends in part on the sensitivity of the particular species to histamine. The mouse, for example, being relatively insensitive is not protected. Moreover anaphylaxis, in some of the species which are not protected, involves active substances other than histamine such as 5-HT. Antihistamines also have a depressant action on the central nervous system.

Mepyramine is absorbed from the gut, producing a maximum effect in one to two hours which lasts three to four hours. Promethazine reaches a maximum effect after oral administration in four to five hours and persists for twenty-four hours. Anthihistamines are partly destroyed in the body and partly excreted in the urine. In the large animals they are given by injection. If these drugs are given by rapid intra-venous injection, a fall in blood pressure may be produced. This is probably related to the local anæsthetic action of the antihistamines and it does not occur when they are injected slowly. The antihistamines are used therapeutically to counteract anaphylactic shock, in various allergic conditions, in laminitis and to antagonise the effects of histamine released by drugs.

Antihistamine drugs are also of value in the prevention of motion sickness (p. 162), although not all compounds are equally suitable. Diphenhydramine, Chlorcyclizine and Pro-methazine are valuable for this purpose. They do not appear to act on the CTZ because apomorphine-induced vomiting was unaffected by pre-treatment with these antihistamines. Simi-larly their effect does not seem to be simple depression of the vomiting centre. Promethazine and Trimeprazine are used as ataractics, whilst Diphenhydramine is an antihistamine with marked depressant actions on the central nervous system. The antihistamines may stimulate the central nervous system. This is particularly likely to be seen in gross overdosage with these drugs. Destructive antagonists of histamine include the enzyme histaminase and are not of therapeutic importance

5-Hydroxytryptamine (5-HT) is a base which resembles histamine. It is present in the tissues and causes contraction of plain muscle in very low concentrations. Most of the 5-HT in the body is made by the hydroxylation and decarboxylation of tryptophan and stored in the argentaffin cells of the intestine. A small amount is present in the brain. When 5-HT is liberated in the body or added to blood *in vitro* it is fixed by the platelets, and when the platelets disintegrate 5-HT is freed. It is also released by drugs such as reserpine and in allergic reactions. 5-HT is destroyed by mono-amine oxidase and excreted in the urine as 5-hydroxyindoleacetic acid (5-HIAA), some of which is conjugated with glucuronic and sulphuric acids. 5-HT is quickly absorbed after parenteral administration but is ineffective when given by mouth.

5-HT stimulates the plain muscle of the arteries, veins, bronchi, uterus and intestine to contract. The sensitivity of plain muscle to 5-HT varies with the species. Avian and rat plain muscle appears very sensitive whilst that from guinea-pigs is relatively insensitive. Sensory nerves are stimulated as are chemoreceptors in the large vessels and lungs, causing a slow pulse and apnœa. The sensory receptors in the intestinal mucosæ are also stimulated, causing peristalsis. It has been suggested that the function of 5-HT in the gastro-intestinal tract is to regulate peristalsis. Ganglionic transmission is improved by small doses and blocked by large doses. The response to 5-HT varies not only between species but between individual members of a species. This variability in response depends partly on the fact that many of the effects produced by 5-HT are reflex due to the compound stimulating receptors to various afferent nerves. Tachyphylaxis is a frequent observation when a series of doses of 5-HT are administered. In tachyphylaxis the response to subsequent doses of similar magnitude shows a progressive decrease. There are a number of drugs which antagonise the effects of

5-HT; some of these act as physiological antagonists, that is they have pharmacological actions which are directly opposed to the actions of 5-HT. Other drugs antagonise 5-HT by acting on the nervous pathway through which the 5-HT is acting. An example of this type of drug is shown when the slowing of the heart, which is produced by 5-HT, is prevented by the prior administration of either atropine or a ganglion-blocking agent. Atropine or the ganglion-blocking drug prevent the effect of 5-HT by blocking the efferent limb of the reflex on which the cardiac slowing depends.

There is, however, a third group of 5-HT antagonists which inhibit the combination of 5-HT with its receptors on either smooth muscle or nervous element. These antagonists are either various ergot alkaloids or derivatives of these alkaloids containing *lysergic acid*. An important member of the latter group is lysergic acid diethylamide (LSD). In man this drug has interesting central actions in that it gives rise to hallucinations, and it is of interest that reserpine, which in man is a potent tranquiliser, depletes the brain of its 5-HT. It has been suggested that 5-HT may be a neurohumor in the central nervous system. A potent antagonist of 5-HT is the lysergic acid derivative Methysergide. However, no antagonist of 5-HT completely blocks all its pharmacological activity.

5-HT is a component of the sting of certain plants. It is involved also in some of the responses to injury and anaphylaxis shown in rats, mice and hamsters. In these species 5-HT is synthesised and stored in mast cells from which it is released together with histamine by injury or in anaphylaxis. 5-HT does not appear to be present in the mast cells of other species.

Angiotensin is a pharmacologically active polypeptide which is formed by the action of the enzyme renin on angiotensinogen. Renin is present in extracts of kidney and, under some circumstances, it may be released from the kidney to act on the angiotensinogen present in the plasma. Angiotensin is the most potent vasopressor agent known and acts by causing an intense vasoconstriction. It has been synthesised and shown to contain ten amino acids. It is probably important in certain pathological conditions.

SHOCK

The use of this term should be confined to cases of peripheral failure of the circulation. In this condition the blood does not return to the heart in sufficient quantities so that there is a fall in pressure in the right atrium It may be due to vasodilatation, loss of blood or loss of plasma or to all these factors A severe injury may be accompanied by hæmorrhage and so cause circulatory failure. This is usually treated by controlling the hæmorrhage and replacing the lost blood with blood if possible or a plasma substitute.

In some conditions the capillaries become more permeable, so that plasma is removed from the blood. This causes œdema, and if it is very marked may be accompanied by a hæmo-concentration and a fall in blood proteins. This increased permeability may be produced by a variety of causes, such as histamine and substances which release histamine, staphylo-coccal toxins, arsenic, extremes of heat or cold and poor circulation in the tissues.

Loss of fluid occurs in diarrhœa, vomiting, pyrexia and in specific diseases such as Grass Sickness in horses. This also leads to a hæmoconcentration. The loss of fluid other than by hæmorrhages is treated by giving fluids by mouth and plasma substitutes, such as Dextran q.v. intravenously. Intravenous salines are not retained in the circulation and tend to exaggerate œdema.

SUGGESTIONS FOR FURTHER READING

ERSPAMER, V. (1966). 5-Hydroxytryptamine and related indolealkylamines. *Handb. exp. Pharmak.*, Suppl., 19.

GLENDINNING, S. A. (1965). Quinidine sulphate for the treatment of atrial fibrillation in 12 horses. *Vet. Rec.*, **77,** 951.

GELL, P. G. H. and COOMBS, R. R. A. (1963). *Clinical Aspects of Immunology.* Oxford: Blackwell.

GLYNN, I. M. (1964). The action of cardiac glycosides on ion movement. *Pharmac. Rev.*, **16,** 381.

KAHLSON, G. and ROSENGREN, E. (1968). New approaches to the physiology of histamine. *Physiol. Rev.*, **48,** 155.

PEART, W. S. (1965). The renin-angiotensin system. *Pharmac. Rev.*, **17,** 143.

SANFORD, J. (1968). The significance of histamine in some animal diseases. *Vet. Rev.*, **19,** 54. [May & Baker].

SILVA, M. ROCHA E (1966). Histamine and antihistaminics. *Handb. exp. Pharmak.* Vol. 28.

WEST, T. C. and TODA, N. (1967). Cardio-vascular pharmacology. *A. Rev. Pharmac.*, **7,** 145.

CHAPTER XV

DRUGS ACTING ON THE RESPIRATORY SYSTEM

THE respiratory centre is controlled in part by the CO_2 tension of the blood; an increase of as little as 0·2 per cent of CO_2 in the alveolar air will double the volume of air respired. A large increase in CO_2 tension produces signs of asphyxia and a decrease causes apnœa. The respiratory centre is not directly stimulated by lack of oxygen, but such a lack makes the centre more sensitive to CO_2. Oxygen lack, therefore, does not cause hyperpnœa if the CO_2 tension is also lowered. In fact in these circumstances oxygen lack causes no very obvious effects excepting a marked cyanosis. Carbon dioxide is the physiological stimulus to respiration and is often useful in treating respiratory failure in small animals. It is supplied in cylinders usually as a 5 per cent mixture with oxygen and is given by intra-tracheal or intra-nasal tube or by means of a suitable mask. Such equipment is very useful in the operating theatre where a few minutes' treatment with an oxygen/CO_2 mixture can be invaluable in stimulating a failing respiration (Fig. 15.1). However, in barbiturate poisoning the sensitivity of the respiratory centre to CO_2 is depressed; under these circumstances the administration of CO_2 is without avail and artificial respiration is the best method of resuscitation.

The respiratory movements are partly controlled through the carotid sinus reflex. A rise in blood pressure in the sinus inhibits respiration and a fall in pressure causes stimulation. Respiratory stimulation is also produced by lack of oxygen or excess CO_2 in the sinus.

Carbon dioxide when inhaled for about one minute produces a brief cerebral depression. This has been used to make pigs unconscious prior to slaughter by bleeding; such animals bleed more thoroughly and bruising of tissues is avoided. Carbon dioxide is used also to render fowls and other small animals unconscious (p. 128). Carbon dioxide decreases the force of contraction of the heart and by a direct action on the blood vessels causes vasodilatation. However, these effects are largely counteracted by the release of adrenaline and noradrenaline by CO_2.

The normal activities of all the tissues of the body depend upon an adequate supply of oxygen. The brain, however, is more susceptible to oxygen lack than any other tissue. Lack

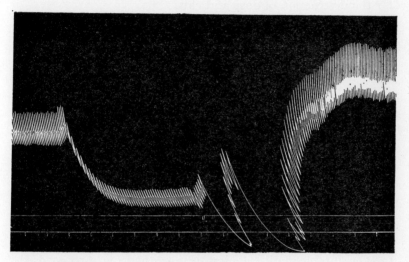

Morph. CO_2
FIG. 15.1

The effect of carbon dioxide on the respirations of a rabbit which have been depressed by morphine. The height above the base line shows the volume of air breathed. Time interval 10 secs.

of oxygen is called anoxia. It may be more correct to use the term hypoxia which means the deprivation of oxygen.

Anoxic anoxia is the state in which the oxygen capacity of the blood is normal but the oxygen supply is inadequate, either because of inadequate ventilation, disease of the lungs or insufficient oxygen in the atmosphere.

Anæmic anoxia exists when the oxygen capacity is reduced, either by lack of hæmoglobin or inactivation of the hæmoglobin, as when it is converted to carboxyhæmoglobin in carbon monoxide poisoning.

Stagnant anoxia occurs in circulatory failure. In this condition the arterial blood is unable to deliver sufficient oxygen to the tissues.

Histotoxic anoxia occurs when the tissues are unable to take and use oxygen from the blood and is produced when the cellular oxidative processes are poisoned by substances such as cyanides. Hydrocyanic acid poisoning is really a form of asphyxiation, and it is, therefore, not a suitable drug to use for the destruction of dogs and cats.

Anoxia gives rise to an increase in the respiratory rate. The extremities are cold and the mucous membranes cyanotic, and there is a depression of the central nervous system similar to that produced by alcohol.

Oxygen

Pure oxygen can be breathed for a few hours without harmful effects, but if this is continued for several days pneumonia and cerebral damage are produced. An atmosphere containing 60 per cent oxygen can be breathed indefinitely without harm. Oxygen at a pressure of four atmospheres kills in a few minutes. This is due to certain enzymes in the brain being poisoned.

The main use of oxygen in veterinary practice is in general anæsthesia. It is best given by intra-nasal or intra-tracheal tube or suitable mask. Unless the anæsthetist is using a closed-circuit apparatus with a CO_2 absorber the oxygen should be given together with 5 per cent CO_2.

Carbon monoxide is an odourless and colourless gas which on inhalation may produce a sudden loss of consciousness. The effects produced by this gas are entirely due to oxygen lack. Carbon monoxide combines with hæmoglobin 200 times more readily than does oxygen; the combination is much firmer and excludes oxygen. The tissues are thus deprived of oxygen and tissue oxidations are inhibited because carbon monoxide also has a high affinity for the respiratory enzymes. The only treatment, which must be prompt, is to give oxygen to remove carbon monoxide from the blood. Under conditions of high oxygen tension, carbon monoxide is displaced from combination with hæmoglobin and, in these circumstances, sufficient oxygen will dissolve in the plasma to maintain many functions. Carbon monoxide as produced by car exhausts or in coal gas is sometimes used to destroy dogs and cats.

Cyanides may be absorbed from the lungs as hydrocyanic acid gas, or after ingestion or in ruminants following the ingestion of plants containing cyano-genetic glycosides. They act by interfering with the tissue oxidations inhibiting oxidative enzymes but not other enzymes. The cyanide ion reacts with trivalent iron, particularly the iron in cytochrome oxidase, and thus gives rise to histotoxic anoxia. Very small doses of cyanides stimulate respiration by stimulating the carotid sinus. This stimulation is probably produced by cyanide blocking oxidative metabolism in the chemoreceptor cells of the carotid sinus and thus acting like a reduction in oxygen tension. This manner of stimulating respiration has long been discontinued because it is of no value when the medullary centres are depressed; moreover, cyanide has well known and marked toxic effects. The treatment of cyanide poisoning must be very rapid if it is to be effective. The object is to form methæmoglobin which competes with cytochrome oxidase for the cyanide, thus freeing the cytochrome oxidase. Methæmoglobin is formed by giving sodium nitrite intravenously. Sodium thiosulphate should be given also by intravenous injection. Sulphur is transferred from the thiosulphate and replaced with cyanide to form thiocyanate in which form the cyanide is unable to combine with iron.

Cobalamin is a member of the group of B_{12} vitamins and has been used to treat cyanide poisoning. It apparently combines with cyanide to form cyanocobalamin (p. 50.)

RESPIRATORY STIMULANTS AND DEPRESSANTS

Stimulation of the respiratory centres is a valuable therapeutic measure in the treatment of respiratory failure, such as occurs during anæsthesia. The most important stimulants are CO_2 and the analeptic drugs which have already been discussed. The sympathomimetic amines act on the respiratory centre and have the added advantage of improving its blood supply.

The respiratory centre is more easily depressed than any other medullary centre and several drugs have this property.

The centres are also made less sensitive to CO_2 stimulation by drugs. Morphine, diamorphine, and the barbiturates are powerful respiratory depressants, as are some of the morphine substitutes such as methadone. Morphine and diamorphine depress the cough centre, and, whilst this is sometimes therapeutically desirable, these drugs are usually avoided because of the restrictions of the Dangerous Drugs Act under which they are scheduled.

Codeine is the drug of choice in the relief of painful coughing, as it depresses the cough centre in doses which have little effect on respiration. This effect of codeine is not antagonised by nalorphine but is in fact augmented. Codeine phosphate and syrup of codeine phosphate are used as depressants of the cough centre in dogs. **Dextromethorphan** is a newer anti-tussive (see p. 111).

DRUGS ACTING ON BRONCHIOLES AND BRONCHI

The function of the bronchial muscles is not fully understood. They are under the control of the autonomic nervous system, being contracted by vagal stimulation and dilated by sympathetic stimulation. Similar effects are, of course, produced by sympatho- and parasympathomimetic drugs. Bronchoconstriction is never required as a therapeutic measure; bronchodilation may be required on occasion. Sympathomimetic amines, atropine, nitrites, papaverine, and xanthine derivatives all produce bronchodilation.

Expectorants

Expectorants are drugs which increase the volume and decrease the viscosity of the bronchial secretion. They are used to relieve coughing and act by stimulating nerve-endings in the stomach and duodenum, causing a reflex increase in secretion of the bronchial glands. The main substances used for this purpose are emetics such as Ipecacuanha, Ammonium bicarbonate and Squill given in sub-emetic doses. Potassium iodide also increases the bronchial secretion and makes it more fluid, and this effect is due to its excretion by the bronchial glands.

Various volatile oils are excreted through the lungs and have some expectorant activity. They include oil of turpentine, balsam of Tolu and balsam of Peru.

Expectorants may be of value in the dog and horse, but it is doubtful if any other species would benefit. Moreover, drugs depending for their action on gastric irritation are unlikely to be effective in ruminants. Disinfection of the respiratory

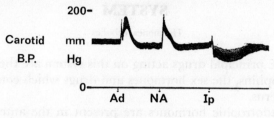

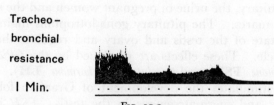

FIG. 15.2

The broncho-dilator action of the sympathomimetic amines is shown. The carotid blood pressure and tracheobronchial resistance were recorded from a sheep which was given successively 1 μg/kg adrenaline, noradrenaline and isoprenaline.

tract would be most effectively carried out by means of suitable antibiotics or chemotherapeutic measures.

In former times drugs were given by intratracheal injection to kill parasites in the respiratory passages. Such measures were of little value and the method seems a good way to produce a broncho-pneumonia.

Bronchial secretions are reduced by atropine, and this fact is made use of in premedication before using a volatile anæsthetic likely to stimulate secretions.

SUGGESTIONS FOR FURTHER READING

DEJOURS, P. (1962). Chemoreflexes in breathing. *Physiol. Rev.*, **42**, 335.
HAUGAARD, N. (1968). Cellular mechanisms of oxygen toxicity. *Physiol. Rev.*, **48**, 315.
LAMBERTSEN, C. J. (1966). Drugs and respiration. *A. Rev. Pharmac.*, **6**, 327.
WIDDICOMBE, J. G. (1963). Regulation of tracheobronchial smooth muscle. *Physiol. Rev.*, **43**, 1.

CHAPTER XVI

DRUGS ACTING ON THE REPRODUCTIVE SYSTEM

Hormones, ecbolics

THE principal drugs acting on this system are the gonado-trophins, the sex hormones and drugs which contract the uterus.

Gonadotrophic hormones are present in the anterior lobe of the pituitary, the urine of pregnant women and the serum of pregnant mares. The pituitary gonadotrophins maintain the normal state of the testis and ovary and regulate the female sexual cycle. These effects are produced by the *follicle stimulating hormone* (**FSH**) and the *luteinising hormone* (**LH**).

FSH stimulates the development of Graafian follicles in the ovary and spermatogenesis in the testis. *FSH* increases the diameter of the seminiferous tubules, but probably both *FSH* and *LH* are essential for complete spermatogenesis. The effect of *LH* may be indirect, acting through the induction of androgen secretion and thus making complete spermato-genesis possible. *LH* stimulates the interstitial cells of the ovary and testis to produce their respective hormones, hence it is also termed the interstitial cell-stimulating hormone (*ICSH*). Provided maturing follicles are present in the ovary, *LH* causes ovulation and luteinisation of the granulosa cells.

Chorionic gonadotrophin is made in the human placenta and appears in the urine during pregnancy. The presence of this hormone provides the basis of various tests for pregnancy, such as the Ascheim-Zondek, Friedman and Xenopus tests. Chorionic gonadotrophin is available for therapeutic purposes. Its effect is mainly luteinising. In female animals this hormone induces ovulation and reinforces the secretion of progesterone by the ovary. It is used to control the time of ovulation in mares because in these animals ovulation normally occurs towards the end of a long œstral period. Chorionic gonadotrophin is used also to induce ovulation in an anovulatory œstrus and for this purpose it is given by intravenous injection. However, the usual route of administering this substance is by intramuscular injection. It is widely used in the treatment of cystic ovarian disease and sometimes in the treatment of retained testicles (cryptorchidism). In male animals chorionic gonadotrophin is used to stimulate the secretion of testosterone by the testes.

Chorionic gonadotrophin has been used to treat anœstrus in cows, but with such variable results that there seems little justification for its continued use.

Serum gonadotrophin

The pregnant mare does not excrete gonadotrophins in the urine, but the serum of such animals (**PMS**) provides a source of gonadotrophin in which FSH is the main hormone. Pregnancy tests in the mare are carried out on the blood serum during the 45th–90th day of pregnancy. Depending on the dose, the administration of serum gonadotrophin will cause one or more follicles in the ovary to develop and rupture, giving rise to a simultaneous oestrus. Ovulation takes place usually 2–5 days after a subcutaneous injection of serum gonadotrophin and it is recommended that mating should not take place at the œstrus induced by serum gonadotrophin because of the risk of multiple pregnancies. It is generally advisable that mating should follow the first spontaneous œstrus which follows the induced œstrus. The administration of serum gonadotrophin causes follicles to develop in the ovary and, if suitably timed, produces œstrus and ovulation. However, an ovarian response may occur without overt œstrus. The response appears to be quantitative but an excessive dose may inhibit ovulation. It is not certain, however, that normal cycles will be resumed; this is particularly the case when the treatment is given outwith the normal breeding season of the species.

Serum gonadotrophin has been used to increase the number of developing follicles and ovulations at œstrus and thus increase the incidence of twins in cattle. It is administered during pro-œstrus, or following manual expression of the corpus luteum to stimulate pro-œstrus so that it reinforces the naturally produced FSH from the anterior pituitary gland. Serum gonadotrophin is used, in conjunction with progesterone or a synthetic progestagen, to induce œstrus in sheep—particularly for controlled breeding out of season. Administered at the end of the progestagen treatment (p. 208) serum gonadotrophin may improve the response of both the percentage of sheep showing œstrus and the number of ovulations induced.

In the male, gonadotrophins may be of some value in the treatment of infertility due to poor libido or low spermatozoa counts in ejaculated semen, but these defects are not commonly due to hormonal deficiency alone.

Methallibure

An interesting recent development in the use of drugs to regulate breeding has arisen from the discovery that certain dithiocarbamoylhydrazine compounds have the pharmacological property of producing a reversible inhibition of pituitary gonadotrophic function. Methallibure is a member of this group which has been used in veterinary medicine to synchronise farrowing in pigs. Although these compounds inhibit all the functions of the anterior pituitary gland, the gonadotrophins appear to be affected at a level of dosage which does not appear to produce any other effects. To synchronise farrowing, methallibure is fed to pigs and after the withdrawal of the drug, œstrus occurs within 4–10 days, 90 per cent of the œstral periods occuring between the fifth and seventh day after withdrawal. Ovulation appears to take place spontaneously during the post-treatment œstrus and artificial insemination on the day following the onset of œstrus produces a high proportion of pregnancies.

Sex Hormones

The sex hormones are chemical substances with the basic structure of steroids. The hormones of the adrenal cortex, cholesterol, vitamin D, the cardiac glycosides and some carcinogenic substances are also steroids The pharmacological differences between these compounds are due to small chemical groups attached to this basic structure (Fig. 16.1). They have, however, some properties in common. For example, they dissolve only slightly in water but are soluble in fats and fat solvents. This property is therapeutically valuable, because if they were water soluble a single injection would flood the body and be quickly inactivated. Since the effect of these hormones takes several days to develop, such a water-soluble compound would be a very inefficient way of administering the drug. These substances are most effective when a low concentration

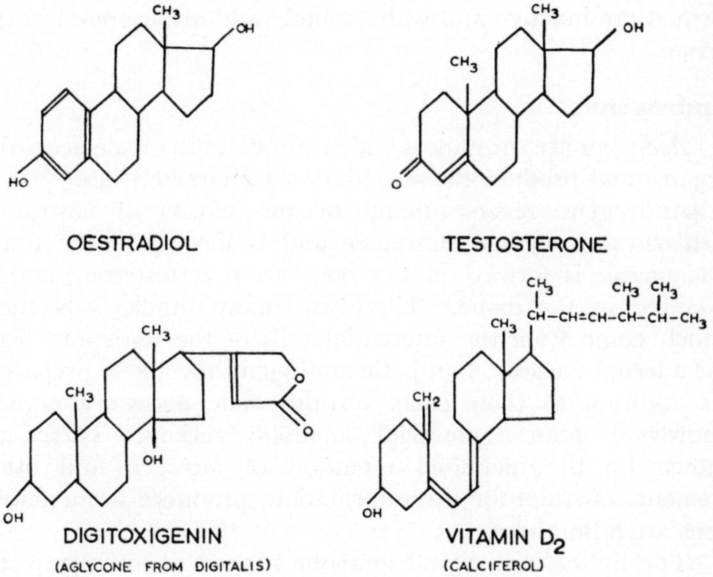

OESTRADIOL   TESTOSTERONE

DIGITOXIGENIN   VITAMIN D₂
(AGLYCONE FROM DIGITALIS)   (CALCIFEROL)

FIG. 16.1

is allowed to act for a long time, and these conditions are most readily obtained by injecting the drug subcutaneously or intra-muscularly in a form from which absorption is very slow. There are a variety of ways in which absorption may be delayed, mixing with a suitable oil, such as arachis oil, has this effect, and by adding palmitic acid, which tends to solidify the fat, absorption is even further delayed. As the esters of some steroids are less water soluble than the parent substance, absorption of the ester proceeds more slowly. Absorption may be prolonged further by introducing the hormone in the form of a compressed tablet inserted surgically into the subcutaneous tissue. Usually the administration of steroid hormones by mouth is rather wasteful, as a large proportion of the dose is excreted in the fæces without having been absorbed. However, the synthetic œstrogens are sometimes incorporated in cattle feed to improve the conversion of food into meat.

Androgens and œstrogens are absorbed from the skin when applied in alcoholic solution. They are also effective when applied locally. After absorption the steroid hormones are partly combined with glucuronic acid, the glucuronides so formed are inactive and water soluble and are excreted in the urine.

Androgens

Androgens are substances which stimulate the male accessory organs and produce the secondary sex characteristics.

Androgens reverse many of the effects of castration *Testosterone* is such a substance and is formed in the testis. *Androsterone* is formed in the body from testosterone and is excreted in the urine. There are many similar substances which come from the interstitial cells of the testis and from the adrenal cortex. Synthetic androgens have been prepared. In addition to their effect on the male accessory organs, androgens possess powerful anabolic actions. These are shown by the increased retention of nitrogen and other elements essential for tissue formation, produced when androgens are administered.

The masculinising and anabolic actions of androgens are assayed in different ways. Masculinising activity, for example, can be assayed by measuring the increased growth of the comb of immature cockerels in response to the androgen. The increase in size of the prostate and seminal vesicles of the castrate rat in response to the administration of androgens can also be used as a measure of masculinising activity. Anabolic activity can be measured by determining the increase in nitrogen retention which takes place when a castrate rat is given androgen or the increase in size of the *levator ani* muscle produced in castrate rats in response to androgen.

Using the two different types of test, it has been possible to prepare compounds in which the virilising and anabolic activities are to a large extent separated. The compound Nor-Ethandrolene (Nandrolone B.P.), for example, has a marked effect on increasing nitrogen retention and the growth and development of bone. It increases also the strength of healing wounds but has very slight masculinising activity and little progestoneal activity.

The negative nitrogen balance and loss of weight produced by the administration of thyroxine can be reversed by Testosterone. Testosterone also prevents the degeneration of muscles which occurs after the motor nerves to the muscle are injured. Laying hens can be protected against spontaneous osteoporosis by the administration of androgens.

A recent development has been the introduction of andro-

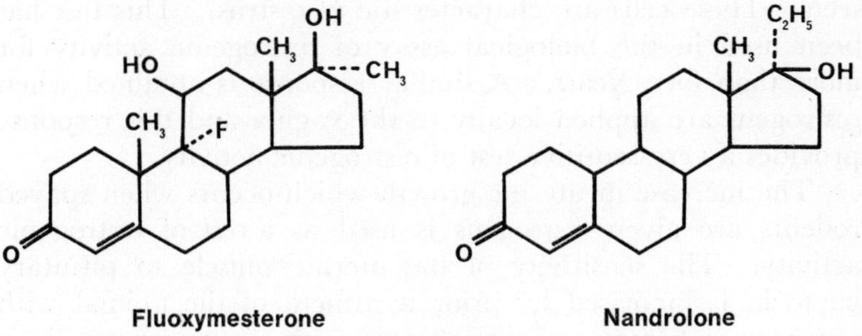

Fluoxymesterone   **Nandrolone**

FIG. 16.2

Two anabolic steroids.

gens with a long action. Some of these are fluorinated compounds, such as fluoxymesterone. This drug has about ten times the virilising activity and twenty times the anabolic activity of methyltestosterone. Androgens do not stimulate the testis of males but take its place, and, if the dose is big enough, actually depress the testis by depressing the anterior pituitary gonadotrophin secretion.

Testosterone is used to aid descent of the testicle but is not as effective as chorionic gonadotrophin. It has been used also to treat mammary tumours in the bitch with equivocal results.

Oestrogens

Œstrogens produce the female characteristics. Acting with other steroids, in particular progesterone, they produce the behavioural and physical effects known as œstrus when mating is permitted. The production of œstrogen in females is mainly cyclical; the periodic ripening of the Graafian follicles, the main source of œstrogen, being controlled by the gonadotrophins secreted by the pituitary gland. The main naturally occurring œstrogens are œstradiol, œstrone and œstriol. Oestradiol is converted in the body into the two other steroids.

Œstrogens stimulate and maintain the tissues of the reproductive tract, stimulating growth of both muscle and epithelium by a direct action. When œstrogens are administered to an ovariectomised rat or mouse and smears taken from the epithelium of the vagina, cornified cells are seen. These cells are characteristic of œstrus. This test has been used in the biological assay of œstrogenic activity for more than forty years. A similar response is obtained when œstrogens are applied locally to the vagina and this response provides a very sensitive test of œstrogenic activity.

The increase in uterine growth which occurs when spayed rodents are given œstrogens is used as a test of œstrogenic activity. The sensitivity of the uterine muscle to pituitary oxytocin is increased by prior treatment of the animal with œstrogen, whereas prior treatment with progesterone diminishes the sensitivity of uterine muscle to oxytocin.

Growth of the mammary glands in both males and females is stimulated by œstrogens. The enlargement of the mammary gland is brought about by an increased growth of ducts and the deposition of fat. In ewes, goats and cows lactation is initiated and maintained. However, this effect in cows is too variable to be used commercially. Low levels of œstrogen activate the lactogenic function of the anterior pituitary but higher levels produce inhibition. Further, lactogenic doses of œstrogen are antagonised by progesterone. Oestrogens are concerned also in the distribution of female fat and sexual changes in the skeleton. They have metabolic actions not unlike those of the androgens, such as increasing the retention of salt, water and nitrogen, in addition to other elements involved in tissue formation. However, the anabolic effects of œstrogens are small compared to those of androgens.

Since the ovaries are not directly affected by œstrogens, these drugs are valueless in producing a normal fertile œstrus.

Moreover, a large single dose, or repeated small doses, may produce cystic ovaries in the cow.

Sex hormones on growth

Androgens are antagonised by œstrogens, and this effect is utilised in the chemical castration of cockerels. Tablets of an œstrogen implanted in the bird's neck improve the conversion of food into flesh and so increase carcase weight without increasing food intake. Œstrogens are used for a similar purpose in cattle, sheep and pigs, being given in the feed or implanted in the base of the ears. This procedure is not free from dangers. Farm animals other than fowls show the growth-stimulating effect of sex hormones through the prolongation of the growth of early maturing parts of the body, and the development of tissues with an early claim on the nutrients, that is the growth of bone and muscle is enhanced. The sex hormones appear to have a specific effect on the appetite of poultry and ruminants. The extra growth in poultry is correlated with the intake of food and there is no increase in nitrogen retention. Hence, the increase in carcase weight in beef animals is brought about by an increase in the amount of body protein and bone, rather than fat, whereas the administration of œstrogens to cockerels produces an increased deposition of fat throughout the body. In the latter animals there is also a lipæmia. This, despite the fact that it occurs in the male, is related to yolk production.

FATE IN THE BODY OF ŒSTROGENS

The naturally-occuring œstrogens appear to be synthesised in the ovary and placenta, the androgen testosterone, amongst other steroids, serving as an immediate precursor. The natural œstrogens are inactivated for the most part in the liver; although some of the œstrogen reaching the liver is excreted in the bile and reabsorbed from the intestine. The endogenous œstrogens are inactivated by conjugation in the body with sulphate and with glucuronide, these conjugates are water soluble and readily excreted by the kidney.

The natural œstrogens are well absorbed from the gut and the reason why their effectiveness when given by this route is limited is probably due to their rapid metabolism in the liver. Certain derivatives of these natural œstrogens are more effective when given by mouth than others; this is because these compounds are more slowly inactivated.

Œstrogens depress the anterior pituitary gland; this causes inhibition of FSH and prolactin accompanied by a secondary degeneration of the gonads. In this way œstrogens actually inhibit the ovary.

SYNTHETIC ŒSTROGENS

Certain simple synthetic substances have œstrogenic activity and these include **Stilboestrol, Hexoestrol** and **Dienoestrol.** The main œstrogens used in veterinary practice are Stilbœstrol and Hexœstrol which have very similar actions. They are active when given by mouth and may be incorporated in the feed. Experiments with rats showed that after subcutaneous injection 80 to 98 per cent was excreted through the bile in the fæces and about 4 per cent in the urine. Rabbits similarly treated excreted 35 per cent in the urine, and it is probable having regard to the toxic effects produced that the fate in sheep and pigs is similar to that in rabbits. This is supported by a study of the distribution of the synthetic œstrogen, hexœstrol. Hexœstrol was synthesised with one of the carbon atoms radio-active. This enabled the distribution of the hexœstrol to be studied with comparative ease and it was shown that the highest concentration occurred in the organs of the reproductive tract and kidney. It was interesting to note that the pituitary gland contained nine times the concentration present in the rest of the brain.

Very large doses of synthetic œstrogen may cause abortion by producing hypertrophy of the uterine mucosa and sensitisation of the uterine muscle to oxytocin. However, the results of this treatment for the induction of abortion are somewhat erratic. Pregnancy following accidental mating is more effectively prevented by the use of œstrogen within 4 days of the mating, when it may inhibit the rate of passage of the fertilised ova down the oviducts, in addition to its effect on the uterine mucosa.

Stilbœstrol is used for its effect on the uterine muscle and mucosa in the treatment of pyometritis and mummified fœtus in the cow. It is used, especially in cattle, to facilitate expulsion of the placenta. The effect is presumably produced by sensitizing the uterine muscle to oxytocin. Œstrogens also help to increase the resistance of the uterus to infection. However, the use of such a drug in pyometritis in bitches increases the risk of toxæmia. It is valuable in the treatment of urinary incontinence and vaginitis in spayed bitches.

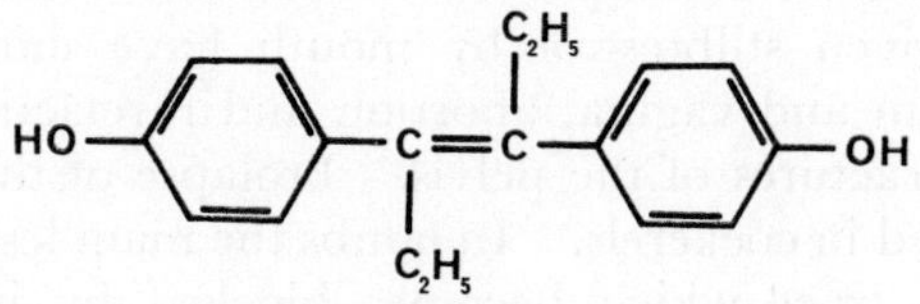

Stilboestrol

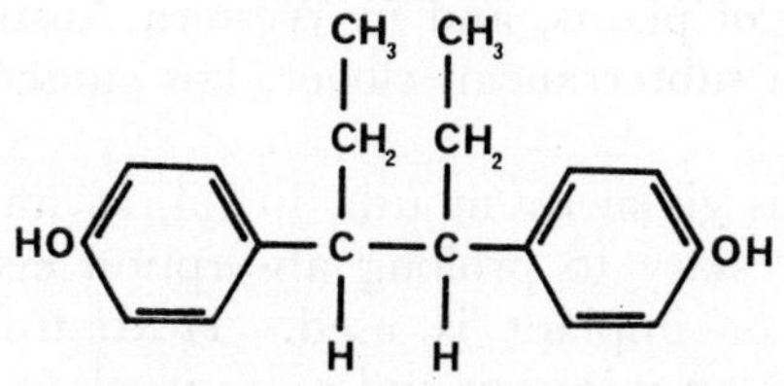

Hexoestrol

FIG. 16.3

Two synthetic œstrogens.

When stilbœstrol has been administered to gilts, the ovulation rate and formation of corpora lutea has been lowered, hence a smaller number of live young has been produced.

The synthetic œstrogens are sometimes given in combination with a synthetic progesterone in a form suitable for oral administration for the purpose of inhibiting ovulation. In the dog, synthetic œstrogens have been used in the treatment of prostatic hyperplasia and certain tumours, such as anal adenomata.

The use of synthetic œstrogens to increase carcase weight has increased the importance of recognising the toxic effects of these substances. The risks associated with feeding œstrogenised food include the contamination of pasture from the drug excreted in the fæces and the absorption of small amounts by persons handling the food. Although stilbœstrol is chemically very stable it is destroyed by soil bacteria in a few weeks. Administration by means of a tablet implant reduces these hazards but introduces new ones. For example, breeding failures have been noted in mink and pigs after feeding capon heads. This is probably due to the head containing a substantial residue of the implant and such offal should be burnt.

Cattle given stilbœstrol by mouth have shown prolapse of the rectum and vagina, abortion and rarefaction of bones, leading to fractures of the pelvis. Prolapse of the cloaca has been reported in cockerels. In lambs the main lesions occur in the urinary tract which becomes blocked by inflammatory changes in the mucous membrane; in addition, prolapse of rectum and vagina may occur.

Compounds with œstrogenic activity have been isolated from a variety of plants, and in Western Australia genistein, an œstrogen in subterranean clover, has caused serious losses of lambs.

Stilbœstrol is given by mouth, in oil, as an injection and when it is necessary to prolong absorption even further the diproprionate or implant is used. Hexœstrol is given by mouth, in oil as an injection and as an implant.

Progesterone

Progesterone is the hormone released by the corpus luteum. It can be synthesised from a substance in soya beans. With the introduction of synthetic analogues of progesterone with a greatly increased potency and a potentially wide use in population control amongst human beings, the assay of progesterone activity has become increasingly important. Progesterone activity can be assayed in a variety of ways. An assay commonly used involves ovariectomised rats pre-treated with œstrogen. The administration of progesterone to such animals causes proliferation of the endometrium which is proportional to the dose of progesterone and can be measured histologically. This test can be simplified by measuring, instead of histological proliferation, increased carbonic anhydrase activity in the endometrium. A test of a different nature involves the effectiveness of the substance under investigation in maintaining pregnancy in ovariectomized rabbits. Rabbits are used because in this species the corpus luteum is the sole source of progesterone. However, the use of these three different tests on the same compounds has given slightly different answers and so they may be testing different kinds of activity.

Although progesterone is well absorbed from the gut it is not very effective when given by mouth, presumably because

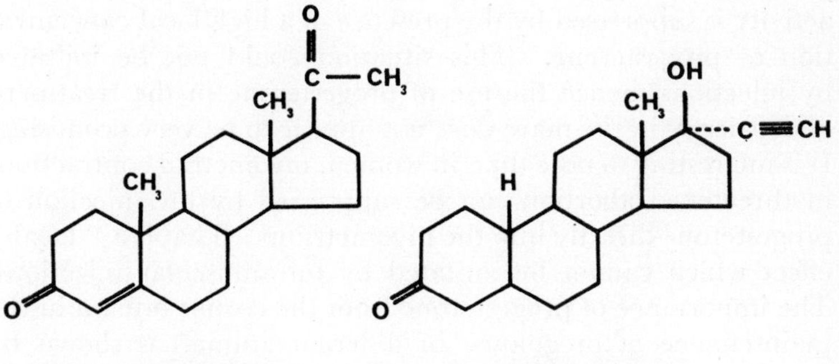

Progesterone   **Norethisterone**

FIG. 16.4

Progesterone and a synthetic progestagen.

of its rapid metabolism. However, some of the new synthetic progesterones are very potent when given orally. In veterinary practice, it is more useful to give parenterally or per vagina. In the body it is converted into pregnandiol which is excreted in the urine as the inactive glucuronide. The tissues affected by progesterone only respond after having been acted on by œstrogens. Thus progesterone increases the thickness of the uterine mucosa and the complexity of the glands after the uterus has been sensitised by œstrogens. It is involved also in the proper development of the mammary glands, acting on them in conjunction with œstrogen. Progesterone depresses the response of the uterine muscle to oxytocin, and in this respect is antagonistic to œstrogen. The characteristic changes which occur in pseudo-pregnancy in the bitch are due largely to progesterone.

The chief function of progesterone is to prepare the uterus

for the fertilised ovum. If pregnancy occurs the uterus becomes insensitive to oxytocin. This is not true of all animals. It does not happen, for example, in the cat. Progesterone has slight androgenic activity and some activity like that of the cortical hormones. Progesterone and its analogues suppress the formation of FSH and LH by the anterior pituitary. This effect is produced by a feed-back mechanism and has been used to suppress œstrus in the bitch and to synchronise œstrus in cattle, sheep and goats, In the mare, progesterone is produced mainly by the placenta and possibly myometrial activity is suppressed by the presence of a high local concentration of progesterone. This situation could not be imitated by injections, hence the use of progesterone in the treatment of deficiency in the mare does not appear to be very promising. It is interesting to note that, in women, myometrial contractions in threatened abortion can be suppressed by the injection of progesterone directly into the myometrium. That is a " local " effect which cannot be imitated by intramuscular injections. The importance of progesterone from the corpus luteum in the maintenance of pregnancy in different animals is shown by whether or not the pregnancy is maintained after ovariectomy. In the mare ovariectomy does not cause abortion but is likely to do so in the sow. The corpus luteum appears to be essential throughout pregnancy in the pig and goat but not in ewe, dog and cat. The use of progesterone together with FSH to produce coincident pregnancies in sheep, cows and sows has been discussed (p. 198). In ewes, a synthetic progestagen may be administered per vagina in the form of an impregnated tampon for this purpose.

Progesterone may be used to treat failure of nidation, for this it is given after ovulation and service. It may be used in the therapy of habitual abortion and nymphomania in cows. In male animals progesterone may produce an azoospermia which is reversible. The synthetic progestagens have been used to supress heat in bitches but unfortunately this treatment was found to increase the incidence of cystic endometrial hyperplasia. *Megestrol*, *Norethisterone* and *Medroxyprogesterone* are all synthetic compounds with high progestonal activity. **Medroxyprogesterone** is used to impregnate tampons which are inserted into the vagina of sheep to control œstrus.

FERTILITY CONTROL

In veterinary practice the usual problem in fertility control is to ensure conception and normal pregnancy. The use, for example, of progesterone analogues and gonadotrophins in the timing of pregnancy in ewes has been discussed. The regulation of farrowing in pigs by drugs which suppress the secretion of gonadotrophins has also been considered.

In man, as is well known, one of the major problems of the world is the regulation of pregnancy so as to prevent the population exceeding the food supply. A considerable amount of work in this field has been carried out and is proceeding with the object of providing cheap and satisfactory methods of controlling pregnancy in man. The chemicals used as contraceptives in man are sometimes of interest in veterinary medicine because the same substances may be of value in the control of malignancy and may also provide a possible alternative to some of the poisons and other objectionable methods at present used to control certain species which may become pests. Seals, for example, are controlled at present either by shooting, or by giving strychnine. These procedures are unsatisfactory and not devoid of cruelty and it seems possible that antifertility drugs could control the seal population in a more humane fashion.

FERTILITY CONTROL IN THE MALE

The chemical control of spermatogenesis can be exercised either by drugs which inhibit spermatogenesis, and are without effect on the endocrine functions of the testis, or by drugs which, by suppressing pituitary gonadotrophin secretion, inhibit both spermatogenesis and the endocrine function of the testis.

Four types of compound have been found to have activity of the first kind, namely nitrofurans, thiophenes, bis (dichloroacetyl) diamines and dinitropyrrole compounds. The nitrofurans are primarily bacteriostatic drugs, and are also used widely in the treatment of coccidiosis. When given orally or parenterally in appropriate doses these drugs cause a degeneration of the seminiferous epithelium resulting in arrest of spermatogenesis : this is reversible. The thiophenes have similar activity but both thiophenes and nitrofurans are regarded as too toxic to use in man for their effect on spermatogenesis. However, a series of bis (dichloroacetyl) diamines have been synthesised which inhibit spermatogenesis reversibly without having any effect on the spermatagonal, Leydig or Sertoli cells. In man these drugs have caused gastric upsets and an increase in the sedimentation rate.

The dinitropyrrole compounds arrest spermatogenesis at the primary spermatocyte stage. A single dose of these drugs will inhibit spermatogenesis for as long as four weeks. It appears that the gonadotrophins are essential for activity of the dinitropyrrole drugs. Salts of cadmium have a specific effect on the elements of the testis, causing degeneration which is usually permanent.

Clomiphene (p. 211) is an anti-œstrogen, which acts by inhibiting the secretion of gonadotrophin by the pituitary gland, and thus interferes with spermatogenesis. It also prevents the development of the very young embryo. Methallibure is a hydrazine compound with similar activity. It has been discussed earlier (p. 198). Higher doses of methallibure are required than is the case with clomiphene.

FERTILITY CONTROL IN THE FEMALE

Since ovulation does not occur during pregnancy, it appeared highly probable that progesterone was involved in the supression of ovulation. When this probability was investigated, it was found that although progesterone would suppress ovulation, a very large dose was required. However, the introduction of the synthetic progestagens with greatly increased potency has provided a method for controlling pregnancy in man and certain of the domesticated animals. The non-steroid gonadotrophin inhibitor, which has already been mentioned (p. 198), is effective in the female in controlling pregnancy.

Other methods used for the chemical control of pregnancy have involved drugs which act by inhibiting the implantation of the embryo, or by destruction of the blastocysts. It has also been found that several anti-progestins interfere with nidation; although these compounds were effective in rats and mice they did not act in rabbits. The non-steroid anti-œstrogen compounds have an antifertility action due to their anti-œstrogenic activity

ANTI-ŒSTROGENS

This term could include androgens and progestins, excepting the latter compounds act with œstrogen to produce the typical pregnancy changes in the vaginal mucosa. There are, however, many compounds which show anti-œstrogenic activity. Their administration to mice prevents the vagina responding to an œstrogen given subsequently. One compound with high activity of this type is **Clomiphene**. This drug inhibits the gonadotrophic function of the pituitary gland. Small doses stop the œstral cycle of rats and large doses inhibit spermatogenesis. The compound does not appear to have progestational or androgenic activity. It will prevent the action of œstradiol on the mouse uterus but does not interfere with pituitary-adrenal or pituitary-thyroid function and may be useful in regulating pregnancy.

Fertility Control in Insects

Certain insects have been eradicated by releasing sterilised members of the particular species into the infested area. The eradication is effected because the sterile insect on mating with its fertile counterpart produces no progeny. This technique has been applied with success in the control of the Screw-worm Fly (*Cochliomyia hominivorax*). The larva of the Screw-worm Fly live on the flesh of mammals and cause a great deal of harm to livestock. The males of this species mate frequently but the females only once, hence, by releasing a number of sterile males, the fly population can be substantially reduced. In the early experiments of this nature the insects were sterilised by irradiation, but now chemicals are used to produce sterility; one of the best of these is 5-fluoro-uracil.

TUMOUR CHEMOTHERAPY

Certain compounds which affect primarily the reproductive system, or are of potential use in the control of fertility, are of value in the treatment of tumours. Androgens, for example, are useful in treating tumours of the mammary gland, and œstrogens have value in alleviating hyperplasia of the prostate and treatment of the anal adenoma. In veterinary medicine the use of these drugs is confined largely to the dog. Therapeutics of this nature, whilst not only being of possible value to the individual animal, have a wider significance in that the dog can provide a useful tool in tumour chemotherapy because the relatively short life of the dog allows natural cases of neoplasia to be treated, and the effects of the treatment studied over the rest of the dog's natural life.

A long-established method of treating malignancy in man and occasionally in animals is to expose the tumour to X-rays. The basis of this treatment is the fact that mitosis is inhibited by X-irradiation. Radio-mimetic drugs are sometimes employed instead of the actual X-rays. Exposure to X-rays affects primarily the bone marrow and lymph glands, lymphocytes disappear from the peripheral blood and this is followed by the disappearance of the other white cells. Exposure to irradiation, or treatment with radio-mimetic drugs, usually causes vomiting, when this is possible, and diarrhœa. If the surface of the body is exposed to X-rays an erythema is first produced, which may be followed by vesication and loss of hair. X-rays were used in the treatment of ringworm to produce depilation but this is an extremely dangerous procedure. Amongst the other effects produced by X-ray is that on the germinal cells, which after exposure produce many more mutations than otherwise. Although some tumours are inhibited by exposure to X-rays, long exposure or, more probably, frequent exposure may produce neoplasia.

Anti-metabolites and Nucleotoxic Agents.—These are of interest because of their possible application in the control of conception and treatment of malignancy. **Spindle poisons** affect the growth of tumours and destroy the rapidly growing conceptus in mice and rabbits. These compounds cause mitosis to be arrested in the metaphase. Colchicine and Podophyllotoxin are drugs with this type of activity.

Chromosomal poisons act at all stages of pregnancy causing complete inhibition of mitosis. They are sometimes referred to as radio-mimetic compounds because they produce similar pharmacological effects to γ-radiations. Mustine (nitrogen mustard), triethylene melamine and busulphan are drugs with this property. They are of some value in the treatment of tumours of connective tissue origin.

Anti-metabolites are drugs which interfere with the function of a natural metabolite usually by combining with a specific enzyme site, and thus preventing access of the true substrate.

Aminopterine, a folic acid antagonist, was found to produce remission in some cases of leucæmia and this observation has stimulated a great deal of activity to produce other compounds of a similar type. Certain pyrimidine analogues have been synthesised which interfere with the synthesis of DNA, and have proved effective in the treatment of experimental tumours, Unfortunately, although this appears to be a promising field for further investigation, the clinical results from the use of these drugs have been disappointing.

ECBOLICS (OXYTOCICS)

Drugs which cause contraction of the uterus are called *ecbolics* or *oxytocics*. A very important drug with this property is **ergometrine,** an alkaloid obtained from a fungus or ergot which grows on rye. The fungus is called *Claviceps purpurea*. It contains several other alkaloids and pharmacologically active substances.

The alkaloids of ergot are derived from lyseric acid and include (in addition to ergometrine) ergotoxine, ergotamine, ergosine, ergocristine and ergotcryptine. Pharmacologically they fall into two groups, one group including only ergometrine and the second group the remainder, of which ergotamine is a typical member. This last group is of very little therapeutic value but has an importance in toxicology. Some forage plants become infected with ergots and when eaten by grazing animals produce toxic effects similar to the effects produced by ergotamine.

P

Ergotamine stimulates contraction in all plain muscle by direct action after a delay of fifteen to thirty minutes. The blood pressure is raised by the contraction of the arteriolar muscle, and if this action is prolonged gangrene of the extremities will be produced. The sphincter pupillæ muscle contracts, giving a very small pupil. The sympathetic nervous system is stimulated by the action of ergotamine on the central nervous system. This effect is of limited duration because the effects of adrenergic nerve stimulation are antagonised by ergotamine.

Ergometrine differs from all the other ergot alkaloids in several respects. It is readily soluble in water and rapidly

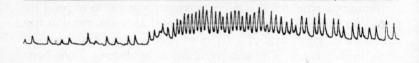

mins

Fig. 16.5

The effect on the uterine contractions of an ovariectomised goat, pre-treated with œstrogen, of the intravenous injection of oxytocin (50 mU). (Courtesy A. Knifton).

absorbed even when given orally to non-ruminants. Ergometrine produces uterine contractions within five minutes and is the most important constituent of crude preparations of ergot. Plain muscles other than the uterus are little affected by this substance, hence it does not cause gangrene. It stimulates the sympathetic system by direct action but does not paralyse adrenergic nerves. The alkaloid is available as the maleate but is usually considered too expensive to use except in the dog or cat.

Extracts of the posterior pituitary gland contain an oxytocic principle, **oxytocin**. For therapeutic purposes, it is preferable to use a synthetic preparation of oxytocin, which is free from pressor activity. *Oxytocin* contracts the uterus by direct action on the muscle. As pregnancy progresses the uterus becomes increasingly sensitive to oxytocin. The uterine cervix can contract independently of the body or cornua. The sensitivity of the body of the uterus to oxytocin increases throughout the second half of pregnancy, the increase accelerating just before parturition, whereas the response of the cervix to oxytocin is high in the œstrogenic phase and low in the luteal phase of the reproductive cycle. Oxytocin increases the rate at which spermatozoa ascend the female reproductive tract. Oxytocin causes vascular plain muscle to relax. This action is particularly marked with avian muscle and is antagonised

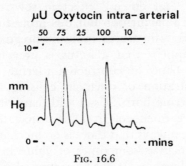

FIG. 16.6

An oxytocin assay using the milk let-down effect in a guinea-pig. (Courtesy A. Knifton).

by the anti-diuretic hormone. The oxytocic principle stimulates the myoepithelial cells of the mammary gland and so produces the " let down " of milk. The effect on the myoepithelial cells of the guinea-pig mammary gland is used in the assay of oxytocin because it is a very specific response. In conducting parallel quantitative assays, other tests include the response of the uterine muscle of guinea-pigs, or rabbits after the muscle has been sensitised by pre-treatment of the animal with an œstrogen. The response of the uterine muscle so treated is less specific but more sensitive than the "let down" effect.

Oxytocin is quickly destroyed in the body by a specific enzyme, and half an administered amount is destroyed within 2–3 minutes in the human, rat, sheep and rabbit. The kidneys and splanchnic organs appear to play an important part in the removal of oxytocin from blood and, in lactating animals, the mammary gland may also be implicated. The specific enzyme, oxytocinase, has so far only been found in the pregnancy plasma of primates and is formed in the placenta. Evidence for the same enzyme being present in the domesticated animals is lacking. The injection of oxytocin given intravenously is the drug of choice to produce the " let down " of milk as it avoids the complications for which the pressor principle is responsible. These complications include cardiovascular collapse rising from the risk of constriction of the coronary arteries. For the effect on the uterus, oxytocin is given intramuscularly, this route may also have to be used to produce the " let down " effect in sows. Oxytocin may be used to induce parturition but this procedure is not devoid of risks. In species in which multiple pregnancies are usual, it sometimes happens that a fœtus is prevented from being delivered by a band of contracted uterine muscle induced by the administration of oxytocin causing the fœtus to be trapped in a uterine horn. Used with caution, oxytocin is of value in the treatment of dystokia associated with uterine inertia providing always that there is no mechanical obstruction to birth. Oxytocin is sometimes of value in assisting in the removal of the placenta. It has been used also in the treatment of bovine mastitis to aid debridement drainage utilising the " let down " effect.

Suggestions for Further Reading

DAWSON, F. L. M. (1966–67). Physiology and pathology of reproduction· Vet. A., **8**, 201.

FOORD, H. E. (1966). Progesterone impregnated tampons in sheep. Vet. Rec., **78**, 461.

JACKSON, H. and SCHNIEDEN, H. (1968). Pharmacology of reproduction and fertility. A. Rev. Pharmac., **8**, 467.

MCLAREN, ANNE. (1968). Advances in Reproductive Physiology, Vol. 3.

POLGE, C., DAY, B. N., and GROVES, T. W. (1968). Synchronisation of ovulation and artificial insemination in pigs. Vet. Rec., **83**, 136.

SCHNITZER, R. J. and HAWKING, F., ed. (1967). Experimental Chemotherapy. Vol. 5. New York: Academic Press.

WOODS, A. J., JONES, J. B. and MANTLE, P. G. (1966). Gangrenous ergotism in cattle. Vet. Rec., **78**, 742.

CHAPTER XVII

DRUGS ACTING ON THE SKIN

THE chief effects which can be produced on the skin by pharmacological means are, cleansing, antisepsis, stimulation, relief of irritation, inflammation and destruction of parasites. The preparations used for these purposes include lotions, powders, ointments, pastes, dips and sprays. Inflammatory conditions of the skin not caused by a pathogenic organism or parasite are of frequent occurrence, especially in dogs, and are sometimes very difficult to treat. Objective evidence of the efficacy of treatment in such conditions is sparse. A method of testing a remedy for this type of condition is to apply the treatment to one side of the animal only, that is where the disease effects both sides, and, using the other side as a control, the local treatment can be assessed.

Cleansing is usually achieved by the use of soap and water; carbolic soap should not be used on dogs as they are often sensitive to it. The synthetic detergents are useful for both cleansing and disinfecting the skin. They should not be used regularly because they remove natural fats and penetrate the epithelium, making the skin liable to infection. Antisepsis is achieved by using an appropriate disinfectant, stimulation by counter-irritation. The relief of irritation sometimes requires a local anæsthetic and inflammation can be relieved by using a corticosteroid. Corticosteroids used locally must be in the active form because they cannot undergo biotransformation until they are absorbed; for example, preparations containing cortisol and not cortisone should be used.

The destruction of ectoparasites involves the use of specific parasiticides. It is sometimes possible to treat parasitic conditions of the skin by giving drugs systemically, for example, ringworm, a disease caused by a fungus, may be treated with griseofulvin given systemically. Certain organophosphorus compounds can be given orally to treat warble fly infestation.

When irritation and itching of the skin occurs, animals usually make matters worse by adding mechanical damage by scratching, biting or rubbing the part. It is known from experiments on man that histamine, histamine liberators, certain proteolytic enzymes and bradykinin when applied locally cause itching or irritation. This observation led to the use of antihistamines as local applications to alleviate pruritis. Unfortunately such local applications were found to be ineffectual.

The absorption of most drugs through the skin takes place very slowly. However, some substances are well absorbed such as lipid soluble substances and their absorption can be accelerated by being applied in a fat solvent.

Dimethylsulphoxide is a widely used industrial solvent. Pure preparations of this water-miscible organic solvent have potential therapeutic uses. It is rapidly absorbed through the skin or gut and excreted in the urine as dimethylsulphoxide or sulphate. A single dose is excreted by the rat in 24 hours, guinea-pigs and rabbits take a little longer. Dimethylsulphoxide has mild antiseptic properties and is a local anæsthetic. As single or repeated doses its toxicity is low. It has some solvent action on collagen and has been used in musculo-skeletal inflammation. However, its main potential use is to transport steroids and large molecules across biological membranes—especially skin.

Occasionally the passage of drugs through the skin has been promoted by electrophoresis. In this technique the drug is driven by an electrical current through the ducts of the sweat glands. It has little practical applicability in veterinary medicine.

The skin of mice is frequently used as the test organ for carcinogenic activity. Many chemicals with carcinogenic activity will show this property when applied to the skin of the mouse over a period of weeks or months.

Powders are used as antiseptics and to relieve irritation. Boric acid is a common antiseptic powder but has a very feeble action. Magnesium trisilicate (talc) is an insoluble inert powder mainly used to allay friction. Talc should not be used to powder rubber gloves or any appliance likely to be introduced into the abdomen as the talc particles act as foreign bodies and cause a tissue reaction. A suitable powder for dusting gloves and instruments is sterile starch powder which is absorbed.

Lotions are preparations containing medicinal substances either in suspension or solution. They are of various kinds, such as antiseptic, irritant, protective and astringent lotions. Protective lotions are probably the most important, the commonest being calamine lotion which acts by depositing calamine, zinc carbonate, on the skin. The drying effect of watery lotions on the skin is reduced by adding 3 per cent glycerin.

Astringent lotions precipitate the proteins of the surface epithelium and thus harden the epidermis. An example of such a lotion is a dilute solution of lead acetate. Alcohol is also a good astringent.

Ointments consist of one or more active ingredients mixed with a fatty base and are intended for application to the skin. The main difference between ointment bases is that some are absorbed through the skin. These include lanoline, lard and emulsifying bases. Soft paraffin and bees-wax are not absorbed. The latter substance is used to stiffen an ointment. Emulsifying bases are of two kinds, those making an oil-in-water emulsion such as " lanette wax " and the water-in-oil emulsion " cold cream " in which the oil forms the continuous phase. Applying an ointment with vigorous rubbing increases the absorption. Sometimes it is necessary to stiffen an ointment. This is done by adding inert powders such as zinc oxide or starch. If the powder represents more than 10 per cent of the preparation it is called a *paste*. Pastes are often preferred to ointments because they are cleaner to apply and less is required.

The application of an ointment or paste is the most popular method of treating a skin disease, excepting where the cause is a parasite for which a specific treatment exists. Sulphur ointment is sometimes used to treat infections of the hair follicles and in some parasitic infestations. It acts by the continuous formation of small amounts of hydrogen sulphide. A useful ointment for treating eye infections is made with yellow oxide of mercury which exerts a mild antiseptic action. Although ointments containing antibiotics and chemotherapeutic agents are very popular, they are not necessarily always better than the older, simpler preparations because they may cause sensitivity reactions and are usually more expensive. The conjunctiva can be protected from irritation, such as may occur when certain volatile anæsthetics are given by mask, by introducing into the eye a few drops of castor oil.

Depilatories are substances which remove hair from the skin. Barium sulphide produces this effect by dissolving the hair shaft and in this way resembles shaving. Exposure to an adequate dose of X-rays produces a slight erythema and loss of hair on the part exposed. Larger doses of X-rays cause permanent damage with ulceration and scarring. Such burns may result from a single large dose or from repeated small doses. The hair does not fall off until about three weeks after exposure, and regeneration takes up to three months. Exposures to X-rays have been used to treat ringworm and some skin tumours.

The elimination of shearing by using drugs to allow sheep to be plucked is now a possibility.

Cyclophosphamide given orally or intravenously produces a thinning of the wool fibre which enables the fleece to be plucked 7 days after administration. It is preferable, however, to wait for 3 weeks before plucking, thus allowing a short growth of new fleece. The drug probably acts by interfering with mitosis and doses which produce de-fleecing do not appear to cause any obvious toxic effects.

Several drugs are used to destroy unwanted living tissue such as warts, horn buds and excess granulation tissue. The mildest of these agents are called *keratolytics*, e.g. salicylic acid, and the strongest *caustics*. Some caustics, such as caustic soda, tend to spread and thus destroy more tissue than intended. Other caustics penetrate too deeply because the compound formed between the caustic and skin protein dissolves in a solution of sodium chloride; mercuric chloride behaves in this fashion. The best caustic is silver nitrate because it is self limiting, being precipitated by sodium chloride. However, it causes a good deal of pain when applied to exposed tissues. Copper sulphate is also used as a caustic but is more painful than silver nitrate.

Styptics are substances used to control small superficial hæmorrhages. They act by precipitating protein. The commonest styptics are alum, tannic acid, ferric chloride and Friar's balsam.

Counter-irritants are agents which cause local vasodilation and increase the blood flow to an affected part. This increased blood flow is presumed to facilitate healing. Counter-irritants stimulate also sensory nerve-endings, thus producing vasodilation by reflexes acting through the posterior roots. This stimulation of sensory nerve-endings can also stimulate medullary reflexes concerned with respiration and circulation.

Rubefacients are substances causing redness of the skin which is accompanied by heat and swelling. These signs are those of early inflammatory change and are produced in a variety of ways. The simplest method is the application of hot water as in hot fomentation; a longer-lasting heat may be applied by a heated poultice. Kaolin poultice (cataplasm of Kaolin) is one of the most convenient. A similar effect is produced by rubbing the affected part with a liniment. *Liniments* are made by incorporating an active substance with an oil. Examples of such preparations are liniments of camphor, ammonia and turpentine. A rubefacient effect can be produced by repeatedly painting the skin with iodine, by applying a mustard plaster, by radiant heat, diathermy short wave and infra-red therapy.

Vesicants or epispastics are agents which cause blisters to form in the skin. They produce first a rubefacient effect which is followed by the exudation of lymph beneath the stratum corneum, raising it to form a blister. The local anodyne effect is followed by pain which subsides when blisters form. The vesicants used in veterinary practice are " green blister " made from cantharides and " red blister " from biniodide of mercury. " Blisters " are used in horse practice to treat chronic inflammatory conditions of the limb joints and tendons. Whether their use is justified other than by custom is open to question.

A more powerful counter-irritant than a vesicant is a *pustulant*. This is a drug which when applied to the skin causes blisters which involve the deeper layers. This blister is accompanied by the migration of leucocytes, suppuration and scarring. These effects are produced by croton oil and tartar emetic, substances which should have no place in

veterinary therapeutics.   The use of the actual cautery or
"firing" is also used to produce counter irritation in horses
but its value is not clear.

SUGGESTIONS FOR FURTHER READING

BARR, M. (1962).   Percutaneous absorption.   *J. pharm. Sci.*, **51**, 395.
KEELE, C. A. and ARMSTRONG, D. (1964).   *Substances producing Pain and Itch.*
   London: Arnold.

CHAPTER XVIII

CHEMOTHERAPY

Drug resistance

THIS term could include the whole of pharmacology but is usually restricted to mean the destruction of obnoxious parasites within the animal body. The most famous name associated with this branch of science is that of Ehrlich, who in fact invented the term " chemotherapy ". His idea was to discover a substance which would combine with the tissues of the parasites and kill them but would not affect the host's tissues. He termed substances which combined with the parasite's tissues " parasitotrophic " and those combining with the host's tissues " organotrophic ". This concept has been modified to a large extent, because it is realised now that the tissues of the host are essential to combat diseases caused by pathogenic organisms.

Ehrlich's histological experiments on the vital staining of tissues led him to study the staining of bacteria. He developed a method of staining the tubercle bacillus with an acid-fast stain which forms the basis of the Ziehl-Neilson stain. Ehrlich also introduced a method of staining bacteria which involved the use of an aniline dye, usually methyl violet. This technique was further developed by Christian Gram and is known as Gram's stain. Whether or not a bacterium is stained by Gram's method indicates to some extent the organism's susceptibility to drugs. Organisms which stain by Gram's method, and usually referred to as Gram-positive, are more sensitive to drugs than Gram-negative organisms. This difference in staining shown by certain bacteria is associated with magnesium ribonucleate which is present in Gram-positive organisms and absent in Gram-negative organisms. The Gram-staining properties of some bacteria of veterinary importance are shown in Table 18.1.

Because a drug in low concentration will kill parasites in test tubes it does not follow that it will be effective in curing

223

animals suffering from disease caused by the same parasites. There are several reasons for this anomaly. For example, some drugs act slowly on the parasite whereas the life of the parasite in the test tube may be too short for the drug to exert its effect. This difficulty may be overcome by improving culture methods and prolonging the *in vitro* life of the parasite.

TABLE 18.1

Bacterial Genera

GRAM-POSITIVE	GRAM-NEGATIVE
Staphylococcus	Pseudomonas
Streptococcus	Vibrio
Micrococcus	Spirillum
Sarcina	Escherichia (Bacterium)
Corynebacteria	Aerobacter
Listeria	Proteus
Erysipelothrix	Haemophilis
Bacillus	Actinobacillus
Clostridium	Neisseria
Mycobacterium	Spirochaetes (where stainable)
Actinomyces	All generic names ending in ella
Nocardia	e.g. Salmonella
Streptomyces.	Shigella
	Klebsiella
	Brucella
	Pasteurella
	Moraxella
	Veillonella.

Another reason for discrepancy between *in vivo* and *in vitro* tests may be due to the conversion of the drug into a therapeutically active substance by the tissues, or, conversely, the body may inactivate a drug shown to have activity *in vitro*.

Whilst test tube tests are valuable in searching for new chemotherapeutic agents, it is not always easy to interpret the results of such tests. They are complicated by the fact that the host's tissues do not behave as a passive vehicle for the parasites but act on them by phagocytosis and by forming antibodies. However, such tests can give fundamental information about the action of some chemotherapeutic agents, especially when the reason for their failure is studied. For example, sulphanilamide stops the growth of streptococci in test tubes but does not kill them, whereas streptococcal infections in animals are cured by this drug. The reason for this difference is that sulphanilamide stops the growth of streptococci in the body and this allows the phagocytes time to remove them.

Chemotherapeutic agents are used in veterinary medicine to treat diseases caused by worms, insects, bacteria and fungi.

DRUG RESISTANCE

Following the introduction by Ehrlich of effective drugs for the treatment of trypanosomiasis, it was noticed that after a period of use these drugs ceased to cure certain cases of trypanosomiasis. Furthermore, arsenical compounds which had been used as dips in the control of certain ectoparasites were found also to have ceased to be effective against some strains of ticks which were formerly susceptible. These are examples of drug resistance. This phenomenon has been observed with many protozoa, bacteria, fungi, viruses and insect parasites. There is as yet no well-authenticated example of drug resistance to anthelmintics. Resistance is partly specific; for example, trypanosomes resistant to suramin are not resistant to organic arsenicals and *vice versa*. However, strains of trypanosome resistant to Homidium are, unfortunately, also resistant to Quinapyramine despite these drugs being chemically quite dissimilar.

Drug resistance has been defined as the temporary or permanent capacity of a cell to remain viable or multiply under conditions which would destroy or inhibit other similar cells. Drug resistance may be either natural or acquired. Natural resistance is intrinsic in the particular species or strain of organism regardless of whether the organism has been exposed to the drug or not. It is the common type of resistance which is shown by staphylococci to penicillin. Certain strains of staphylococci produce the enzyme penicillinase which destroys penicillin; these strains tend to predominate following the elimination of penicillin-sensitive strains of staphylococci.

Acquired resistance develops as a result of the exposure of the organism to the drug either in a test tube or in the animal. Acquired drug resistance in bacteria has been classified as being due to (a) an insusceptible metabolism, (b) an impedance of uptake or penetration of drug into the cell, and (c) destruction of the drug. This classification may also be applied to other types of organism. Some drugs kill or inhibit micro-organisms by interfering with the parasite's metabolism, and certain organisms develop resistance to a particular drug by evolving an alternative metabolic process.

Some antibacterial agents act by blocking the access of the organism to an essential metabolite. These organisms may develop resistance to this type of drug by making excessive quantities of the metabolite and so overcoming the block. An example of this occurs when certain strains of bacteria are exposed to a sulphonamide but are not killed and eventually become resistant to it. This resistance, in some cases, is due to the bacteria acquiring the ability to make very large amounts of para-amino benzoic acid, a competitive inhibitor of sulphonamides.

Impaired penetration is a common cause of drug resistance in protozoa; for example, the dyestuff parafuchsin will cause the disappearance of trypanosomes from the blood of an infected mouse without killing them all. The surviving trypanosomes re-appear in the blood after about one week. If the treatment is repeated the trypanosomes are eventually unaffected by parafuchsin. They have become parafuchsin resistant. If resistant and non-resistant strains of trypanosomes are placed in test-tubes containing a solution of parafuchsin the normal strains adsorb the drug whilst the resistant strains do not. Several trypanocidal agents behave similarly. Drug resistance due to destruction of the drug is shown in bacteria; for example, some bacteria secrete an enzyme penicillinase, and if exposed to sub-lethal amounts of penicillin produce more enzyme and so destroy more penicillin. Resistance to dicophane (DDT) shown by some strains of house-fly (*Musca domestica*) is due to the presence in the fly of the enzyme DDT-dehydrochlorinase.

TRANSFERABLE RESISTANCE

This is a relatively new phenomenon which was first noticed by the Japanese worker Watanabe and his colleagues. Most of the information about transferable resistance has been obtained by work on the **Enterobacteriaceae** (*Salmonella, Escherichia, Shigella*).

It has been shown that resistance to antibiotics can be transferred from one organism to another by so-called resistance factors or R factors. The R factor consists of R-determinants which are genetic features and RT (resistance transfer) factors which are present in the bacterial cytoplasm. The RT factor is involved in the transference of resistance from one organism to another. An example of this is shown in experiments on the bacteria commonly involved in intestinal infections in domesticated animals, such as calves. These organisms, for example the *Salmonella typhimurium* organism, may cause disease in man. Strains of this organism are often found to be resistant to the following combinations of antibiotics; streptomycin, tetracycline, the sulphonamides; or chloramphenicol, streptomycin, tetracycline, sulphonamides; or streptomycin, tetracycline, neomycin, kanomycin and the sulphonamides. In addition to the drugs mentioned these strains of organisms are often resistant to furazolidone.

When 4,700 cultures of *S. typhimurium* were examined, it was found that 36 per cent were of Phage type 29, and of this 36 per cent only 2·4 per cent were resistant to drugs. One third of the 36 per cent Phage type 29 were of human origin and two thirds of animal origin, mainly calves. The experimental work to show the presence of the transfer factor was carried out by taking a drug-sensitive strain of Phage type 29 *S. typhimurium* which had the transfer factor and adding this to a strain of *Escherichia coli* which had the non-transferring R-determinant for resistance to the synthetic penicillin Ampicillin. The R factor was formed by the entry of the transfer factor RT from the drug-sensitive *S. typhimurium* type 29 into the Ampicillin-resistant *E. coli*. The RT factor combined with the R-determinant producing an R factor which can be transferred to the final recipient which, in the case under consideration, would be the type 29 *S. typhimurium*. This organism would then become Ampicillin-resistant, resistance having been transferred from the *E. coli*.

SUGGESTIONS FOR FURTHER READING

ANDERSON, E. S. (1965).   Transferable drug resistance.   *Br. med. J.*, **2**, 1289.
KUSHNER, D. J. (1964).   Microbial resistance to harsh destructive environmental conditions. In *Experimental Chemotherapy*, ed. Schnitzer, R. J. and Hawking, F. Vol. II.   New York: Academic Press.

OPPENOORTH, F. J. (1965). Biochemical genetics of insecticide resistance. *A. Rev. Ent.*, **10**, 185.

ROLLO, I. M. (1966). Antibacterial chemotherapy. *A. Rev. Pharmac.*, **6**, 209.

SCHNITZER, R. J. (1962). Drug resistance in chemotherapy. In *Experimental Chemotherapy*, ed. Schnitzer R. J. and Hawking, F., Vol. I. New York: Academic Press.

WALTON, J. R. (1968). Infectious drug resistance. *Vet. Rec.*, **82**, 448.

CHAPTER XIX

CHEMOTHERAPY OF BACTERIAL INFECTIONS

SULPHONAMIDES

DESPITE the introduction, in the early years of this century, of drugs effective against pathogenic protozoa and spirochætes, the treatment of acute bacterial infections was symptomatic until the mid 1930s. In fact many authorities felt that only in sera and vaccines lay any hope of combating such diseases, and the announcement by Domagk in 1935 that mice, treated with an azo dyestuff " Prontosil ", survived many times the lethal dose of hæmolytic streptococci, was received with some scepticism. In the same year Trefouel, Trefouel, Nitti and Bovet showed that para-amino benzene sulphonamide had the same effect and concluded that prontosil was broken down to this simpler compound in the body. However, it was the publication of the results of an extensive clinical trial one year later which established the drug. Puerperal septicæmia in women is caused by hæmolytic streptococci. Colebrook and Kenny treated alternate cases of this disease with para-amino benzene sulphonamide, the remaining cases receiving the same care but not the drug. The death rate in the cases receiving the sulphonamide was 3 per cent and in the others 20 per cent. These facts placed the value of the drug in this and similar infections beyond question.

Thousands of compounds modelled on sulphanilamide have been made and some are of greater value. Drugs in which the amino group is substituted are broken down in the body to a form with a free amino group because this group is essential for anti-bacterial activity. Prontosil is an example of this type of compound as are *Succinylsulphathiazole* and *Phthalylsulphathiazole*. The last two compounds are very poorly absorbed from the gut, but the Succinyl and Phthalyl groups are split off in the intestine liberating sulphathiazole to exert its

229

antibacterial activity. Sulphanilamide will be considered in detail to provide a basis for discussing the other more therapeutically important sulphonamides.

Sulphanilamide is completely absorbed from the small intestine and distributed throughout the whole of the body water. It is acetylated in part mainly in the liver. The acetylated compound has no bacteriostatic powers. The degree of acetylation varies between species, the domestic animals can be arranged in descending order of acetylation thus: cow, rabbit, sheep, horse, cat. The dog does not acetylate sulphonamides. Both free and acetylated sulphonamides are excreted in the urine, and about one-third of the dose is destroyed in the body.

Sulphadimidine is acetylated to a less extent than sulphanilamide and excreted more slowly. Moreover, although the main route is by way of glomerular filtration, the amount reabsorbed by the tubules varies with each sulphonamide. Sulphacetamide is not reabsorbed to any appreciable extent.

Binding with the plasma proteins takes place to a varying extent with all the sulphonamides. The binding is not firm and the bound sulphonamide is released continually. It is usually considered that only the unbound fraction is available for urinary excretion and antibacterial action.

Sulphanilamide may be used locally as it dissolves slowly in serum and so maintains a steady concentration. The other sulphonamides are too insoluble except as the sodium salts which are strongly alkaline. The alkalinity of the soluble sodium salts of sulphonamides may cause considerable tissue damage and pain if they are injected subcutaneously. The intravenous route is safest for parenteral administration but care must be taken not to allow the solution to leak around the vein. *Sulphacetamide* is an exception in forming a sodium salt which is nearly neutral and is suitable to use as an antiseptic in the eye.

Sulphanilamide prevents the growth of certain bacteria and so allows the phagocytes of the body to destroy them. This bacteriostatic effect is antagonised by para-amino benzoic acid or material containing it, such as pus, necrotic tissue, extracts of micro-organisms and yeast. Para-amino benzoic acid will antagonise 1600 times its weight of sulphanilamide. Substances such as methionine have a similar but weaker effect. Certain drugs such as procaine which have a free amino group attached to a benzene ring will also produce antagonism. It is probable that sulphanilamide acts by competing for the same enzyme receptors on the bacteria as para-amino benzoic acid.

Para-amino benzoic acid is probably essential for the

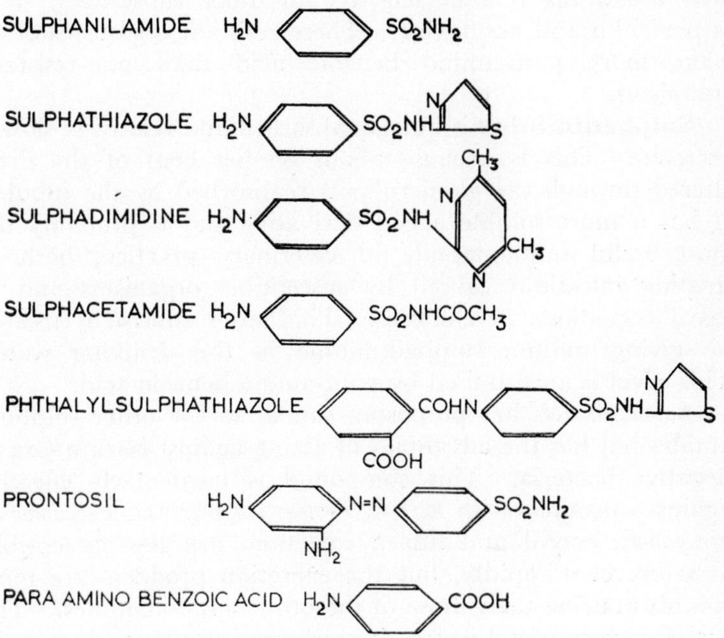

FIG. 19.1

Structural relationship between some sulphonamides of veterinary importance and para-animo benzoic acid

organism to make folic acid. Sulphanilamide may undergo part of this synthesis but not all and so blocks the metabolic pathway. Folic acid antagonises sulphanilamide but not competitively, since folic acid is the product of the enzyme reaction sulphanilamide inhibits. Sulphanilamide inhibits the enzyme carbonic anhydrase which, amongst other important actions, appears to be involved in the formation of egg shells, hence hens on sulphanilamide lay soft-shelled eggs. The other sulphonamides do not have this action.

The difference between the various sulphonamides are

quantitative rather than qualitative. They are very active against *hæmolytic streptococci*, less so against *pneumococci* and even less against *staphylococci*. The *anthrax bacillus*, *Brucella abortus* and *Streptococcus fæcalis*, are unaffected by sulphonamides.

Organisms exposed to sulphonamides but not killed by them may become resistant to these drugs. Fortunately, such organisms remain sensitive to other substances, such as penicillin and acriflavine. These resistant organisms often make more para-amino benzoic acid than non-resistant organisms.

Sulphadimidine is quickly absorbed and relatively slowly excreted. This is because about 80 per cent of the drug filtered through the glomerulus is reabsorbed by the tubules. It has a more soluble acetyl derivative and is probably the most useful sulphonamide in veterinary practice, both in treating infections caused by susceptible organisms and in cæcal coccidiosis in chickens. This latter disease is treated by giving sodium sulphadimidine in the drinking water. This effect is antagonised by para-amino benzoic acid.

Sulphafurazole has properties similar to the other sulphonamides but has the advantage of acting against certain Gramnegative bacteria. This compound is particularly effective against infections with *E. coli*. *Proteus vulgaris* and *Pseudomonas aeruginosa*, coccal and mixed infections are less susceptible. It is excreted rapidly, but the excretion products are more soluble in urine than those of the other sulphonamides. This makes it very useful in treating urinary infections.

Succinylsulphathiazole and **Phthalylsulphathiazole** are poorly absorbed from the gut. This is probably because these compounds are almost completely ionized in the gut. With succinyl sulphathiazole 0·1 per cent is un-ionized at pH 7, whereas sulphanilamide is un-ionized at pH 7, hence it is sulphanilamide which is almost completely absorbed. Succinyl and Phthalylsulphathiazole are slowly hydrolysed in the intestine to liberate sulphathiazole and are useful in treating intestinal infections.

A development of recent years has been the introduction of sulphonamides which are well absorbed from the gut and slowly excreted. These compounds give a concentration of sulphonamide in the plasma which will persist at a reasonably high level for one or more days, hence they have potential advantages in veterinary therapeutics. However, generally speaking, they should not take the place of the quickly absorbed and quickly excreted sulphonamides in the treatment of acute infections as their persistence in the body is a disadvantage if there are any toxic effects. Moreover, towards the end of their time in the body, the concentration may fall below a bacteriostatic level and yet be sufficient to allow resistant strains of organisms to develop.

Sulphamethoxypyridazine is a member of this group. It may be given by all routes but the same objections to parenteral administration exist as with the other sulphonamides. The explanation of the persistence in the body of this compound is partly because of the proportion which is bound to plasma proteins, and partly due to the very effective tubular reabsorption of the free drug. Of the animals so far studied, protein binding is highest in the cow.

Sulphamethylphenazol is a sulphonamide which persists in the body substantially longer than does sulphamethoxypyridazine.

The low solubility of the acetyl derivatives in acid or neutral fluids such as dog or cat urine may cause the deposition of crystals of these compounds in the renal tubules. This may produce renal irritation leading to hæmaturia and even anuria. A plentiful supply of liquids together with sodium citrate or bicarbonate to make the urine alkaline will reduce this risk. The urine of herbivores is usually alkaline. In an attempt to reduce the likelihood of a crystalurea, mixtures of sulphonamides have been used. The basis of the employment of such mixtures depends on the fact that substances can exist in solution without interfering with each others solubilities, hence it is possible by using a mixture of sulphonamides to obtain a higher concentration of total sulphonamide without reaching a level at which any individual sulphonamide would crystallize out. Such mixtures commonly contain three sulphonamides usually including sulphacetamide and sulphadimadine. Cyanosis may occur during sulphonamide therapy due to the formation of sulphæmoglobin or methæmoglobin; this is rarely serious. The most serious complication is the production of an agranulocytosis due to bone marrow damage, and characterised by the disappearance of polymorphonuclear leucocytes from the blood. This is a rare complication, especially when the treatment lasts less than ten days as is usual in veterinary practice.

SUGGESTIONS FOR FURTHER READING

HAWKING, F. and LAWRENCE, J. S. (1950). *The Sulphonamides*. London: Lewis.
NEIPP, L. (1964). Anti-bacterial chemotherapy with sulphonamides. In *Experimental Chemotherapy*, ed. Schnitzer, R. J. and Hawking F., Vol. II. New York: Academic Press.

CHAPTER XX

CHEMOTHERAPY OF BACTERIAL INFECTIONS

ANTIBIOTICS

THIS term is used to describe substances produced by micro-organisms which inhibit bacteria. The first useful antibiotic was penicillin, and the astonishing success of this substance stimulated an intensive search for other antibiotics; only a few of those discovered have proved clinically useful.

Penicillin

In 1877 Pasteur and Joubert discovered the fact that certain common air bacteria stopped the growth in culture of the anthrax bacillus. The most important of these air bacteria was *B. pyocyaneus* from which in later years the enzyme pyocyanase was extracted. However, this growth inhibiting property was of no clinical value because the substance responsible was too toxic to use on animals.

In 1928 Fleming found that the growth of staphylococci was inhibited when the cultures in which they were growing became contaminated with the mould *Penicillium notatum*. A substance inhibiting their growth passed into the medium; Fleming called this substance penicillin and showed that it was non-toxic and could be used successfully as an antiseptic. Unfortunately, early attempts to purify this substance failed, and it was not until 1940 that Florey, Chain and their colleagues succeeded in isolating a concentrated preparation of penicillin which was stable when dried. They were able to extract penicillin because when it is acid it passes into an organic solvent from which it can be recovered by shaking with water and alkali.

Several strains of *P. notatum* and various culture media

have been used to produce Penicillin, and it was soon realised that a number of penicillins were produced. They differ in their activity on micro-organisms and in the rate of absorption and excretion.

Penicillin chrysogenum is used now rather than *P. notatum* because it gives a better yield. In the presence of phenylacetic acid *P. chrysogenum* produces benzylpenicillin and in the presence of phenoxyacetic acid, phenoxymethyl penicillin. A great advance resulted from the discovery that a strain of *P. chrysogenum* produced 6 amino-penicillanic acid, the nucleus of penicillin, which permitted the synthesis of a large number of new penicillins. Some of these compounds have great therapeutic value. These manufactured penicillins are usually called semi-synthetic.

Benzylpenicillin is widely used in veterinary therapeutics. It forms calcium and sodium salts which are very soluble in water and a procaine salt which is relatively insoluble. The potency of penicillin can be expressed either in terms of the weight of the pure substance or with reference to a standard preparation. The standard consists of pure sodium benzyl-penicillin and contains 1670 units per mg.

The sodium and calcium salts of penicillin are stable when dry but aqueous solutions lose their strength. Penicillin is destroyed by acids, alkalies and heat. The optimum pH is 6·5, but solutions at this pH are stable for only about one week even when kept at 4° C. Oily solutions are quite stable. Some organisms which are often present in non-sterile distilled water secrete an enzyme penicillinase which quickly inactivates penicillin. It is important that solutions of penicillin should be sterile. Since penicillin is destroyed by acids it cannot be given orally.

Aqueous solutions of penicillin are quickly absorbed after subcutaneous or intramuscular injection and quickly removed from the body, about 60 per cent of a single dose being excreted in the urine, most of this taking place in the first hour. This rapid urinary excretion shows that the renal tubules excrete a considerable proportion; glomerular filtration as the sole mechanism would be slower. After absorption, penicillin can be detected in bile and saliva. It enters the fœtus across the placenta but only a little passes into serous sacs. Penicillin does not enter the cerebro-spinal fluid, and when given parenterally only small amounts are secreted in milk. Attempts to prolong the effect of a single dose have been directed at either delaying absorption or blocking tubular excretion.

Absorption is prolonged after a suspension of the insoluble procaine penicillin in oil or water has been injected intramuscularly or subcutaneously. A further delay in absorption can be produced by adding a water repellant such as aluminium stearate. Preparations such as these only provide a low blood level of the drug and are useless when high concentrations are required.

The excretion of penicillin can be delayed by giving at the same time substances such as diodone and para-amino-hippuric acid which are excreted by the tubules. *Probenecid* is the most effective drug of this kind and acts by blocking the mechanism which controls the tubular excretion of penicillin and reabsorption of uric acid but does not affect other renal functions.

Penicillin is most effective against Gram-positive bacteria such as *Staphylococci, Streptococci, Leptospira, Anthrax, Actinomyces, Clostridium tetani* and *Cl. welchi*. It is ineffective against Gramnegative bacteria, *E. coli, Brucella abortus, viruses, protozoa* and *moulds*. Penicillin is a bactericidal antibiotic. The primary mechanism of its action is due to interference with the formation of the bacterial cell wall which it does by inhibiting the synthesis of a muco-polypeptide. It has no effect on formed cell walls, hence it is only active against actively growing bacteria.

Early studies showed that giant forms of bacteria were produced when they grew in concentrations of penicillin, insufficient to kill them. When *Staphylococcus aureus* grew in the presence of penicillin, uridine diphosphate derivatives of muramic acid and muramic acid peptides accumulated. It was then observed that the cell walls of Gram-positive bacteria contained a muramic acid derivative and certain amino acids in the same proportions as they occurred in the aforementioned peptides. This led to the idea that these peptides were the precursors of the cell wall. Penicillin was found to inhibit the incorporation of four cell wall amino acids into the cell wall fraction of *S. aureus* but not into cytoplasmic proteins. Lastly, a good correlation was found between the growth inhibiting concentrations of various penicillins and the inhibition of mucopeptide synthesis in *S. aureus* and *Escherichia coli*.

Certain non-sensitive bacteria and some penicillin-resistant strains of otherwise susceptible bacteria secrete an enzyme penicillinase which destroys penicillin. Acquired resistance may be induced in some bacteria as a result of exposure to penicillin stimulating the production of penicillinase. Unlike the sulphonamides the action of penicillin is not impaired by blood, pus, tissue autolysates or large numbers of bacteria.

Penicillin is notable for its lack of toxic effects although crude preparations may contain impurities. An untoward effect may arise in veterinary practice due to the widespread use of penicillin as an intramammary injection. Milk containing penicillin is unsuitable for cheese making as the bacteria responsible are often sensitive to penicillin, and milk after intramammary injections may contain enough to prevent the cheese bacteria acting. Very large doses given parenterally may produce the same effect by some of the penicillin being excreted in milk. Intramammary injections of antibiotics to cows may cause illness in babies whose diet consists largely of milk. Milk should not be fed to babies for at least 48 hours after the last intramammary injection. The presence of penicillin in milk is detected by means of a dye test. The dye used is triphenyltetrazolium chloride (T.T.C.). This dye changes from colourless to red in the presence of a growing organism (*Str. thermophilus*). This organism fails to grow in the presence of antibiotic and hence the dye fails to change in colour. This test will detect 0·05 i.u./ml. of penicillin.

SEMI-SYNTHETIC PENICILLINS

Benzylpenicillin has the following shortcomings: (1) it is unstable in acids and, therefore, cannot be given orally. This is, however, of little importance in veterinary medicine. (2) Penicillinase-producing organisms are resistant and such organisms are not uncommon. (3) It is active against only a narrow range of organisms. Since the introduction of penicillin into medicine, a search has been made for derivatives which

overcame these various drawbacks. The first disadvantage
was overcome fairly quickly by a relatively simple modification
of the benzylpenicillin molecule and Phenoxymethylpenicillin
was introduced. This derivative has a sole virtue of being

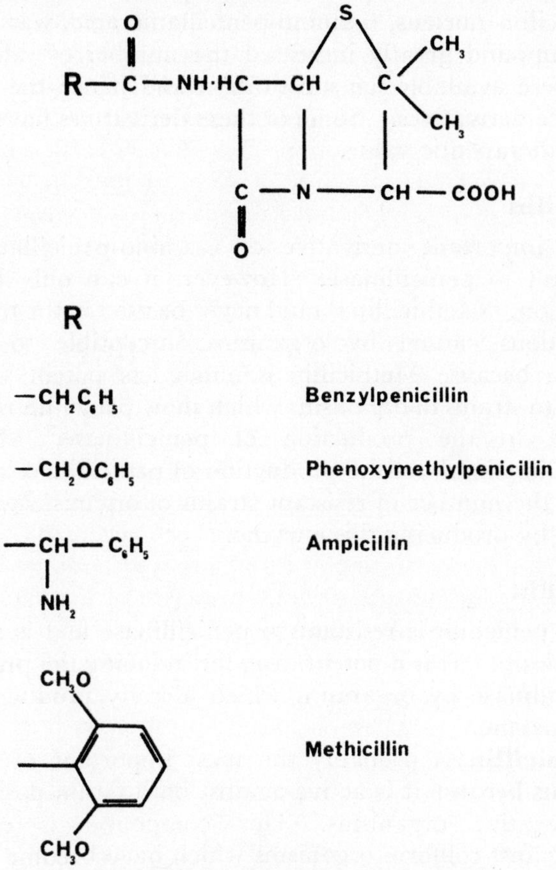

R

—CH₂C₆H₅   **Benzylpenicillin**

—CH₂OC₆H₅   **Phenoxymethylpenicillin**

—CH—C₆H₅   **Ampicillin**
  |
  NH₂

                            Methicillin

FIG. 20.1
The formulæ of some penicillins.

stable in acid medium and hence is suitable for oral administration to dogs and cats. **Phenethicillin potassium**
was developed as an improvement on Phenoxymethylpenicillin.
This derivative is also acid stable and gives almost twice the
concentration in blood after oral administration. It is

slightly resistant to penicillinase and is used in veterinary medicine in the treatment of mastitis when the disease is due to strains of streptococci and staphylococci which are susceptible to this antibiotic.

The search for new penicillins was greatly facilitated when the penicillin nucleus, 6-amino-penicillanic acid, was isolated. This compound greatly increased the number of side chains which were available for substitution and hence the number of possible derivatives. Some of these derivatives have proved of great therapeutic value.

Methicillin

This important derivative of 6-amino-penicillanic acid is resistant to penicillinase. However, it can only be given by injection. Methicillin should never be used in the treatment of infections caused by organisms susceptible to benzylpenicillin because Methicillin is much less potent and may give rise to strains of organisms which show penicillin resistance not due to the production of penicillinase. Moreover, Methicillin stimulates the production of penicillinase and may increase the number of resistant strains of organism which are resistant by producing this enzyme.

Cloxacillin

This penicillin is resistant to penicillinase and is stable in acid medium. It is a potent drug for inducing the production of penicillinase by organisms which already produce a little of this enzyme.

Ampicillin is probably the most important of the new penicillins because it is active against both Gram-positive and Gram-negative organisms. This compound is especially useful against coliform organisms which have become resistant to tetracyclines, and strains of *Proteus*, *Pseudomonas*, *Salmonella*, *Shigella* and *Pasteurella* which are not readily treated by other antibiotics. Ampicillin is less potent than benzyl-penicillin against bacteria susceptible to the latter drug. Ampicillin is not resistant to penicillinase and is, therefore, not active against organisms which owe their penicillin resistance to the production of this enzyme. It is acid stable.

Benethamine penicillin is a long-acting preparation which, given by intramuscular injection as an insoluble suspension, slowly releases benzylpenicillin.

Benzathine penicillin has similar properties. However, benzathine penicillin is acid stable and can be given to dogs and cats by mouth.

Streptomycin

Streptomycin was discovered in a search for antibiotics active against Gram-negative bacteria. Hydrogenation produced dihydrostreptomycin which has similar properties but is more toxic to the cochlea nerve and should be used with great care.

Streptomycin causes damage to bacterial cell membranes, inhibits the synthesis of protein by bacteria and causes a breakdown of RNA. It is not yet clear which of these actions is the primary action. The most attractive theory suggests that streptomycin by combining with the ribosomes of sensitive bacteria affects the attachment of messenger RNA, and hence protein synthesis. Streptomycin is poorly absorbed from the intestine and is not inactivated in the gut. It has been used to modify the gastro-intestinal flora of poultry, pigs and ruminants, Administration may be also by intramuscular injection or local application. Between 50 and 60 per cent of the absorbed drug is excreted by glomerular filtration through the kidneys. About a third of the drug is bound to protein and hence cannot pass through the glomerulus and between 2 to 5 per cent is excreted in the bile.

Streptomycin is active against most penicillin-sensitive organisms, and some Gram-negative bacteria including *Brucella abortus, E. coli, Proteus sp.* and *Pseudomonas pyocyanea.* It acts also against *Mycobacterium tuberculosis,* but this is only of importance in human medicine as veterinary policy is directed to the eradication of this disease.

The great disadvantage of this antibiotic is the ease with which restraint strains are produced, and its use should be restricted to the treatment of infections such as those caused by *Proteus sp.* for which no other antibiotic is suitable. Prolonged treatment with streptomycin may cause renal and hepatic damage and, in dogs and cats, cerebellar and labyrinth disturbances.

Neomycin

Neomycin is obtained from *Streptomyces fradiæ* and is a water-soluble basic compound. This antibiotic is similar to streptomycin chemically, pharmacologically and in anti-bacterial activity. It is active against *Streptococci*, *Staphylococci*, *Anthrax*, *E. coli* and *Proteus* and this activity is unaffected by pus. Neomycin is poorly absorbed from the gut. In some severe infections by bacteria resistant to other antibiotics it may be given by intramuscular injection, intramammary injection or applied locally. It has proved useful in enteritis in foals and calves and in some cases of bovine mastitis.

Novobiocin

This antibiotic which is related chemically to dicoumarol resembles benzylpenicillin in its antimicrobial activity. There is some evidence that novobiocin acts by interfering with bacterial cell membrane synthesis but this is by no means established. It can be used in the treatment of systemic infections and locally. In veterinary therapeutics its main use is in the form of an intramammary injection along with other antibiotics for the treatment of mastitis. It is used in this way to treat staphylococcal infections which are resistant to other antibiotics. In the treatment of infections with *P. vulgaris*, particularly those involving the urinary tract it is to be preferred to neomycin because it is safer. This antibiotic is also active against Gram-negative cocci but it induces resistance in micro-organisms very readily.

TETRACYCLINES

The *tetracyclines* were discovered as a result of a search for antibiotics active against a wider range of bacteria than penicillin. **Chlortetracycline** was obtained from *Streptomyces aureofaciens*, **oxytetracycline** from *Streptomyces rimosus* and **tetracycline** is semi-synthetic. In recent years a new family of **demethyltetracyclines** have been introduced. The tetracyclines form odourless, yellow bases, insoluble in water but soluble as the hydrochloride. Solutions lose their activity in a few days.

These drugs inhibit a wider range of Gram-positive and Gram-negative organisms than penicillin or streptomycin, being bacteriostatic rather than bactericidal. They are less potent than penicillin but have an additional property of acting against certain protozoa such as the *Anaplasma* and *Theileria*, as well as *Rickettsia* and some large viruses. The tetracyclines only inhibit rapidly growing organisms and can give rise to resistant strains, but less readily than streptomycin and erythromycin. Unfortunately, when resistance to one tetra-

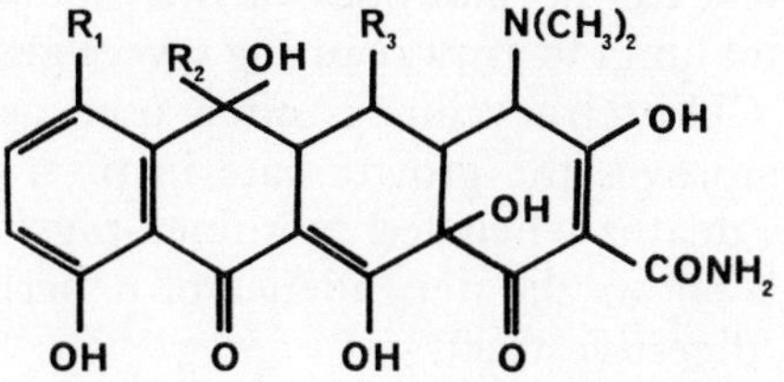

	R_1	R_2	R_3
Tetracycline	H	CH_3	H
Chlortetracycline	Cl	CH_3	H
Oxytetracycline	H	CH_3	OH
Demethylchlortetracycline	Cl	H	H

FIG. 20.2

The formulæ of some tetracyclines.

cycline develops, the organism is usually resistant to all the tetracyclines; this is called cross-resistance. *Proteus* and *Pseudomonas* organisms are unaffected by the tetracyclines.

The tetracyclines may be given by mouth except to ruminants. In carnivores a peak concentration in the blood occurs in two to four hours after oral administration and lasts about six hours. They are widely distributed, entering the CSF and crossing the placenta. Excretion is partly in the urine and bile and part is destroyed in the body. An oral dose takes three to four days for its excretion. The daily dose should be divided and given six-hourly. The tetracyclines are bacteriostatic excepting in concentrations higher than are produced in the tissues by the usual therapeutic doses. Their mode of action has not yet been established, although it has been shown that they interfere with protein synthesis by bacteria.

They have also a chelating action in binding the metallic ions, calcium, magnesium and manganese, and so inhibit a number of essential enzyme systems. Moreover, because of this chelating property the tetracyclines are deposited in bones and teeth as a bright yellow fluorescent calcium complex. There is some evidence that in young animals this deposition of the tetracyclines may affect the growth of teeth and bones.

The oral administration of these drugs even in dogs and cats may suppress the normal flora of the digestive tract and allow moulds and fungi to grow, causing severe gastro-intestinal disturbances. Chlortetracycline is often used as a food supplement. It improves the growth rate in pigs, chickens and rats, but causes deaths when fed to guinea-pigs over a period of weeks. This shows the dependence of a herbivore on the bacteria of the digestive tract.

The tetracyclines are irritant, and if it is necessary to inject them subcutaneously the injection should incorporate procaine hydrochloride. Apart from these risks the tetracyclines have a low toxicity.

Demethylchlortetracycline is a member of the group of demethyltetracyclines which have been introduced into therapeutics. It is well absorbed from the gut and persists in the body for nearly twice as long as the other tetracyclines. This persistence is not due to protein binding because the proportion of demethylchlortetracycline which is protein bound is not substantially different from other tetracyclines. It is equally active to the other tetracyclines but may have some action on *Ps. aeruginosa* and *P. vulgaris*. In man photosensitisation has been reported as occuring after the administration of this tetracycline.

Methacycline is a synthetic derivative of oxytetracycline. It gives a higher concentration of antibiotic in the blood than demethylchlortetracycline and is more slowly excreted in the urine. The persistence in the body may be due to the fact that a greater proportion of methacycline is bound to plasma protein. This compound has a similar range of antibacterial activity to demethylchlortetracycline. However, the most important use of methacycline in veterinary medicine is probably in the treatment and prevention of chronic respiratory disease (CRD) in poultry, as it appears to be particularly effective against the mycoplasma.

CHLORAMPHENICOL

Chloramphenicol was first isolated from *Streptomyces venezuelæ* as a crystalline compound, which proved to have a simpler structure (Fig. 20·3) than most antibiotics and was soon synthesised. It is poorly soluble in water but dissolves in several organic solvents. Readily absorbed after oral administration, chloramphenicol persists in the blood for several hours; in man, most is excreted in the urine conjugated with glucuronic acid but 10 per cent is excreted unchanged. It can be found also in milk, bile and CSF. However, in the rat most of the drug is excreted in the bile as the glucuronide which on entering the gut is acted on by intestinal organisms which hydrolyse the glucuronide, thus regenerating the antibiotic. In view of this marked discrepancy between the fate in the body in man and in the rat, it is unfortunate that similar information is not available for the domesticated animals.

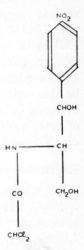

FIG. 20.3
Chloramphenicol.

Chloramphenicol is active against many Gram-positive and Gram-negative organisms, Rickettsia and large viruses. The organism involved in swine erysipelas, *Erysipelothrix rhusiopathiæ*, is unaffected by chloramphenicol. It is bacteriostatic rather than bactericidal, acting by inhibiting the synthesis of protein by bacteria. Chloramphenicol has an antagonistic action when used in conjunction with either penicillin or streptomycin. This is because chloramphenicol inhibits bacterial growth, whereas the other antibiotics act on the growing bacterial cell wall. However, the effect of chloramphenicol is additive to that of other antibiotics with bacteriostatic action such as the tetracyclines. Since it is a non-irritant substance it is suitable for local application. These local applications are used in foot-rot in sheep and

R

mastitis in cattle. Suitable preparations containing chloramphenicol penetrate the cornea and are used in the treatment of infections of the eye. Apart from the risks associated with the oral administration of antibiotics, chloramphenicol may depress the function of the bone marrow and cause aplastic anæmia.

THE MACROLIDE ANTIBIOTICS

This large group of antimicrobial agents are called Macrolides because one of their chemical characteristics is the possession of a large lactone ring. They are active against most Gram-positive organisms and, in addition, the *Mycoplasma* (PPLO; pleuropneumonia-like organisms), Rickettsia and certain large viruses. The macrolides are mainly bacteriostatic but, depending on the number of microorganisms and concentrations of antibiotic, they may be bactericidal. There is some degree of cross-resistance between the various members of this group. The macrolides of veterinary importance include **Erythromycin, Spiramycin, Oleandomycin** and **Tylosin**.

Erythromycin

Erythromycin is an antibiotic obtained from *Streptomyces erythreus*. It is selective in action. The susceptible organisms of veterinary importance include *Streptococci, Staphylococci, Corynebacteria, Erysipelothrix, Clostridia, B. anthracis*, and *Brucella abortus suis*. The *Salmonella, Escherichia, Proteus* and *Br. abortus* are not susceptible. This antibiotic is used only when penicillin-susceptible strains have developed resistance to penicillin. Resistance to erythromycin develops quickly. It is relatively non-toxic.

Erythromycin when given by mouth to dogs and cats is rapidly absorbed, giving effective blood levels for six hours. It is widely distributed and excreted in the urine and bile. Since erythromycin is destroyed by acid gastric juice it is given as enteric coated pills or a suspension of an insoluble preparation. It is too irritant for parenteral administration, although it is sometimes stated that it can be given to all species by intramuscular injection and to poultry subcutaneously.

Oleandomycin is used mainly for the treatment of infections due to staphylococci and streptococci which are resistant to penicillin. It is relatively non-toxic and when given by mouth to rabbits produces a peak concentration in the serum after one hour but the level falls to a low concentration in five hours.

Spiramycin has a range of antibacterial activity similar to that of the other macrolides but has greater *in vivo* activity. This is probably because spiramycin persists longer in the tissues and at higher concentration than the other macrolides. Spiramycin is probably concentrated and excreted in the bile, hence the fæces have antibiotic activity The main use in veterinary medicine of this drug is in the prevention and treatment of mycoplasmosis (*M. gallisepticum*) in turkeys. It is also used in the treatment of mastitis due to penicillin-resistant staphylacocci.

Tylosin is a macrolide antibiotic which is absorbed from the gut and excreted in the urine and in bile. It is not very toxic and is active against a large number of gram-positive organisms, a few gram-negative organisms and the mycoplasma (PPLO). The main use of this drug in veterinary medicine is in the prevention and treatment of chronic respiratory disease (CRD) caused by mycoplasma in poultry. Tylosin is given for this purpose in the water or poultry feed. It is useful also in the treatment of vibrionic dysentery in pigs.

POLYPEPTIDE ANTIBIOTICS

Polymyxins

Polymyxins are polypeptide antibiotics like neomycin and bacitracin and are obtained from *Bacillus polymyxa*. There are several polymyxins. They are basic polypeptides which give salts with mineral acids which are water-soluble and stable.

Polymyxin B is the least toxic and only member of the group suitable for clinical use. It is water-soluble, stable in acids and destroyed by alkalies. It has a selective action on Gram-negative bacteria especially *E. coli, Hæmophilus, Salmonellæ, Pasteurellæ, Brucellæ, Shigellæ,* and *Vibrio*. It is also active against many strains of *Pseudomonas æruginosa* but its activity against *Brucella* is limited. The *Staphylococci, Streptococci, Corynebacteria, Proteus, Clostridia* and *Anthrax* are unaffected by this antibiotic. In general Polymyxin is regarded as too toxic to administer parenterally and it is used mainly as a local application. It is not absorbed from the gut and is used very occasionally in the treatment of certain intestinal infections. In rare cases of infections of the urinary tract, where the organism is not sensitive to any other antibiotic, it is justifiable to give polymyxin by intramuscular injection. It is excreted in the urine. Polymyxin is strongly bactericidal, and its effectiveness depends on the number of organisms present. Polymyxin is a surface-active agent and substances which are antagonistic to the cationic detergents also inhibit polymyxin. This activity does not completely explain the antibacterial action of polymyxin which is restricted to Gram-negative organisms whereas the cationic detergents are effective against both Gram-positive and Gram-negative organisms. The action of polymyxin is first to disorganise the bacterial cell membrane causing a leakage of intracellular material and secondly to inhibit oxidative metabolism. The surface activity shown by polymyxin on bacterial cells can also affect the cells of the host, and polymyxin is known to cause the release of histamine from cells containing this active substance. Resistance to polymyxin is infrequent, hence this drug is often combined with other antibiotics. Polymyxin is used in veterinary therapy in local applications to the skin, mucous membranes, the external ear and intramammary injections.

Bacitracin

Bacitracin is an antibiotic obtained from a strain of *B. subtilis*. This bacterium was found on the infected wounds of a patient, Miss Tracy, after whom the antibiotic was named. It is active against Gram-positive organisms including some *Clostridia* and *Actinomyces bovis*. It is poorly absorbed from the gut and in fact is destroyed in the alimentary tract. Bacitracin is used only as a local application; given intramuscularly it may cause kidney damage.

Nystatin and Griseofulvin are antibiotics active against yeasts and fungi and are considered later (p. 317).

Framycetin is an antibiotic similar in structure and activity

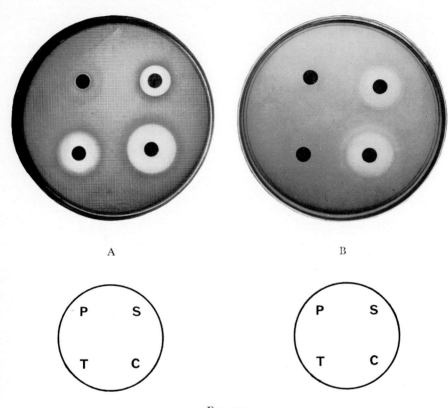

A   B

FIG. 20·4

An antibiotic sensitivity test.

Dish A: *Staph. pyogenes)aureus)*   Dish B: *Proteus mirabilis*

Key to antibiotic discs: P=benzyl penicillin; S=streptomycin; C=chloramphenicol; T=tetracycline.

The clear zone around the disc indicates antibiotic sensitivity. (*Courtesy M. E. Davies.*)
This strain of Staph. pyogenes is resistant to benzyl penicillan,

to neomycin. Given in the drinking water, it has been effective in the treatment and prevention of coccidiosis in chickens.

CHOICE OF ANTIBIOTICS

The *selection* of antibiotic or sulphonamide depends on the infecting organism and its sensitivity to the various drugs. However, it is often essential to begin the treatment without this knowledge, and it is necessary to act on the assumption that the organism will be sensitive to antibiotic or sulphonamide. Should there be no response to treatment within two days, or laboratory tests show the organism more sensitive to another drug, the treatment can be changed accordingly The most commonly used test for determining the sensitivity of a pathogenic organism to antibiotic is to spread the infective material on a suitable plate of agar culture medium and to place on the surface discs of filter paper which have been soaked in the various antibiotics under test. When an organism is sensitive to an antibiotic, tested in this way, there is a clear zone around the filter paper indicating the absence of bacterial growth. The size of the clear zone does not necessarily indicate relative potency of the antibiotic as the clearing can be influenced by factors such as the size of the inoculum and the rate at which the antibiotic diffuses through the agar. However, it serves as a crude test of sensitivity and the results of such tests should be treated in this light. It is sometimes possible by the use of tests of this kind to determine in a matter of a few hours whether or not a particular organism is antibiotic sensitive and, using such relatively rapid tests, to initiate treatment, in cases such as bovine mastitis, sufficiently quickly to prevent the loss of a quarter of the udder.

Antibacterial drugs fall into two categories when classified according to their mode of action, that is they can be considered as either bacteriostatic or as bactericidal agents. In general, it is better to use a bactericidal rather than a bacteriostatic antibiotic. However, even when using such a compound complete bactericidal action may be cancelled by the presence, of organisms which are sometimes called " persisters ". These organisms represent a small proportion of dormant bacteria which, although potentially sensitive to the drug,

survive the effect of the bactericidal drug and may give rise
to a subsequent infection. Such organisms are common
in old bacterial populations, inside cells and in pus. The
common bactericidal antibiotics are penicillin, cloxacillin,
methicillin, streptomycin and polymyxin. The sulphonamides,
the tetracyclines, chloramphenicol, ampicillin, erythromycin
and novobiocin are bacteriostatic agents.

The importance of the phenomenon of antibiotic resistance
has already been discussed. There are, however, two further
categories of resistance worth mention, the phenomenon of
so-called multiple resistance and that of " one step " resistance.
It has been shown in the laboratory by repeated exposure of
organisms to drugs that the induction of resistance to penicillin
is a slow or step-wise process, whereas the repeated exposure
of organisms to an antibiotic, such as streptomycin, results
in a very rapid increase of resistance; this is sometimes called
multiple resistance. The drugs against which multiple
resistance is most likely to occur are streptomycin, erythromycin, and novobiocin. It is considered usually a sound general
principle that the drugs which show multiple resistance
should be used in conjunction with at least one other drug
which is effective against the particular organism to be treated.
This procedure is adopted because it is hoped that the second
drug of the combination will affect not only all the organisms
sensitive to the first drug, but will include a small proportion
of the mutants which are naturally resistant to the first drug.
The site of the infection together with the fate of the drug in the
body and the possibility of producing undesirable side effects
have also to be considered in selecting the drug. Sometimes
antibiotics may act synergistically; those acting as bactericides, such as penicillin, bacitracin and neomycin, may
potentiate each other, but when combined with the tetracyclines and chloramphenicol which are bacteriostatic may
produce antagonism. This can be appreciated when one
considers that a bactericidal drug, such as penicillin, which
exerts its effect on actively growing organisms cannot do so
if the growth of the organism is suppressed by a bacteriostatic
agent. The difficulty of measuring the effectiveness of antibiotic combinations clinically, coupled with the risk of producing drug-resistant strains, make it advisable to begin

treatment with one antibiotic and to change only when laboratory tests or lack of clinical response show it to be unsuitable.

EFFECTS OF ANTIBIOTICS ON GROWTH RATE

Very small amounts of antibiotics when fed to chickens produce an increase in growth. Food conversion is increased and a reduction in mortality in growing chickens is also produced. It is now common practice to add an antibiotic to poultry foods. Similar but more variable results have been obtained with fattening pigs. In ruminants antibiotics in food may be used up to the onset of rumination to produce a similar effect.

There have been a number of theories which attempt to explain the growth-promoting action of antibiotics but the evidence, so far, is inconclusive. It has been suggested that the growth-promoting antibiotics affect the intestinal flora in such a way as to increase the synthesis of certain growth factors essential to the host. Another suggestion has been that these antibiotics, by inhibiting certain organisms which compete for growth factors produced in the gut allow these growth factors to become available to the host. A third theory proposes that the antibiotics act by inhibiting organisms which produce toxic substances deleterious to the host. A further theory which is supported by some experimental evidence implicates pathological changes in the intestinal epithelium. In this theory it is suggested that, in the absence of antibiotics, organisms in the gut cause damage to the epithelium which impairs absorption. The antibiotics by inhibiting these organisms prevent the damage and thus facilitate the absorption of nutrients. In support of this theory, it has been shown that the intestinal epithelium of antibiotic-fed animals is thinner than in untreated animals. However, probably the most widely accepted explanation of the growth-promoting activity of antibiotics is that these drugs produce this effect by curing sub-clinical infections. These infections are not such as to produce obvious clinical signs of disease but are, nonetheless, present, hence are termed sub-clinical. The best evidence for this type of drug-promoting action has been obtained from experiments with chickens. It has been shown that the droppings of untreated fowls apparently contain growth-suppressing agents which are not present when antibiotics are added to the diet. Moreover, the better the general management and hygiene of the animals the less effect antibiotics have on food conversion and mortality.

Procaine penicillin, chlortetracycline and oxytetracycline are used in poultry and the tetracyclines are fed to pigs and calves. There are no ill-effects on sows or suckling pigs. However, resistant strains of *E. coli*, a cause of scouring in calves and pigs, have been found on farms using antibiotic feed supplements and this may be the main risk. It is desirable therefore to restrict the antibiotics in the food to a single substance so as to leave the others as effective antibiotics available to the veterinary surgeon for therapy. The discovery of transmissible resistance has added emphasis to the importance of restricting the use of antibiotic additives to the food.

SUGGESTIONS FOR FURTHER READING

EDWARDS, S. J. (1964–65). Antibiotics as supplements in the food of calves. *Vet. A.*, **6**, 22.
ENGLISH, P. B. (1965). Antibiotics in veterinary practice. *Aust. vet. J.*, **41**, 80.
GALE, E. F. (1963). Mechanism of antibiotic action. *Pharmac. Rev.*, **15**, 481.
SCHNITZER, R. J. and HAWKING, F. (1964). *Experimental Chemotherapy*, Vols. II and III. New York: Academic Press.
STRATTON, J. (1964–65). Sulphonamides, antibiotics. *Vet. A.*, **6**, 268.

CHAPTER XXI

CHEMOTHERAPY OF PROTOZOAL INFECTIONS

PROTOZOA are the causal agents of many diseases of domestic animals, and drugs are available for both the prevention and treatment of several of these diseases. Probably the commonest protozoal diseases in the United Kingdom are caused by coccidia, and although most species of domestic animal are affected it is a particularly serious problem in poultry.

COCCIDIOCIDAL AND COCCIDIOSTATIC DRUGS

There are many species of coccidia of which those of importance in veterinary medicine infest the epithelium of the gut, biliary tract or the urinary system, causing damage to capilliary vessels and a consequent loss of blood. The organism is transmitted from animal to animal by fæcal contamination and thus attention to hygiene is important in the control of this disease.

The sulphonamides were the first effective drugs used in the treatment of coccidiosis in chickens (*Eimeria tenella*) and are still valuable for this purpose. The sodium salts of either *sulphadimidine* (0·2 per cent) or *sulphapyrazine* (0·1 per cent) are given in the drinking water. The therapeutic effect depends upon the maintenance of an effective concentration of sulphonamide in the blood which is similar to that required in bacterial infections, 5 to 10 mg./100 ml. blood. Para-amino benzoic acid antagonises this effect of the sulphonamides.

THE NITROFURFANS

One of the earliest coccidiostatic agents introduced into veterinary medicine was a member of the group of mononitro

253

compounds, the **nitrofurans**. The nitrofurans also show marked antibacterial activity against a wide range of organisms.

Nitrofurazone is a nitrofuran used to prevent and treat cæcal coccidiosis in chickens. It is less effective in duodenal coccidiosis or in coccidiosis in turkeys. This drug is effective also in infections due to Gram-positive and Gram-negative organisms and is used externally to treat such infections. When used to prevent cæcal coccidiosis it is given in the dry mash because it is insoluble in water. Five parts nitrofurazone

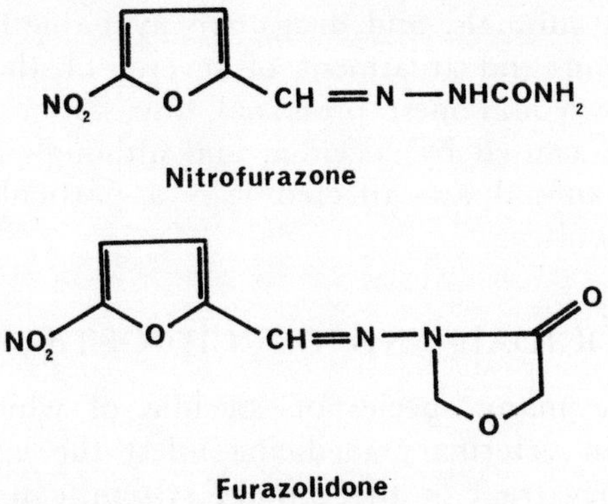

NO_2 — O — CH = N — NHCONH$_2$

Nitrofurazone

NO_2 — O — CH = N — N — O

Furazolidone

FIG. 21.1A, B
The formulæ of two anticoccidial agents.

per 1000 parts feed do not interfere with growth. However, toxic effects may arise due to errors in mixing or feeding or to individual birds being especially susceptible. Birds so affected lose their appetite and appear bedraggled and motionless, small numbers show excitement. On post-mortem a patchy enteritis and cardiac degeneration are found. Toxic signs and pathological changes are occasionally produced by feeding at the rate of one part per thousand. A particularly important toxic effect is the reversible arrest of spermatogenesis which is associated with testicular changes and occurs after the prolonged prophylactic use of nitrofurazone. Ducklings appear to be particularly susceptible to its toxicity. Resistant strains of coccidia have appeared after the prophylactic use of nitrofurazone.

Furazolidone is a nitrofuran which is active against a

number of pathogenic protozoa, in particular, *coccidia*, *hexamita*, *histomonas* and *trichomonas*. It is effective also against many Gram-positive and Gram-negative organisms and, in particular, it is used to control the mortality in fowl typhoid (*Salmonella gallinarum*) and pullorum disease (*S. pullorum*). It has an inhibitory action on the protozoa causing blackhead in turkeys (histomoniasis), and is used also for the treatment of infectious sinusitis in turkeys. A preparation is available which can be injected into the sinuses. This drug should not be fed to breeding stock because changes in the testicular tissue may be produced, although egg production and the fertility of eggs are unaffected. Calves are particularly susceptible to nitrofuran poisoning. Although furazolidone is effective in producing a clinical cure of certain Salmonella infections of large animals, a bacteriological cure does not always occur and organisms may persist especially in the gall bladder. Moreover, certain Salmonella of the large animals present a potential hazard to humans and it is doubtful whether the treatment of animals used for food is justified.

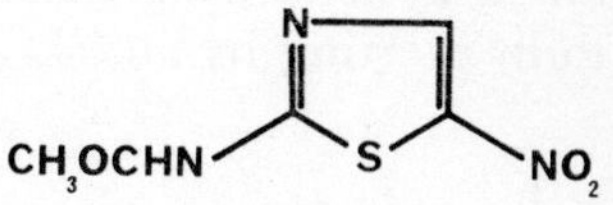

Acinitrazole has replaced aminonitrothiazole for the treatment and prevention of blackhead (histomoniasis) in turkeys. This is because acinitrazole is almost free from toxic effects even when fed to breeding birds over long periods. For the prevention of histomoniasis, acinitrazole is given continuously in the feed.

Acinitrazole

FIG. 21.2

The formula of an antihistomoniasis drug.

DINITRO COMPOUNDS

Nicarbazin is a complex of two chemical compounds used in the prevention of coccidiosis in poultry. The morbidity and mortality from *Eimeria acervulinum*, *E. necatrix* and *E. tenella* and from mixed infections are prevented. Moreover, strains of coccidia resistant to other coccidiostatic drugs may be susceptible to nicarbazin. The drug is fed continuously as 0.0125 per cent of the ration. It is usually diluted with an inert vehicle before mixing with the food. The administration of nicarbazin may reduce egg production and the hatchability of fertile eggs. It may increase the incidence of eggs with mottled yolks but it does not appear to affect the quality of the semen.

Vitamin Antagonists

Amprolium hydrochloride is a coccidiostatic agent whose action depends on the fact that it is antagonistic to aneurin, hence, high concentrations of aneurin prevent amprolium exerting its anticoccidial activity. It is considered that

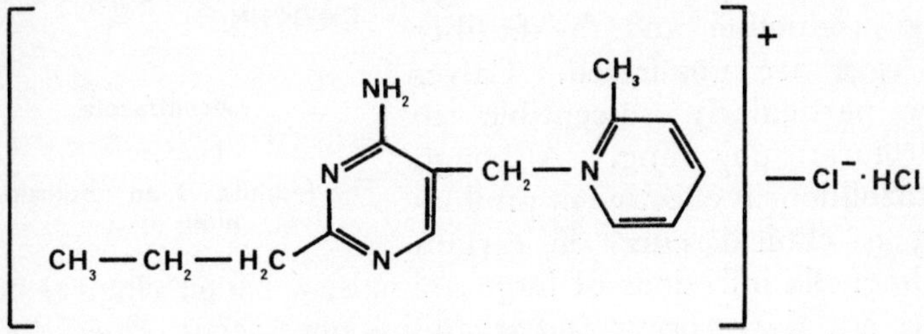

Amprolium chloride hydrochloride

Fig. 21.3

amprolium, by antagonising aneurin, denies aneurin to the coccidia and since the requirements of the coccidia for aneurin are greater than those of the host, the coccidia suffer more from this deprivation. Amprolium is used prophylactically to prevent coccidiosis in chickens and turkeys and for this purpose it is given mixed in the feed as a continuous medication. Amprolium is often combined with other coccidiocidal and coccidiostatic agents such as sulphaquinoxaline and sulphadimidine. The toxicity of Amprolium is due to the antagonism of aneurin and the signs of Amprolium poisoning are those of aneurin deficiency. Although in the concentrations usually fed, amprolium has no effect on the fertility of poultry, a proportion of the chickens hatched from eggs produced by hens treated with this drug may be weak.

Diaveridine is an analogue of the antimalarial pyrimethamine and like this compound is a folic-folinic acid antagonist. Although diaveridine possesses bacteriostatic properties, it is primarily a coccidiostatic agent used to prevent coccidiosis in poultry. It is given together with sulphaquinoxaline because there is a degree of synergism in the coccidiostatic action of these two drugs. This synergism results from each of the two drugs influencing a different phase of the folic acid metabolism of the coccidia. The sulphonamide interferes with the p-aminobenzoic acid metabolism which is concerned in the production of folic acid

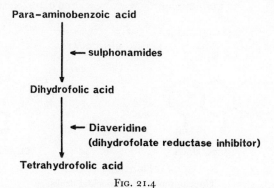

Para–aminobenzoic acid

← sulphonamides

Dihydrofolic acid

← Diaveridine
(dihydrofolate reductase inhibitor)

Tetrahydrofolic acid

FIG. 21.4

A diagram to illustrate the points at which sulphonamides and dihydrofolate reductase inhibitors such as diaveridine interfere with the formation and metabolism of folic acid by micro-organisms.

whereas Diaveridine interferes with the actual folic acid metabolism. The life cycle of the parasite is not completely interrupted by Diaveridine and sufficient coccidial development takes place to produce a high degree of immunity in birds exposed to infection whilst these drugs are being given. Diaveridine itself has a very low toxicity. This toxicity is increased by the addition of the sulphonamide but not until four times the recommended prophylactic dose is given. Egg production, fertility and hatchability appear to be unimpaired by diaveridine.

Ethopabate is a para-aminobenzoic acid antagonist which is coccidiostatic against most coccidia with the important exception of *Eimeria tenella*. Ethopabate potentiates pyrimethamine, a folic-folinic acid antagonist and may be combined with it or with its analogue Diaveridine in a coccidiostatic mixture.

THE QUINOLATES

Methyl benzoquate is a comparatively new coccidiocidal agent which appears to act when the sporozoites penetrate the epithelial cell. It is active against all the common species of coccidia which infest poultry and no ill effects have appeared

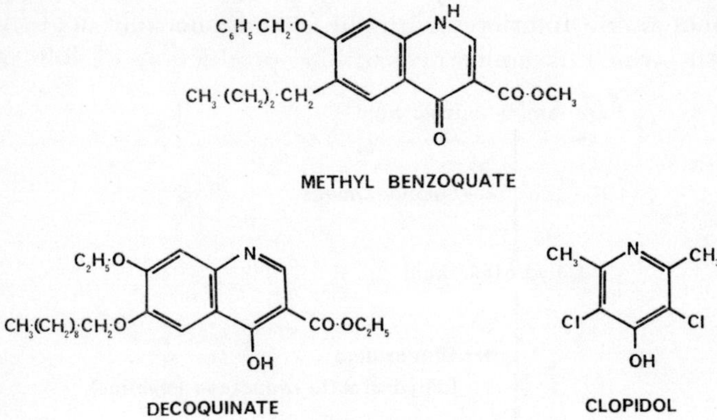

METHYL BENZOQUATE

DECOQUINATE   CLOPIDOL

FIG. 21.5
Three quinolate coccidiocidal drugs.

after the continuous feeding of this drug. It is claimed that **Methyl benzoquate** is more active than other anticoccidial agents on a weight basis. Less than 0·3 per cent of an oral dose is absorbed hence no residues of this drug are found in the tissues. Chemically Methyl benzoquate is a quinolate. Two other quinolates introduced recently are *Decoquinate* and *Clopidol*. These quinolates resemble Methyl benzoquate in coccidiocidal activity.

BABESIOCIDAL DRUGS

The babesia or piroplasmas are protozoal parasites which multiply in the red blood cells of various mammals or birds and are transmitted by ticks. They cause disease in the domesticated animals as, for example, in British Redwater (*Babesia divergans*). A useful drug in the treatment of this disease is **Quinuronium Sulphate**, a compound of quinoline and urea (Fig. 21.6). It is effective against all babesia but does not completely eradicate all the parasites, and animals which clinically appear to have recovered may still harbour parasites. This drug must be given by subcutaneous injection as it is dangerous to inject it intramuscularly or intravenously. Shortly after the injection the animal salivates, defæcates and may stagger and fall. The drug causes a fall in blood pressure, increases intestinal contractions and salivation. Species differ in their susceptibility to these side effects and,

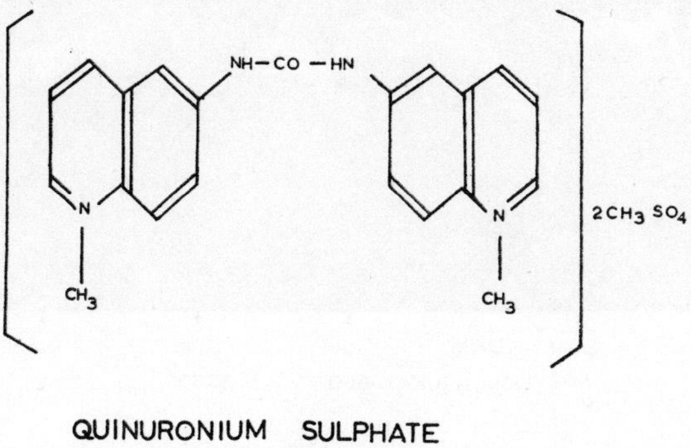

QUINURONIUM   SULPHATE

FIG. 21.6

Quinuronium sulphate.

arranged in decreasing order of susceptibility, they are dog, horse, cattle, sheep and pig. These effects are due mainly to the potent anticholinesterase activity of Quinuronium and they can be alleviated but not completely prevented by giving a large dose of Atropine before the administration of Quinuronium (Fig. 21.7). Quinuronium also releases histamine and depresses cellular oxidation but these various actions probably do not account for all the pharmacodynamic effects of this drug.

Amicarbalide (3 : 3-diamidinocarbanilide) has replaced quinuronium to a large extent for the treatment of babesiasis. However, it is less effective against *B. canis* but compares favourably against other species. Amicarbalide is much less toxic; for example the L.D.50 of Amicarbalide in mice is 15 times that of Quinuronium. Moreover, the only untoward effect reported as occuring in animals treated with amicarbalide has been a mild ataxia. Amicarbalide given by intramuscular injection caused only a transitory swelling, but a severe local reaction followed the subcutaneous injection of this drug. Some of this reaction may be due to the histamine releasing action of amicarbalide. It has been suggested, however, that certain strains of *Babesia* are resistant to Amicarbalide and this may reduce the usefulness of the drug.

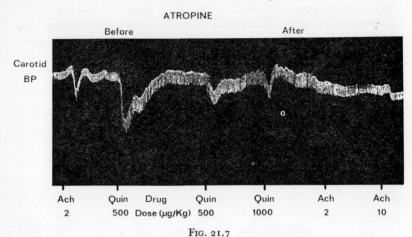

ATROPINE

FIG. 21.7

The effect of atropine on the fall in blood pressure produced by quinuronium. The effect on the blood pressure of a sheep of the administration of acetylcholine and quinuronium is shown before and after atropine. (*Courtesy of P. Eyre.*)

Phenamidine has been used occasionally to treat babesiasis in horses and dogs.

Diminazene is an active babesiacidal agent but is more often used for its trypanocidal actions and is considered later (p. 265).

TRYPANOCIDAL DRUGS

The trypanosomes are flagellates which live in the blood and tissues of vertebrates and are particularly important because they cause disease in livestock. They are transmitted by tsetse flies (*Glossina*). Since the recognition of these protozoa as pathogenic organisms, attempts have been made to devise drugs to kill them. The discovery by Ehrlich that certain dyestuffs, first used as stains, had a specific affinity for these parasites led eventually to the discovery of the trypanocidal action of the organic arsenicals. In recent years many hundreds of compounds have been tested for trypanocidal actions, and substances which are more effective and less toxic than the organic arsenicals are now available.

Quinapyramine

It has been shown that quinapyramine has moderate trypanocidal activity *in vitro* in addition to its *in vivo* action against these parasites, but the most significant property of this drug lies in its power to destroy the infectivity of trypanosomes. This is shown by its action in mice infected with trypanosomes. The trypanosomes in the mice continue to multiply for one to two days after treatment with quinapyramine. However, during this period these trypanosomes are no longer infective and after this initial multiplication the trypanosomes in the blood diminish and ultimately disappear. Quinapyramine has a curative action against infections of *T. congolense* and *T. vivax* in cattle. This drug will cure *T. evansi* in horses and is the only effective drug against *T. simiae* in pigs. *Quinapyramine* is available as the chloride and as the methyl sulphate (Fig. 21.8) The chloride is only 0·12 per cent soluble in water whereas the methyl sulphate is 33 per cent soluble. The difference in solubility is reflected in the rates of absorption, the methyl sulphate being quickly and the chloride slowly absorbed from sites of subcutaneous or intramuscular injection. The slightly soluble chloride forms a depot in the tissues from which absorption proceeds over several weeks. Quinapyramine chloride is unsuitable as a general prophylactic in cattle and it is better to use the so-called " Pro-salt ". This " Pro-salt " is a mixture of two parts quinapyramine chloride and three parts quinapyramine methylsulphate and is used because the initial sterilizing action of the methylsulphate on the trypanosomes is required. It has been found that the trypanosomes appearing towards the end of a period of prophylactic treatment are resistant to the drug. Therefore, unless the challenge to the prophylaxis is very light the period between prophylactic doses should not be more than 2-3 months. Trypanosomes which have become resistant to Quinapyramine are usually resistant also to Homidium and Prothridium but not to Diminazene or to Suramin. There is evidence that the more trypanosomes there are present the more drug will be required.

S

Toxic effects are not uncommon after the administration of quinapyramine. The maximum dose of the methylsulphate is 5 mg./kg. and this produces increased salivation, sweating, tremors, even loss of consciousness and sometimes death two to six hours after the injection. These untoward effects may be due in part to released histamine since quinapyramine is a drug with this property; there may be also an anticholin-

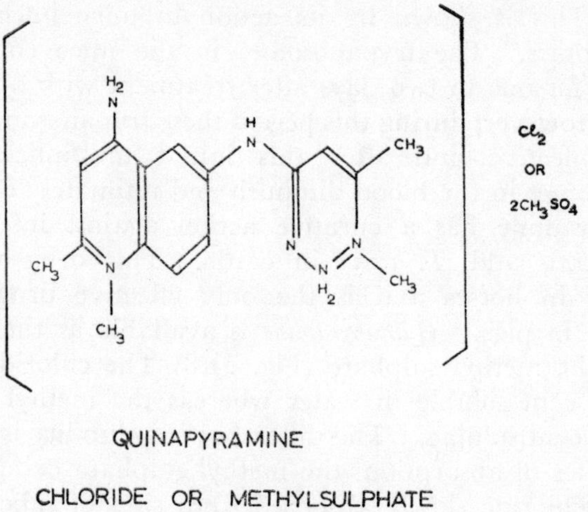

QUINAPYRAMINE

CHLORIDE OR METHYLSULPHATE

FIG. 21.8

Quinapyramine.

esterase action. Some animals develop a gastro-enteritis forty-eight hours after the injection and may die six to twelve days later. The local reaction produced by the injection is rarely serious, excepting in the horse. In this species the local reaction, which may be severe, can be reduced by dividing the dose and injecting in two or three different sites. The quinapyramine chloride in the " Pro-salt " causes a hard swelling at the site of injection which may persist for months or even years.

PHENANTHRIDINIUM COMPOUNDS

In 1938 trypanocidal activity was discovered in a series of Phenanthridinium compounds (Fig. 21.9), and in 1944 one of these, *Dimidium bromide*, was shown in field tests to be effective against *T. congolense*. However, animals treated with this drug showed delayed toxic effects which presented a serious disadvantage. The methyl group of Dimidium was replaced by an ethyl group giving a less toxic trypanocide which is called *Homidium*. In recent years two other Phenanthridinium derivatives have been introduced for their trypano-

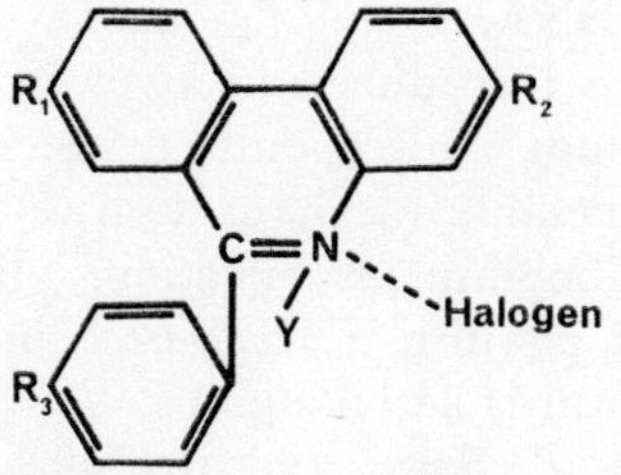

	R_1	R_2	R_3	Y
Dimidium	NH_2	NH_2	H	Me
Homidium	NH_2	NH_2	H	Et
Prothridium	—NH 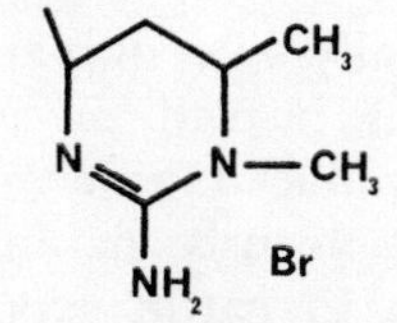	NH_2	NH_2	Me

FIG. 21.9

Some phenanthridinium trypanocidal compounds.

cidal properties, Prothridium which has a pyrimidine moiety as in Quinapyramine and Metamidium which has a substituent which corresponds to the meta version of Diminazene. Homidium is eliminated fairly rapidly from the body but Prothridium and Metamidium persist and are of value in prophylaxis. The Phenanthridinium compounds are active mainly against *T. congolense* and *T. vivax* but are not equal and even different strains of *T. congolense* vary in their response to these trypanocidal compounds.

The mode of action of the Phenanthridiniums is not understood but an interesting hypothesis has been put forward. It has been suggested that the Phenanthridinium compounds

are fixed by the trypanosomes in very small amounts and this
small amount of drug inhibits the factor required for division
of the trypanosomal cytoplasm. When the store of this factor
has been exhausted, the trypanosomes cease to multiply and
disappear. This factor may be a substance required for the
synthesis of DNA as it is known that Homidium inhibits the
synthesis of DNA in a flagellate *Strigomonas oncopelti* and moreover, the antibacterial activity of this Phenanthridinium
compound is antagonised by DNA.

Homidium bromide was introduced in 1952 to replace
dimidium bromide. Homidium causes only transient liver
damage but there is an appreciable local reaction at the site
of either intramuscular or subcutaneous injection. It is ten
times as active as dimidium against *T. congolense* infections
in mice. In the field homidium is active against *T. congolense*
and *T. vivax*, less so against *T. brucei* and inactive against
T. evansi. Homidium is rapid in action and acts prophylactically for about a month. Less local reaction is produced
by intramuscular than subcutaneous injection. It is dangerous
to give intravenously.

Prothridium is chemically like quinapyramine but has a
phenanthridinium nucleus instead of a quinoline nucleus.
This compound was introduced as a prophylactic drug, a
single dose given subcutaneously or intramuscularly, it is
claimed, gives protection to cattle exposed to a moderate
infection for six to eight months. However, resistance to
Prothridium appears to occur fairly readily. This prophylactic
action in cattle probably depends on the persistence of the
deposit of the drug at the site of subcutaneous injection and
this may last for several weeks. About half the Prothridium
present in the blood is bound to plasma protein which explains
in part the persistence in the body of this compound. After
absorption the highest concentration of the drug is found in
the liver and a substantial proportion is excreted in the bile.
Occasionally cases of delayed poisoning have been reported
following the administration of Prothridium. *Metamidium*
is a Phenanthridinium compound introduced for its prophylactic properties. It owes its prophylactic activity to being
deposited at the site of subcutaneous or intramuscular injection
from which there is a slow absorption.

THE DIAMIDINES

Trypanosomes require a great deal of glucose for their activities and their multiplication *in vivo* is decreased by the administration of insulin. A guanidine which lowers the blood sugar called *Synthalin* was tested and found to be trypanocidal *in vivo*. However, this drug was an equally effective trypanocide *in vitro* thus demolishing the hypothesis of trypanocidal activity being related to hypoglycæmia. However, this discovery led to the study of a series of related Diamidine compounds such as Propamidine, Pentamidine, Phenamidine

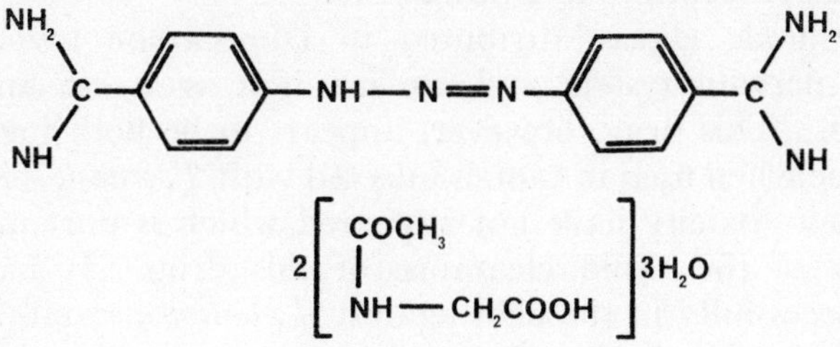

Diminazene Aceturate

FIG. 21.10

and Diminazene. Metamidium, which has been discussed with the Phenanthridium trypanocides has the meta version of Diminazene as a substituent of the Phenanthridinium nucleus.

The Diamidines are not well absorbed from the gut. After intraperitoneal or intravenous injection the concentration in the blood falls rapidly. Propamidine and Pentamidine are retained in the body for a relatively long period probably due to their fixation in the liver.

Diminazene is an active trypanocide, babesiocide and bactericide which appears to act directly on the parasites. This drug kills a number of different bacteria but is particularly active against *Brucella* and *Streptococci*. In trypanosomiasis a single dose of Diminazene usually gives a clinical cure within 24 hours and recovery is followed by a degree of premunity. It is given by subcutaneous or intramuscular injection and produces a local reaction at the injection site. In cattle most of a single dose of Diminazene is metabolised or excreted in the urine within 24 hours. Experimentally, sub-effective doses of this drug fail to produce resistance in *T. congolense;* hence, Diminazene differs from other Diamidines in this respect. The rapid clearance of Diminazene from the body probably accounts for the relative freedom from producing resistant strains. Recently, however, reports have been made of the existence of certain strains of trypanosomes which are resistant to this drug. It is interesting to note that, despite the similarities in chemical structure between Diminazene, Homidium and Metamidium, trypanosomes resistant to the last two compounds remained susceptible to Diminazene.

The toxic effects attributed to Diminazene involve the central nervous system and are manifest as ataxia and convulsions. This drug, however, appears to be both ineffective and toxic when used in camels infected with *T. evansi.* Reports of chronic toxicity have not appeared which is unremarkable in view of the rapid clearance of this drug. It has been used successfully in the field against *T. congolense* and *T. vivax* infections.

PROPHYLACTIC COMPLEXES

Suramin is one of the older trypanocides which is still used against *T. evansi* infections in camels. It is effective also against *T. brucei, T. equinum* and *T. equiperdum* but not against *T. congolense, T. vivax* or *T. simiæ.* This substance is given by intravenous injection, because it is too irritant for intramuscular or subcutaneous injection. Suramin is exceptional amongst the trypanocides in being an acidic substance, hence it combines firmly with the plasma proteins and persists for many weeks in the body. Since Quinapyramine, the Phenanthridiniums and Diminazene are basic substances the acidic Suramin will combine with them to form an insoluble complex. These complexes, when injected, form depots from which absorption proceeds very slowly. They are of particular value in prophylaxis. An important disadvantage possessed by these Suramin complexes is the intense local irritation they produce which may be sufficiently severe to cause sloughing and loss of the deposit. There is, of course, no longer any prophylaxis if the deposit has been lost. The complex which appears to cause the least irritation is that between Prothridium and Suramin. Protection of seven months' duration has been obtained using a suramin-homidium complex. Suramin may cause degenerative changes of the liver, kidneys and, especially in horses, the adrenals.

ORGANIC ARSENICALS

Arsenic as the trioxide was used by David Livingstone to treat trypanosomiasis in horses, but this drug did not produce a lasting cure and often killed the horses as well as the protozoa. However, in 1906 Thomas found that *Atoxyl*, a pentavalent organic arsenical, cured trypanosomiasis in rats. About this time Ehrlich was examining a long series of trivalent arsenical compounds of benzene and found that compounds in which the benzene had an amino group attached in the para position were most effective. Ehrlichs' research culminated in the discovery of Arsphenamine, which he called Salvarsan. This drug was used for many years to treat syphilis in man. Some organic arsenicals are occasionally used to treat trypanosomiasis in domestic animals. Fig. 21.11 shows the formulæ of the organic arsenicals of veterinary importance.

Tryparsamide, a pentavalent organic arsenical, is used in the treatment of trypanosomiasis and histomoniasis. It is given parenterally. *Acetarsol*, also a pentavalent compound, is used together with arecoline in dogs infested with tapeworms. *Arsenophenylbutyric acid* is a trivalent compound used against *T. equiperdum*, the cause of Dourine in horses, and *Neoarsphenamine*, also a trivalent compound, is used in Dourine and histomoniasis; both these drugs are given parenterally.

The activity of all organic arsenicals is due to the trivalent form.

Pentavalent organic arsenicals are reduced in the body to the active arsenoxide, the reaction being slowly reversible. After an intravenous injection pentavalent compounds are excreted nearly completely in the urine within twenty-four hours. The trivalent compounds are excreted more slowly. This slower excretion is due to the trivalent compounds being rapidly fixed by the tissues. They disappear from the bloop within a few minutes. The tissue fixation delays their excretion so that nearly seven days are required for a single dose to be cleared.

Arsenic trioxide was widely used formerly as a "tonic" and in skin disease. It is now of importance because of its toxicology and use in some countries as a dip against ticks. Arsenic

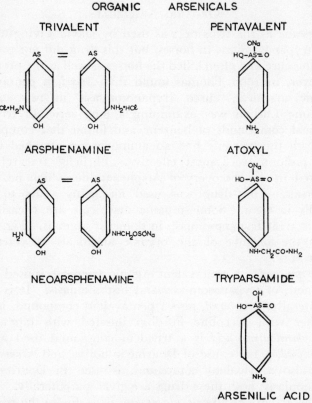

FIG. 21.11
Organic arsenicals of veterinary importance.

causes an acute gastro-enteritis and death from shock. It acts by poisoning oxidative enzymes in the body, in particular those with thiol groups. Many heavy metals and metalloids, such as mercury and arsenic, have a high affinity for thiol compounds, probably combining with them by displacing hydrogen, and various thiol compounds act as antidotes to arsenic.

Although the use of inorganic arsenic as a " tonic " has been discontinued because of the lack of clear evidence of its value, certain organic arsenicals are being introduced to increase the growth rate of animals such as pigs and poultry. Organic arsenicals are chosen because they are safer than the inorganic compounds, and the most active for this purpose are *Arsenilic acid*, 3-nitro-4-hydroxyphenylarsonic acid and atoxyl. Chickens given these drugs showed a 20 per cent increased weight gain. This gain is, however, less than that produced by feeding chlortetracycline and Vitamin B_{12}. Turkey poults have shown a gain of 19 per cent. The drugs are given at the rate of 0·0025 per cent in water or 0·005 per cent in the food. In addition to the increased weight gain, chickens fed these compounds started egg laying two to twenty-four days earlier than untreated control chickens. The feed conversion efficiency was improved and fewer deaths occurred in the treated birds. The result of feeding these organic arsenicals to pigs was more variable. This variation may be explained by the fact that arsenicals suppress chronic enteritis in pigs and, therefore, will show an increased gain in weight only in pigs suffering from this condition. *Sodium aminoarsenate* is used for the treatment of enteritis in pigs. Pigs are more susceptible to arsenic poisoning than poultry. Affected animals show incoordination of gait, blindness and frequent uncontrolled micturition. Animals should not receive any arsenical compound during twelve days before slaughter. The liver and kidneys are sites where arsenic is fixed; the concentration in the muscles is only a fraction of that in the liver. As these offals are often incorporated into foodstuffs, it is important that sufficient time should elapse after use of arsenicals for the concentration in these tissues to have fallen to levels which are commonly found in untreated animals.

ANTIDOTES TO HEAVY METALS

Dimercaprol is a thiol compound which combines with arsenic and so prevents arsenic from combining with thiol groups in the tissues. The arsenic so combined cannot inhibit sulphydryl enzyme systems and exert its toxic actions.

Arsenic forms a very stable five-membered ring by combining one atom of arsenic with two thiol groups on adjacent carbon atoms. Dimercaprol provides two thiol groups on

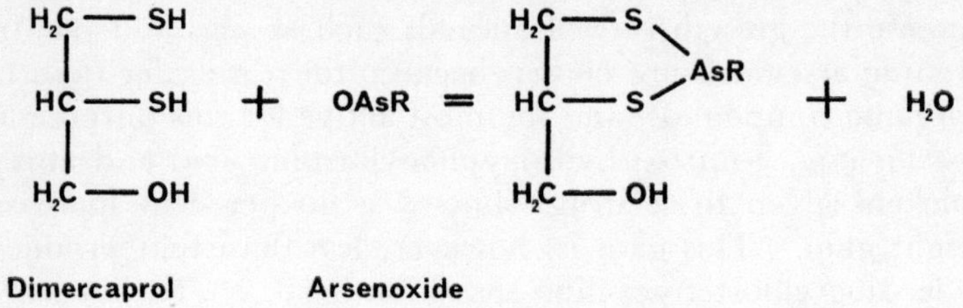
H₂C — SH
HC — SH
H₂C — OH
+ OAsR =
H₂C — S
HC — S
AsR
H₂C — OH
+ H₂O
Dimercaprol
Arsenoxide

FIG. 21.12
The chelation of an arsenoxide.

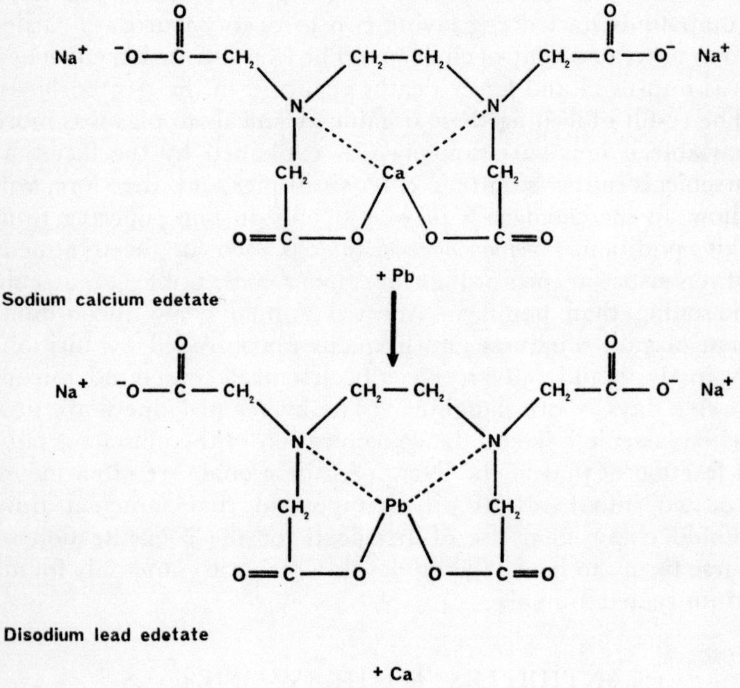
Sodium calcium edetate
+ Pb
Disodium lead edetate
+ Ca

FIG. 21.13
The chelation of lead.

adjacent carbon atoms, with which arsenic and certain other metals such as cadmium and mercury combine to form a poorly dissociable chelate. It can be used, therefore, in the treatment of poisoning by these metals. However, Dimercaprol itself is oxidised in the tissues, thus releasing the metal from the chelate. It is essential, therefore, that the treatment must ensure the continuous presence of Dimercaprol. Moreover, treatment must be prompt because the extent to which an enzyme can be reactivated depends on the length of time it has been inactivated. The dose of Dimercaprol is limited by its toxicity which is exerted mainly on the central nervous system and shows as tremors and convulsions. In animals capable of doing so, vomiting may occur. Dimercaprol may cause damage to capillaries.

Sodium calcium edetate forms a stable soluble metallic chelate with divalent metallic ions which have a higher affinity for chelation than calcium. The main use of this drug is in the treatment of lead poisoning. Its effect in mercurial poisoning is poor and it is valueless in arsenical poisoning. Sodium calcium edetate has so low a dissociation that the calcium is not precipitated by oxalate or carbonate but may be replaced by ions such as lead, which are bound even more strongly than calcium. This drug is injected intravenously 33 mg./lb./day, being given in divided doses. The heavy metal appears in the urine as the chelate, none being free as ions of the heavy metal, hence none can react with the tissues and cause damage. Sodium calcium edetate is relatively non-toxic.

SUGGESTIONS FOR FURTHER READING

JOYNER, L. P. (1965–66). Chemotherapy of protozoal infections. *Vet. A.*, **7**, 299.
SCHNITZER, R. J. and HAWKING, F. (1962). *Experimental Chemotherapy*, Vol. I. New York: Academic Press.
SOFFER, A. (1964). *Chelation Therapy*. Springfield, Illinois: Thomas.
STEPHEN, L. E. (1963). Chemotherapy of *Trypanosoma simiae*. *Vet. Bull.*, **33**, 599.

CHAPTER XXII

CHEMOTHERAPY OF HELMINTH INFECTIONS

ANTHELMINTICS

THE drugs in this group kill or remove parasitic worms from the animal. As no single drug is effective against all worms it is convenient from a therapeutic point of view to consider worms as falling into three groups—cestodes, nematodes and trematodes. The first and second group are, respectively, the tapeworms and roundworms which live mainly in the alimentary canal. The third group represents the flukes which live mainly in the biliary tract. Some nematodes live in the lungs and in other tissues.

Although some anthelmintics have been used since the earliest times, one of the first attempts to study their action was made in 1884 by von Schroeder, who investigated the effect of various drugs on ascarids *in vitro*. This type of experiment was elaborated by various people in the past thirty years. The elaborations usually involved hanging segments of worm in a constant-temperature bath in physiological saline and recording the movements of the worm on a smoked drum. It was found that some known anthelmintics stopped the movements but others were without effect. This kind of experiment is therefore of little value in discovering whether a new chemical will be a good anthelmintic, but may be useful in studying how various known anthelmintics work.

Female worms in the gut or bile ducts lay eggs which are passed out with the fæces. This fact has been made use of in testing anthelmintics since if a worm is killed it can no longer lay eggs. However, as drugs exist which merely inhibit egg-laying, the results of such tests of anthelmintic activity can be misleading. The best evidence of anthelmintic activity is supplied by using the " Critical Test " devised by a United States veterinarian named Hall, in 1918. In this test, which was intended for assessing the activity of anthelmintics against gastro-intestinal worms, each animal infested with the worm or worms under study is given the drug; after dosing, the fæces are collected and the worms in the fæces counted and identified. The host animal is then killed and the gut examined. The worms remaining in the host are counted and identified. Adding together the worms of each species found in the fæces to those remaining in the gut gives the number of worms in the host at the time of treatment. The worms in the fæces together with dead worms in the host expressed as a percentage of the initial infestation shows the efficiency of the particular anthelmintic for the worm infestation studied. The efficiency of an anthelmintic should be in the region of 90 per cent. A deficiency of this test is that it fails to take account of worms killed in the first part of the gut being digested and therefore not appearing in the fæces. With suitable modification this test can be applied to study drugs acting on liver flukes and lung worms.

The critical test used directly on parasitised animals of the species in which the anthelmintics are ultimately intended to be used is expensive and time-consuming. It is not well adapted to the development of new anthelmintics. To overcome this difficulty laboratory rodents infected with their specific helminths have been used. Such animals are sometimes called the " Primary Screen ". These screening tests are based on the belief that parasites which are systematically related have similar chemotherapeutic responses. Unfortunately this belief is not wholly true but is, nonetheless, a useful working premise. It has been shown, for example, that a nematode of mice, *Nippostrongylus muris*, the trichostrongyles of sheep and cattle and the hookworms of the dog all respond to bephenium compounds, hence mice infected with *Nippostrongylus* provided a suitable primary screen for anthelmintics against certain worms infesting ruminants and dogs. Unfortunately a similar relationship does not apply to phenothiazine or certain organophosphorus compounds.

Male fern and dichlorophen are active against a tapeworm of mice, *Hymenolepis nana*, and the larger tapeworms of domesticated animals, and this mouse parasite can be used for screening Tænicides. However, hexachlorophene is active against the chicken tapeworm *Ræillietina cesticillus* and not against *H. nana*. It is advisable, therefore, where possible, to test drugs which are being developed for their anthelmintic activity against a diversity of parasitic helminths in the primary screen. However, a secondary screen, whereby the drug is tested against the parasite in its normal host, is necessary before proceeding to clinical trials.

In a clinical trial the parasitised animals are divided by a process of randomisation into two groups, one group receives the drug and the other group is left untreated. After a suitable interval, all the animals in both groups are killed and the number of worms remaining in each animal counted, the various species present being enumerated separately. It is thus possible to determine the proportion of each species of worm removed by the drug under test. However, before the drug can be marketed, it is necessary to carry out toxicity tests and any drug to have prospects of wide use as an anthelmintic must have a very low toxicity to the host animal. It is now advisable to obtain information about the possibility of residues of the anthelmintic remaining in the tissues of the host, since many of the species in which anthelmintics are used are animals whose carcase and organs are likely to be used for human consu ption.

DRUGS ACTING ON TAPEWORMS

Arecoline hydrobromide given to dogs by mouth has been shown by the Critical Test of dosing infected dogs, killing them after an interval and searching the gut for tapeworm heads, to be a most effective anthelmintic. This drug stimulates the secretions of glands and plain muscles innervated by the parasympathetics. The anthelmintic effects are probably due to a combination of increased intestinal secretions and movements together with some action on the worm. This latter action is shown by the fact that arecoline given by mouth is between 75 and 80 per cent effective, given by subcutaneous injection only 0·1 per cent of the worms are expelled. Arecoline has a depressant effect on segments of tapeworms suspended in an isolated organ-bath. It is used only in dogs, and it is usually given after withholding food overnight. Vomiting after dosing only reduces the efficiency of the drug if it takes place within the first two minutes after administration.

This drug is an effective anthelmintic only when it produces purgation. Unfortunately purgation may sometimes be severe and this constitutes a marked disadvantage to the use of this drug. It is a most effective drug for use against *Echinococcus granulosus*, a tapeworm of dogs with public health importance as man can provide an intermediate host with serious consequences.

Preparations are available in which acetarsol, a pentavalent organic arsenical, has been added to arecoline. There is no evidence that such preparations are more effective than arecoline. They are more expensive.

Arecoline should never be administered to cats, as in this species the gastro-intestinal stimulation is particularly severe and may cause death.

Dichlorophen is used to treat dogs and cats affected with tapeworms. This drug is also fungicidal and bacteriostatic. The tapeworm becomes detached from the intestinal wall within 30 to 40 minutes after dosing, it then disintegrates in the gut, hence treated animals do not pass segments of worm in the fæces.

The main advantage in the use of dichlorophen is that it is unnecessary to withhold food before administering the drug. Dichlorophen does not cause the very severe purgation which may be produced by arecoline. Unfortunately, dichlorophen is relatively ineffective against *E. granulosus* and *Dipylidium caninum*. It has, moreover, other disadvantages; vomiting, colic and occasionally diarrhœa may be produced. Furthermore the dose is very bulky and this presents difficulties in administration. This drug is alleged to be more effective in cats than dogs; it is no doubt preferable in cats. The fringed tapeworm of sheep is not affected by dichlorophen.

Bunamidine hydrochloride (N : N-Di. butyl-4-hexyloxy-1-naphthamidine HCl) has been shown by critical tests to be effective in the treatment of infestations with *T. pisiformis*, *D. caninium* and *E. granulosus* in the dog and *Hydatigena tæniæformis* in the cat. Dogs infected with *Echinococcus* and treated with this drug show a few scolices embedded in the gut and it is not clear, unless time is given, whether these scolices will develop and prove viable. The drug is given in cachets or tablets and it seems important that when tablets are given the formulation should be such as to allow the rapid disintegration otherwise the effectivity of the drug is decreased. When bunamidine is given as a drench, inflammation of the buccal mucus membrane is caused. The only toxic effects of consequence so far described have been vomiting and diarrhœa in certain dogs.

Quinacrine hydrochloride, originally an anti-malarial drug, has been used to treat dogs infected with tapeworms. This

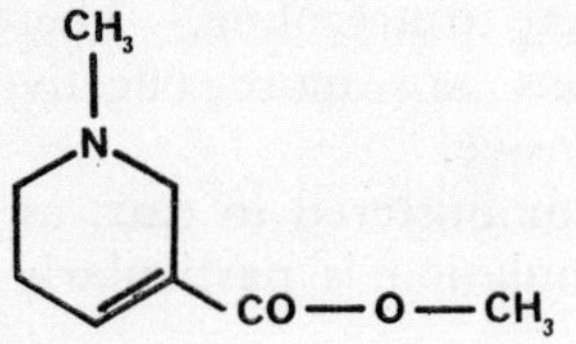

Arecoline 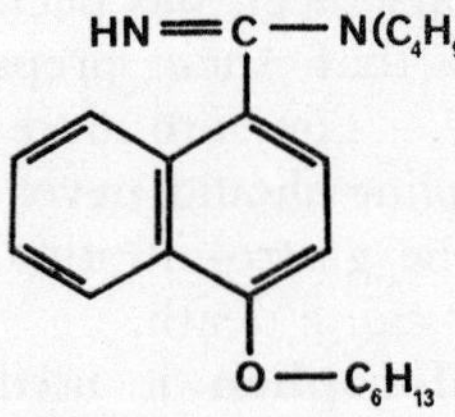   Bunamidine

FIG. 22.1
The formulæ of two tæniacides[1]

drug does not kill the worm but stimulates it so that it is detached from the mucosa. The worm is then easily expelled from the animal by a purge; the worm segments are stained yellow. It is effective against *Dipylidium caniniom* and *Tænia pisiformis*. About 1 per cent of dogs treated with quinacrine show nausea and vomiting.

Niclosamide has been introduced for the treatment of *T. pisiformis* in dogs and *T. tæniæformis* in cats. It is effective also in sheep infected with *Moniezia* species. The published evidence on this drug is less satisfactory than that for bunamidine; the criterion of cure in dogs and cats treated with this salicylamide has been the absence of tænia from the fæces during the six-week period after treatment. This evidence is much less satisfactory than the rigid application of a critical test involving a search of the gut for scolices. Moreover, this drug does not appear to be effective in the treatment of *Echinococcus*. As yet there have been no published cases of toxic effects from the use of this drug.

Lead arsenate is effective against tape-worms of the *Monezia* species in lambs, calves and kids, but is valueless against the fringed tapeworm. This drug is given by mouth in a gelatin capsule and this is followed by a suitable dose of castor oil. It has been found too toxic to use in poultry.

Felix mas, the extract of male fern, is an obsolete tænicide which was widely used in dogs. It is a thick dark green liquid whose active principle is filicic acid. The main importance of this drug now lies in its toxic effects. These include jaundice, gastro-enteritis, optic neuritis and may include coma, convulsions and heart failure. It is sometimes used to treat cattle and sheep with liver fluke but is apt to cause similar toxic effects.

Pelletierine tannate is used occasionally to treat dogs and cats suffering from tapeworms. It is similar in action to arecoline.

SUGGESTIONS FOR FURTHER READING

HATTON, C. J. (1965). A new tæniacide, bunamidine hydrochloride. *Vet. Rec.*, **77**, 408.

LAPAGE, G. (1968). *Veterinary Parasitology*, 2nd Ed. Edinburgh: Oliver & Boyd.

MÖNNIG, H. O. (1968). *Helminths, Arthropods and Protozoa of Domestic Animals*, 6th ed. by E. J. Soulsby, London: Bailliere, Tindall & Cassel.

STANDEN, O. D. (1963). In *Experimental Chemotherapy*, ed. Schnitzer, R. J. and Hawking, F., Vol. I. New York: Academic Press.

T

CHAPTER XXIII

CHEMOTHERAPY OF HELMINTH
INFECTIONS

DRUGS ACTING AGAINST ROUND WORMS

PHENOTHIAZINE

Despite its limitations, phenothiazine is still an important drug acting against roundworms in sheep, horses and, to a lesser extent, cattle. In the pure state is exists as a green-yellow powder which easily oxidises. It is stable when dry, but moisture quickly starts the oxidation. The commercial product contains various oxidation products, but these are of less anthelmintic importance than the size of the phenothiazine particles.

Phenothiazine is widely used against stomach worms in ruminants such as *Hæmonchus*, *Ostertagia* and *Trichostrongylus*. Nodular worms in cattle, sheep and pigs of the *Œsophagostomum* species, the colon worm, *Chabertia ovina* in sheep, *Strongyles* in horses and *Heterakis* in poultry are also susceptible. It is not an effective treatment for worms of the *Cooperia Bunostomum* and *Nematodirus* species. In horses, phenothiazine given in combination with piperazine has been shown particularly effective against *Trichonema*, *Strongylus vulgaris* and *S. edentatus*. Phenothiazine is used also in combination with various organophosphorus compounds in the treatment of nematode infections of sheep. This combination allows a smaller dose of organophosphorus compound to be used without reducing the effectivity of the mixture and thus reduces the risk of toxicity.

Phenothiazine is given by mouth as a compressed tablet or suspended in water with a suitable dispersing agent. Because of difficulties of estimation its fate in the body is incompletely known; an appreciable amount is absorbed, some being excreted in the urine as a conjugate and some as phenothiazone

278

and as phenothiazine sulphoxide (Fig. 23.1). Sheep convert the sulphoxide into phenothiazine and phenothiazone.

Phenothiazone has no appreciable anthelmintic action; phenothiazine sulphoxide is an effective anthelmintic, but the dose is as big as that of phenothiazine so it is unlikely that the activity of phenothiazine depends on its conversion to the sulphoxide. There is some evidence that certain parasites

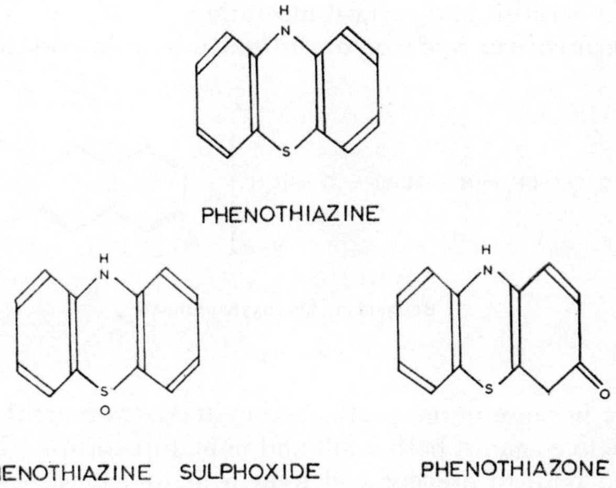

PHENOTHIAZINE

PHENOTHIAZINE SULPHOXIDE   PHENOTHIAZONE

FIG. 23.1
Phenothiazine and two metabolites.

have a special affinity for phenothiazine and absorb it through their cuticle. Phenothiazine inhibits glycolysis and the egg-laying of worms. This last feature may mislead if the criteria of cure is the absence of worm eggs. However, it is used to reduce the larvæ on a pasture by keeping the host animals on a small continuous dose of phenothiazine.

The fact that phenothiazine can be used continuously for long periods without untoward effects shows its comparative safety. However, it may give rise to toxic signs. Generally speaking young animals of any species are more susceptible than the older and amongst the domestic species, sheep are the most resistant to poisoning and the horse least. In the horse, hæmoglobinurea and jaundice may occur. Since the excretion of phenothiazine imparts a red colour to the urine and to milk, it is important that a red colour in the urine is not mistaken for hæmoglobin.   The milk is preserved because of the antispetic action of phenothiazone.

A serious consequence of the administration of phenothiazine is in the production of photosensitisation in calves. This is due to the sulphoxide which is a photodynamic agent. In calves the sulphoxide is not completely converted in the liver to phenothiazine as it is in sheep.   The affected animals usually show a keratitis and corneal ulceration.

Bephenium hydroxynaphthoate is an important anthel-

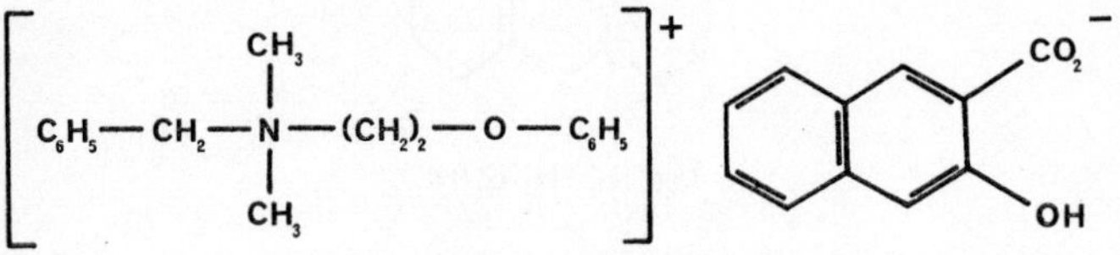

Bephenium hydroxynaphthoate

Fig. 23.2

mintic because of its specific action in *Nematodirus* infestations. It is active against both adult and immature forms.   This drug is used both to prevent and treat nematodiriasis, being given for prophylaxis at intervals of three weeks and for treatment as a single dose.   The drug is given as a drench made with water and a dispersing agent.   It is active also against *Cooperia sp.*, *Trichostrongylus sp.*, *Ostertagia sp.*, *Hæmonchus contortus* and in the treatment of dogs infested with hookworms. It appears to be free of toxic effects.

Thiabendazole is a very effective anthelmintic against worms of the *Strongyloidea*, *Ascaroidea* and *Trichinelloidea*.   In sheep and goats it has been shown to be more than 95 per cent effective against *Hæmonchus*, *Ostertagia*, *Trichostrongylus*, *Cooperia*, *Nematodirus*, *Bunostomum*, *Strongyloides*, *Chabertia* and *Oesophagostomum*.   It is very effective also in the treatment of horses infected with *Strongyles*, *Ascarids* and *Oxyurids*.

Thiabendazole is larvicidal and inhibits helminth egg production.   This drug has no residual action and it has been recommended that administration should be continuous or the dose repeated every six weeks in spring and summer.

The high effectiveness of this drug and in particular the larvicidal action may, by removing the worms so completely, make the host susceptible to re-infection and prevent the development of immunity. Thiabendazole appears free from toxic actions.

The fate in cattle, goats and pigs has been studied by the use of thiabendazole labelled with [14]C. Thiabendazole was rapidly absorbed from the gut, the highest concentration in the blood occuring between 4 and 7 hours after dosing. Nearly all the drug was metabolised; the only metabolite identified being 5-hydroxythiabendazole. This occurred as either the

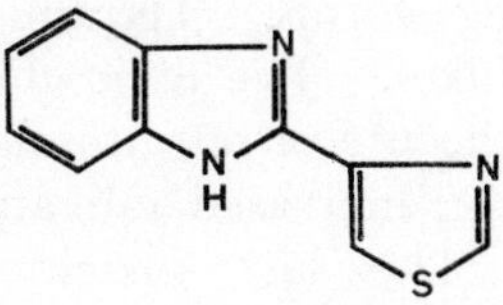

Thiabendazole

FIG.23.3

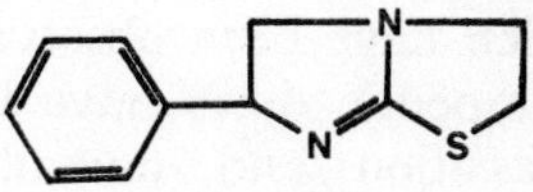

Tetramisole

FIG. 23.4

glucuronide or the sulphate. Within 3 days of administration approximately 6 per cent of the dose was excreted in the urine and 20 per cent in the fæces. Thirty days after administration no residue of thiabendazole or metabolite could be detected in the tissues, although calves dosed with this drug showed traces of radio-activity not in the form of thiabendazole two months after dosing.

Parbendazole is an anthelmintic similar to thiabendazole used to treat round worm infestations of the sheep's gastro-intestinal tract.

Tetramisole is an anthelmintic recently discovered which appears to have activity against the greatest variety of nematode species which infest the domesticated animals of any drug so far introduced. It is effective against nematodes of chickens, sheep, cattle, pigs, horses, dogs and cats and a single dose is usually effective. This drug can be administered orally or in the feed, or by subcutaneous, intramuscular or intra-peritoneal injection.

When tested *in vitro* tetramisole has been shown to have

a paralysing effect on nematodes and, on treating an animal infested with nematodes, the worms which are most rapidly expelled appear in the fæces alive; worms expelled later are decomposed and may not be apparent in the fæces. Tetramisole is less active against immature worms than adults in comparison with thiabendazole which is active against larval forms in addition to mature worms. However, the main advantage of tetramisole over other anthelmintics is in the treatment of animals in which both the gastrointestinal tract and bronchial passages are infested with nematodes. Tetramisole is effective against nematodes of the gastrointestinal tract as well as those species which infest the lungs whereas thiabendazole has little action against lung worms. Tetramisole has no action against tapeworms or flukes. The toxic effects which have been observed following the use of tetramisole at therapeutic doses have been depression, increased salivation, defæcation and muscular tremors. The low toxicity of tetramisole gives it a distinct advantage for use in the treatment of lung worm infestation over *Cyacetazide*. Cyacetazide was introduced specifically for the treatment of lung worms of cattle, sheep and pigs. It does not kill the worm but renders it inactive and susceptible to removal by the bronchial cilia, and coughing. Although cyacetazide can be given by mouth or subcutaneous injection the latter route gives rise to local irritation, lacrimation and salivation, and overdosage causes convulsions. The toxic effects of cyacetazide are due to pyridoxine (B_6) fixation, and hence the specific antidote is to give pyridoxine intravenously. However, it seems probable that this drug will be used decreasingly in future years.

Pyrantel tartrate is a widely used anthelmintic which has activity against infestations by *Nematodirus*, *Ostertagia* and *Hæmonchus*. It has a depolarising action and probably produces paralysis of the worm by causing a contracture of the worm muscle. This drug also has local anæsthetic activity. When given by mouth about one third of the dose is absorbed and approximately a quarter of this is excreted in the urine, the remainder of the absorbed fraction is metabolised, some to urea and carbon dioxide. It does not leave residues in the tissues and is fairly free from toxic effects even in pregnant animals.

ORGANOPHOSPHORUS ANTHELMINTICS

Haloxon is an organophosphorus compound with a high degree of anthelmintic activity against nematodes of sheep and cattle. The adult forms of *Hæmonchus, Ostertagia, Trichostrongylus, Cooperia, Strongyloides, Nematodirus* and *Bunostomum* are particularly susceptible. Haloxon is active also against *Capillaria sp.* in poultry, although *Heterakis* infestation in birds is unaffected by Haloxon. This drug provides an effective treatment for horses infested with *Ascarids, Oxyurids, Triodontophorus sp., Trichonema sp.* and *Strongylus vulgaris*. The other horse strongyles are less susceptible but it is effective against bots (*Gastrophilus sp.*). *Ascaris lumbricoides* and *Œsophagostomum sp.* in pigs and *Ancylostomes* and *Ascarids* in carnivores are also eliminated by Haloxon. This drug is palatable when given in the feed and can be administered thus to horses, pigs and poultry. It has larvicidal activity.

Haloxon differs from closely related organophosphorus compounds in causing only slight depression of mammalian red cell cholinesterase, i.e. acetylcholinesterase. Toxic effects have appeared when ten times the therapeutic dose has been given. These effects consisted of anorexia, diarrhœa and death after several days. However, a proportion of sheep and poultry treated with therapeutic doses have shown posterior ataxia. Atropine has not proved an effective antidote to the toxic effects of Haloxon, which is not surprising in view of the failure of this drug to depress acetyl cholinesterase.

Geese are very susceptible to Haloxon poisoning and fortunately 2-PAM is an effective antidote. Goose brain cholinesterase apparently forms a stable phosphoryl derivative with Haloxon and it is claimed that this is unique amongst vertebrates. Certain nematodes which are susceptible to Haloxon have cholinesterases which form stable compounds with this drug whereas other nematodes which are insusceptible and mammals have cholinesterases which form unstable compounds with Haloxon. This observation may explain the mode of action of this drug and also its freedom from toxic effects in the host animals (see Fig. 24.3).

Metriphonate is an organophosphorus compound with anthelmintic and insecticidal properties. The latter effects are obtained by either local application or oral administration. The effect of the drug by either of these routes of administration is of short duration because it is broken down on the skin as well as in the body. It can be used in the treatment of warble fly but treatment should be avoided in the months of December, January and February because at this period the migrating larvæ are situated along the spinal cord and if killed in this situation may give rise to a reaction which could have serious consequences.

It is effective in the treatment of nematode infestations in cattle for which purpose it is given as a drench. Worms of the following species are susceptible to Metriphonate: *Cooperia*, *Bunostomum*, *Trichuris*, *Hæmonchus* and *Œsophagostomum* species. It is of little use in the treatment of nematode infestations in sheep and goats because in these species the effective dose of metriphonate approaches the toxic dose. The toxic effects of this drug are due to the inhibition of cholinesterase and, since it is relatively quickly metabolised, recovery takes place in a few hours. Atropine provides a specific antidote. The dose of atropine in the treatment of organophosphorus poisoning is 4-5 times the usual therapeutic dose.

OTHER NEMATOCIDES

Diethylcarbamazine acid citrate is a derivative of piperazine (Fig. 23.5). It is the most active and least toxic piperazine used to combat infestations with microfilaria. After small doses of this drug 90 per cent of the microfilaria rapidly disappear from the blood; however, a few persist even after big doses are given. Unfortunately this drug has little effect on the adult *Dirofilaria immitis* of dogs. When tested against other helminth parasites it was found to be about 100 per cent effective against ascarids in dogs and cats. For this purpose it is given by mouth in gelatin capsules to avoid buccal irritation, and it is unnecessary to starve or purge the host. The main disadvantage is a tendency to cause vomiting and loss of appetite. It also acts against hook worms and tapeworms, and, when given by intramuscular injection, it is effective in the treatment of chronic parasitic bronchitis in calves and sheep. This bronchitis is caused by roundworms in the bronchi, *Dictyocaulus viviparus* in calves and *D. filaria* in sheep. Diethylcarbamazine is rapidly absorbed from the gut and its metabolites are excreted in the urine; 70 per cent of the dose can be accounted for in this way within the first 24 hours after administration. It is of low toxicity, although drug sensitisation has been reported in dogs treated with diethylcarbamazine, and as this condition is probably due to released histamine an appropriate treatment might be to give an antihistamine. *Methyridine* was the first drug which could be given to sheep and cattle subcutaneously to remove

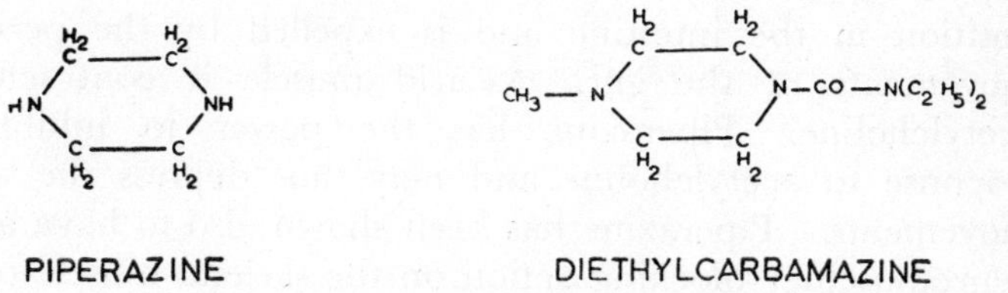

PIPERAZINE   DIETHYLCARBAMAZINE

FIG. 23.5
Diethylcarbamazine and piperazine.

nematodes present in the abomasum and small intestine. It is effective against *Ostertagia*, *Trichostrongyles*, *Cooperia*, and *Nematodirus* and has some effect against *Monezia*, a tapeworm of ruminants and the lung worm *Dictyocaulus* in sheep and cattle.

Subcutaneous injections of this drug give a local reaction which is particularly serious in the horse and it should not be used in this species. Methyridine paralyses the worms, probably by a depolarizing action similar to that produced by decamethonium. It is both secreted into, and absorbed from, the alimentary tract. It is absorbed even through the skin. Methyridine has a toxic action which is additive to that of the organophosphorus compounds and diethylcarbamazine and should not be given until two weeks after the administration of either of these latter drugs.

Piperazine

One of the most important anthelmintics developed in recent decades is Piperazine. The use of this drug was suggested by a pharmacist of Rouen for the treatment of ascaris infection in man. Fortunately the drug was known to be reasonably safe, having been used for many years in the treatment of gout. It is a safe and effective anthelmintic against *ascarids*, *oxyurids*, the nodular worms (*Œsophagostomum*) and *Strongylus vulgaris*. It is ineffective against the other horse strongyles, *S. equinus* and *S. edentatus*, and against *Hæmonchus contortus*. The trichostrongyles, hookworms and tapeworms, are also unaffected by piperazine.

Piperazine is readily absorbed from the gut, between 30 to 40 per cent is excreted in the urine in the first twenty-four hours and the remainder metabolised. It appears to act by depressing motility so that the worm cannot maintain its position in the intestine and is expelled by the peristaltic movements of the gut. Ascarid muscle is contracted by acetylcholine. Piperazine has the power to inhibit this response to acetylcholine and may thus depress the worms' movements. Piperazine has been shown also to have a weak neuromuscular blocking action on the skeletal muscle of cats.

It is interesting to note that d-tubocurarine blocks the contraction shown by ascarid muscle to acetylcholine. The ascaris during its normal metabolism produces large quantities of succinic acid, but in the presence of piperazine this succinate production is reduced and this effect is parallel to the acetylcholine blocking action. Worms at all stages of development in the gut are affected but larval forms in the tissues are not. A single dose of piperazine is usually sufficient, but the dose may be repeated if necessary because of the relative freedom from side effects.

Piperazine is given by mouth as the adipate, citrate, hydrate, phosphate or as a complex with carbon disulphide. It is used against *Parascaris equorum*, *Trichonema* and *Oxyuris equi* in the horse, *Ascaris lumbricoides* and the *Œsophagostomum* in pigs and *Ascarids* in dogs. Poultry infested with *Ascaridia* and *Capillaria* are given piperazine hydrate in the feed or water. However, the activity of the various salts of piperazine is due entirely to the piperazine base. Horses are usually given the drug by stomach tube or bran mash; other animals receive it in the form of drenches, tablets, capsules or in the feed.

Thenium closylate is a drug with marked anthelmintic

activity against hookworms in dogs. It is, however, only slightly active against dog ascarids and is given combined with piperazine to treat weaned puppies and dogs infested with both hookworms and roundworms. This combination is usually given as a layered tablet with the Thenium on the inside because it is a bitter-tasting compound. Food is withheld from the dog overnight and the dose is divided into two parts and given separately. Unweaned puppies should be removed from the bitch and fed protein hydrolysate until three hours after treatment. Toxic effects shown as the result

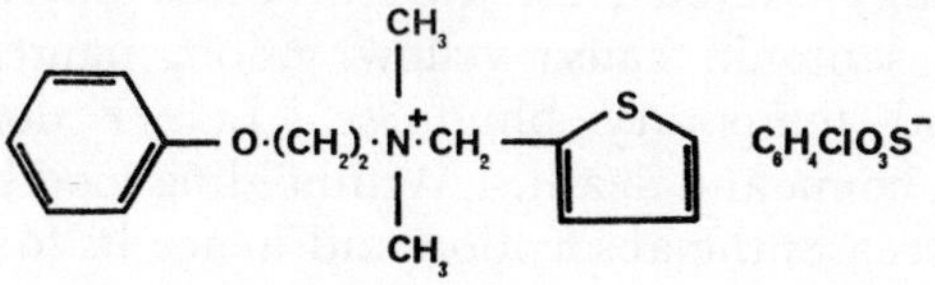

Thenium closylate

Fig. 23.6

of treatment with thenium include vomiting, diarrhœa and muscular weakness.

Sodium fluoride was extensively used to remove ascarids from pigs but has been replaced by piperazine which is as effective and much less toxic.

Cadmium oxide and *anthranilate* were used as ascaricides in pigs but have been replaced by piperazine. *Tetrachlorethylene* was used to treat nematode infestations in sheep, dogs and cats. When used in ruminants it was given by mouth after closing the œsophageal groove with 1 per cent copper sulphate or 10 per cent sodium bicarbonate. In small animals it was given in a gelatin capsule and followed by a saline purge. *Oil of chenopodium* was used for many years in the treatment of ascarid infestations and it is occasionally found as part of a proprietary mixture. It may give rise to toxic effects, being particularly poisonous to cats. The toxic signs include gastroenteritis, muscular incoordination, coma and convulsions. Occasionally dogs treated with this drug develop a permanent deafness.

Barium antimonyl tartrate forms a specific treatment for Gape worms in poultry. The worm (*Syngamus trachea*) is poisoned by contact with this drug. The birds are placed in a closed box and a fine powder of barium antimonyl tartrate is blown in at the rate of 1 oz. per 8 cubic feet. Three exposures are given with intervals of five to fifteen minutes between them, taking a total of thirty minutes for the treatment. During the exposure the box is rocked, making the birds flutter, stirring the powder and causing them to inhale it.

Santonin was used formerly to combat ascarid infestations. It is important now only from a toxicological point of view. In the body santonin is converted into a yellow compound and is not completely excreted for two to three days. Moderate amounts of santonin cause yellow vision, nausea, muscular twitches and temporary blindness. Larger doses produce convulsions, coma and death. Withholding food before giving santonin increases the absorption and hence its toxicity.

DRUGS ACTING ON FLUKES

Carbon tetrachloride

The most practicable method for the control of *Fasciola hepatica* infection in domesticated animals is still the regular use of anthelmintics. Carbon tetrachloride has long been known to be an effective drug against adult liver flukes and its efficiency against immature flukes increases as the dose rate is increased. Pharmacologically, carbon tetrachloride resembles chloroform. After absorption from the alimentary canal it is excreted mainly by the lungs because it is a volatile drug. Some is excreted in the urine, but only 50 per cent of a single dose can be accounted for, as carbon tetrachloride. There is evidence of the excretion of carbon tetrachloride in the bile, but since it has been shown that therapeutic doses damage the liver the anthelmintic action may in fact be due to the liver damage produced by the drug. Only mature flukes are susceptible unless the drug is given in very large doses (0·4 ml./kg.) This makes it necessary to repeat the dose after an interval of one month to give the larvæ time to mature. Carbon tetrachloride is usually considered too dangerous a drug to use in fascioliasis in cattle. However, it is effective against hookworm and ascarids in the dog.

In the United Kingdom it is usual to administer carbon tetrachloride in gelatin capsules. It may be given orally dissolved in liquid paraffin. Carbon tetrachloride has been given also by subcutanteous or intramuscular injection and it has been shown that this route of administration is highly effective. This may be due to the fact that the part of the liver affected by fascioliasis has a better developed arterial blood supply than other parts of the liver and this may allow more carbon tetrachloride to be carried to the fluke-infested parts when the drug is given parenterally than after oral administration. Injections are irritant.

Toxic effects are, unfortunately, not uncommon, even in sheep treated with this drug, and these may be aggravated under various circumstances. Debilitated animals are usually more susceptible. However, since fascioliasis causes debility, it is difficult to avoid treating debilitated animals. Feeding oil cake increases the risk of poisoning, probably due to the additional protein the damaged liver has to metabolise. Such supplementary feeding should stop ten days before the treatment. Calcium deficiency accentuates carbon tetrachloride poisoning. The signs of acute poisoning are those of hypocalcæmia, and treatment, the parenteral administration of calcium borogluconate. Lactating and pregnant ewes are also rather susceptible to tetrachloride poisoning, probably because of the increased demands on their calcium reserves. The chief toxic effect of carbon tetrachloride is the production of fatty changes in the liver.

In view of the various factors which may influence the toxicity of carbon tetrachloride it is generally considered advisable before treating a whole flock of sheep with this drug to carry out what is sometimes called " trial dosing ". This procedure involves administering the drug to a small number of sheep from the flock and carefully observing these animals to see whether any untoward effects develop before proceeding to treat on a larger scale.

Carbon tetrachloride has been used experimentally to produce liver damage, hence this phenomenon has received considerable attention. It appears that various lipoproteins are formed in the liver and extruded into the plasma. The fatty changes which are observed in the liver after exposure to carbon tetrachloride are due to a block of the secretion of triglycerides by the hepatic cells which thus accumulate in the cell. For many years it was thought that the toxicity of carbon tetrachloride was due to its solvent action on the lipids of the cell membrane but as many other compounds which were just as good non-polar solvents as carbon tetrachloride did not show the same degree of liver damage this hypothesis was not tenable. Evidence has accumulated which supports the hypothesis that the oxidation of carbon tetrachloride was involved in some way with its toxic action. It is known, for example, that certain antioxidants protect the liver against damage by carbon tetrachloride and it is now thought that the toxicity of carbon tetrachloride depends to a considerable extent on the cleavage of the carbon to chlorine bond. The hypocalcæmia which is sometimes a consequence of treatment with carbon tetrachloride might be due in part to the accumulation of calcium in the liver. The calcium content of the liver mitochondria may rise to many times the normal level after exposure to this compound.

Although carbon tetrachloride is a reasonably efficient fasciolicide its toxic effects have led to a search for fasciocidal drugs free from this disadvantage and in recent years a number of active agents have been introduced. The available evidence indicates that the new drugs are not completely effective against immature flukes nor are they substantially better than carbon tetrachloride against mature flukes. In the treatment of fascioliasis in sheep, the cost of the drug is an important consideration and it does not appear that carbon tetrachloride will be replaced completely in the near future.

Hexachlorophane was introduced as a remedy for fascioliasis a little over ten years ago. It is given in an oily base by subcutaneous injection or orally dissolved in oil, as an aqueous suspension or in propylene glycol. The subcutaneous injection of this drug often gives rise to a large painful swelling. The effectivity of this drug against immature flukes is not substantially better than that of carbon tetrachloride and in cattle it does not appear to be a great improvement on the established drug hexachlorethane, although it has the advantage of not tainting the flesh or milk. Hexachlorophane has caused death due to biliary occlusion and occasionally produced signs of intoxication. This drug is probably excreted in the bile but more knowledge is required about its fate in the body and in particular what residues are likely to remain. It is a potent bactericide and is used in surgery to disinfect the hands.

Oxyclozanide is a relatively recent introduction into the field of fasciocidal remedies. The main advantage of oxyclozanide over carbon tetrachloride or hexachlorophane is

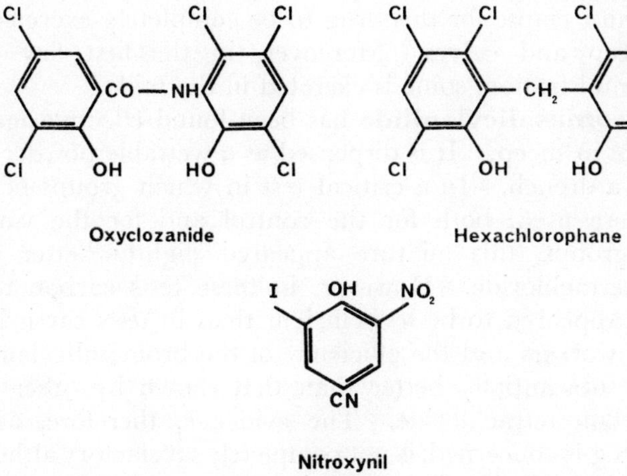

Oxyclozanide   Hexachlorophane

Nitroxynil

FIG, 23.7

Three fascioliacidal agents.

that it appears to be less toxic. This drug is chemically related to hexachlorophane. The main toxic effect described as arising from this drug has been a slight scouring. Oxyclozanide does not taint milk although the milk yield is reduced, particularly when scouring occurs. Oxyclozanide appears to produce a lymphocytopænia. Residues of oxyclozanide have been detected in the tissues of sheep fourteen days after the administration of a single dose. It is recommended that animals treated with this drug should not be slaughtered until at least fourteen days have elapsed since the last dose.

Nitroxynil is a drug used in the treatment of fascioliasis which is more active after intramuscular or subcutaneous injection than after oral administration. Like the other fasciocidal agents it is more effective against the older fluke than the less mature. Deaths have occurred in sheep when twice the effective dose has been given. There is slight local reaction at the site of the injection and, as this drug is a yellow dye, the wool at the site may be stained.

In experimental animals nitroxynil has been shown to raise the blood pressure, increase the respiratory rate and cause a rise in body temperature. Since chemically it is a close relative of dinitrophenol which has well-known stimulating effects on metabolism, nitroxynil may act similarly. Over a month must elapse for this drug to be completely excreted by both sheep and calves. Moreover, in the first few days after administration, some is excreted in the milk.

Tribromosalicylanilide has been found effective against liver fluke in sheep. It is dispensed as a wettable powder and given as a drench. In a critical test in which groups of sick sheep were used, both for the control and for the various treated groups, this mixture appeared slightly better than carbon tetrachloride. However, in these tests carbon tetrachloride appeared to be less efficient than in tests carried out by other workers and the efficiency of the bromosalicylanilide was not substantially better than that shown by other tests with carbon tetrachloride. The evidence, therefore, as far as this drug is concerned, is not completely satisfactory although it is probably more efficient against immature flukes than is carbon tetrachloride.

Two recent introductions into the field of fasciocidal agents are *Clioxanide* and *Nichlopholan*. These drugs resemble nitroxynil in activity, but may be slightly more active and less toxic.

Hexachloroethane is used to treat cattle infested with liver fluke, as it is less liable than carbon tetrachloride to produce toxic effects and is equally effective. The white crystals of hexachloroethane smell like camphor and are given by mouth, usually suspended in water with a suitable dispersing agent. However, only mature flukes are affected by hexachloroethane.

It is slowly absorbed and excreted. A substantial proportion is excreted in the exhaled air and also in the bile; some is excreted in the urine. Tetrachloroethylene and Pentachloroethane are two of the main metabolites of hexachloroethane in the sheep. Substantial amounts can be detected in the tissues 10 days after administration. Although hexachloroethane is less toxic than carbon tetrachloride it also causes appreciable liver damage in therapeutic doses.

Various other untoward effects sometimes occur and some animals show signs of intoxication and muscular incoordination. These toxic effects are amenable to treatment with calcium borogluconate given parenterally. Hexachloroethane taints the milk and may also cause loss of appetite and diarrhœa. A high protein diet pre-disposes the animal to these various toxic effects. Flukes in the rumen, abomasum and duodenum of cattle are also susceptible to hexachloroethane.

Tetrachlorodifluoroethane has been given by all routes of administration as a 50 per cent solution in liquid paraffin. It has been claimed to be an effective cure for fascioliasis but the evidence is incomplete.

Carbon disulphide is given to horses to remove bots (gastric myiasis) and ascarids. It is effective against the stomach worm in pigs. This volatile, irritant liquid is most effective when given after food has been withheld. Unfortunately, fasting increases the drug's toxicity. The toxic effects produced include laryngeal spasm and depression of the central nervous system.

SUGGESTIONS FOR FURTHER READING

BORAY, J. C. and HAPPICH F. A. (1968). Standardized chemotherapeutical tests for immature and mature *Fasciola hepatica* infections in sheep. *Aust. vet. J.*, **44**, 72.

BORAY, J. C., HAPPICH, F. A. and ANDREWS, J. C. (1967). Comparative chemotherapeutic tests in sheep. *Vet. Rec.*, **80**, 218.

GIBSON, T. E. (1962). *Veterinary Anthelmintic Medication.* Commonwealth Agric. Bureau., England.

GIBSON, T. E. (1965–66). Anthelmintics. *Vet. A.*, **7**, 291.

GIBSON, T. E. (1966–67). Anthelmintics. *Vet. A.*, **8**, 264.

STANDEN, O. D. (1963). Chemotherapy of helminthic infections. In *Experimental Chemotherapy*, ed. Schnitzer, R. J. and Hawking, F., Vol. I. New York: Academic Press.

CHAPTER XXIV

CHEMOTHERAPY OF INSECT INFESTATIONS

INSECTICIDES

DRUGS used to kill insect parasites on the surface of the body, on plants and on inanimate objects are termed insecticides. Insects are important in veterinary medicine, as they not only produce pathological effects by damaging the tissues but act as the transmitting agents in certain specific diseases. Lice, fleas, keds, ticks, mange mites and ringworm fungi are important skin parasites in veterinary medicine and are destroyed by the application of sprays, dips, lotions or ointments containing the active ingredients.

Insecticides are said to have a " knock down " effect when insects are immobilised immediately on contact. Insects may recover from this immobilisation. Insecticides whose effect persists for several weeks are said to have a " residual action ". Insecticides which act when the insect eats them are called " stomach poisons ", and those acting when the insect gets some on its cuticle are " contact " poisons. Contact poisons usually are soluble in the lipoid which is present in the insect cuticle and are soluble in fats and fat solvents.

Sulphur, oil and inorganic arsenic have been used against insects from the earliest times. However, more recently a number of chlorinated hydrocarbons have been shown to possess powerful insecticidal properties.

Chlorinated Hydrocarbon Insecticides

Dicophane (DDT), a chlorinated hydrocarbon, exists as white, pleasant-smelling crystals soluble in organic solvents but not in water. It is a stable, non-volatile compound usually requiring to be mixed with a " wetting " agent.

Dicophane was used extensively as a dusting powder or

in aqueous suspension against most external parasites of animals; however, it has been superceded to a considerable extent. The solutions of dicophane in oil used for spraying dairies and similar structures must not be used on animals.

The main use of this drug is as a residual insecticide for the control of house flies, stable flies, buffalo flies, tsetse flies

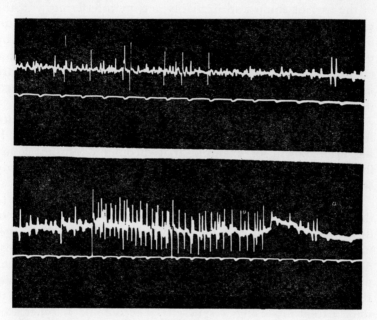

FIG, 24.1

Action potentials recorded from a cockroach nerve, Upper tracing untreated insect, lower tracing after treatment with dicophane. (Adapted from Brown, A. W. A. 1963, *Chemical Injuries* from: *Insect Pathology*, Vol, I, ed. E. A. Steinhaus, Academic Press: New York, London.)

and mosquitoes. Dicophane is active against flies, lice and fleas. It is valueless against mange mites.

Dicophane acts on insects mainly as a contact poison but may act also as a stomach poison on ingestion by the insect.

The drug is particularly well absorbed by the insect's chitinous cuticle, and the susceptibility of the insect to the poison depends largely on this relatively selective absorption.

The main difference between the response of insects and mammals to dicophane is due to the failure of mammals to absorb this compound through the skin, unless it is in an oily solution, and to the increased susceptibility of insect nerves (Fig. 24.1).

Dicophane appears to act by interfering with the transmission of the nervous impulse. It increases the negative after-potential of the insect nerve but does not affect the nerve of the frog or squid and probably acts by interfering with the efflux of potassium from the nerve. The sensory and motor fibres of the insect's peripheral nervous system are affected by dicophane, causing the insect to become excitable, lose coordination and develop convulsive movements which are followed by general paralysis and death. Some insects develop a resistance to dicophane.

Most of the resistance to dicophane is due to the presence in the insect of a specific enzyme DDT dehydrochlorinase. It has been shown, for example, that dicophane-resistant house flies have very high concentrations of this enzyme in the body whereas susceptible strains do not.

However, this enzyme is not the sole cause of resistance to dicophane. It has been shown, for example, that nerves of flies resistant to dicophane only produce motor discharges in the presence of high concentrations of this drug; whereas nerves from susceptible flies produce motor discharges in the presence of comparatively low concentrations of dicophane. Resistance due to dehydrochlorinase can be overcome to some extent by using a synergist. Dicophane is synergistic with N-di-n-butyl-p-chlorobenzene sulphonamide because this latter compound specifically inhibits the dehydrochlorinase.

When dicophane is absorbed by mammals the central nervous system is mainly affected. The animals show convulsions of cortical or cerebellar origin, the spinal cord and myoneural junctions being unaffected. The myocardium is sensitised so that ventricular fibrillation may develop and liver damage may also occur.

Dicophane may be absorbed from the mammalian gut when in the presence of fat and fat solvents. After absorption it is found in all the tissues but especially in fat, where it is stored. An animal may store several lethal doses without showing signs of poisoning until or unless it has to draw on the fat depots and so bring enough dicophane into the circulation to produce the characteristic toxic effects. About half the accumulated dicophane is stored for more than three months. The milk fat is a major excretory route for dicophane. Lactating animals excrete dicophane in the butter fat and this constitutes a public health hazard, especially to infants. The dicophane stored in fat represents about one-quarter the amount absorbed. Most of the metabolites of dicophane are excreted in the bile.

Dicophane is metabolised by mammals and some insects to DDA (Bis (p-chlorophenyl) acetic acid) and some is converted

DDA
Dichlorodiphenylacetic acid

DDD
Dichloro-di(p-chlorophenyl)ethane

Dicophane (DDT)

FIG, 24.2
Dicophane and two major metabolites.

to DDD (2, 2-bis (p-chlorophenyl) 1, 1-dichloroethane). The compound DDD is also insecticidal. This latter conversion which can be accomplished by invertebrates and micro-organisms can cause DDD to be found when Dicophane was the insecticide primarily used. DDD is found in high concentration in the adrenal and can cause damage to this gland. Derivatives of DDD have been used to produce pharmacological adrenalectomy. Dicophane is not well metabolised by soil organisms and hence can persist on pastures.

Dicophane has interesting actions on certain liver enzymes reminiscent of the activity of phenobarbitone in affecting drug metabolism. It causes hepatomegaly and this increase in size of the liver is associated with an increase in the activity of certain liver enzymes and a decrease in the activity of others. This observation may be of importance in that most drugs are metabolised by the liver enzymes hence the presence of dicophane may affect the metabolism of other drugs.

Methoxychlor is one of the least toxic of the halogenated hydrocarbon insecticides. It exists as a white crystalline solid, soluble in organic solvents, and is used as a dusting powder or with a wetting agent as a suspension.

This drug is not stored in the tissues because it is rapidly metabolised, hence only traces are excreted in the milk. Methoxychlor has a faster " knock-down " effect than dicophane but not so fast as pyrethrum. Its residual action resembles that of dicophane. It is less toxic than dicophane and does not damage the liver. Only small amounts of methoxychlor are stored in the fat and these are eliminated in ten weeks.

Benzene hexachloride as the gamma isomer is a widely used insecticide. This white crystalline powder has a slightly musty odour which prevents its use around meat, eggs and milk intended for human consumption.

Moreover, possible hazards due to the presence of residues in meat and milk have led to the use of this drug being curtailed in the U.S.A., Australia and New Zealand. Technical quality of benzene hexzchloride contains the β isomer which persists in the body very much longer than the γ isomer. It is nearly insoluble in water but dissolves in alcohol and is available as a " wettable " powder, an emulsion, a dusting powder and in solution. Benzene hexachloride is ten to twenty times as toxic to insects as dicophane, and although its insecticidal action is slow, it is faster than that of dicophane.

Resistance to benzene hexachloride has been observed on several occasions and studied in some detail in house flies. Resistance to this drug appears to be directly proportional to the rate at which the flies metabolise the compound. It is also inversely proportional to the rate at which the drug is absorbed through the cuticle.

Benzene hexachloride is absorbed to a limited extent from the skin, respiratory tract and gut, absorption being increased by fats and fat solvents. After absorption the drug accumulates in fatty tissue and is slowly excreted in the urine, fæces and milk.

This drug has a similar effect on the central nervous system to dicophane, producing convulsions which may be controlled by sodium pentobarbitone and calcium boro-gluconate given intravenously. The pathological changes produced by benzene hexachloride are similar to those of dicophane, excepting the liver damage is greater and the renal tubules are involved. Calves under three months old, emaciated sheep, cats and turkeys are especially susceptible to poisoning by benzene hexachloride. It is used to kill mange mites, fleas, lice and ticks.

Chlordane acts both as a stomach and contact poison to insects. It is a viscous, odourless, amber liquid, insoluble in water but soluble in fats and fat solvents. In the presence of alkalies this compound is dehalogenated and so inactivated. It is more volatile than dicophane and does not persist for more than four weeks. Chlordane has a similar effect on mammals to dicophane but is only three-fifths as toxic. The vapour of chlordane is more toxic because it may be absorbed through the intact skin.

Dieldrin is a stomach and contact insect poison. Its use is not permitted in the United Kingdom. It is particularly effective against the larvæ of the sheep blowfly (*Lucilia*), persisting in the fleece for four months. Dieldrin is active also against screw worms (*Calliphora*) and lice but less active than gamma benzene hexachloride against ticks, mange mites and keds. Insects resistant to dicophane and benzene hexachloride are often susceptible to dieldrin. The persistence of dieldrin in the fleece is due to its diffusion along the wool fibre into the growing zone. Dicophane and similar compounds do not have this property. Aldrin and toxaphene are insecticides similar to dieldrin. Aldrin is used as a sheep dip and its effects last about three months.

In the mammalian body aldrin is converted into dieldrin. The restrictions which apply to dieldrin apply also to aldrin. Fish and birds are particularly susceptible to poisoning by these chlorinated hydrocarbons.

Toxaphene is four times as toxic as dicophane and not suitable to use on dogs. Its main use is as a spray or dip for cattle. Toxaphene is a yellow waxy solid insoluble in water but soluble in fat solvents. It is probably the most toxic chlorinated hydrocarbon insecticide. On absorption it is fixed by the tissues and takes three or four months for elimination. It causes chronic poisoning due mainly to liver damage.

ORGANOPHOSPHORUS INSECTICIDES

The persistence in the body of most of the chlorinated hydrocarbon insecticides led to the search for less persistent, equally potent and more specific drugs. Although some of the most toxic chemicals known are organophosphorus compounds developed for use as war gases it has been possible to prepare organophosphorus compounds with insecticidal properties which are substantially less toxic than the chlorinated hydrocarbons.

Several theories have been propagated to explain the action of these insecticides; none is completely satisfactory. Although an explanation in terms of cholinesterase inhibition has not been established conclusively this seems to be the most likely. Moreover, it is this inhibition of cholinesterase which is responsible for most of the toxic effects these compounds produce in mammals. All organisms so far studied have been shown to hydrolyse organophosphorus compounds but differ markedly in the rate at which this hydrolysis proceeds. In mammals the insecticidal organosphorus compounds are hydrolysed rapidly whereas in insects the hydrolysis takes much longer; the insecticide malathion is degraded sixteen times faster by the mouse than by the house fly. The products of the hydrolysis of organophosphorus compounds are usually non-toxic and do not inhibit cholinesterase. Certain organophosphorus compounds only inhibit cholinesterase after they have been converted into an active compound; this is the case with the phosphorothionates.

Parathion was the first organic phosphorus insecticide used in agriculture. It is a rapid-acting contact insecticide whose activity persists for several days. The toxicity to mammals is high, and it is essential for them to avoid external contact with this drug or its inhalation.

Malathion (O, O dimethyl dithiophosphate of diethylmercapto succinate) has a high toxicity to insects and a relatively low toxicity to mammals. Its activity against flies persists for three weeks.

Resistance to malathion is encountered not infrequently and in many instances has been shown to be due to the insect

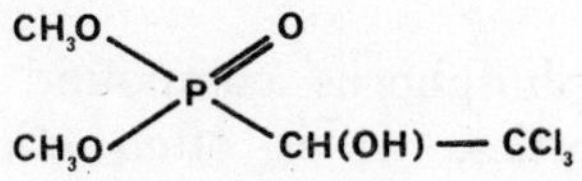

CH₃O large structure

Metriphonate

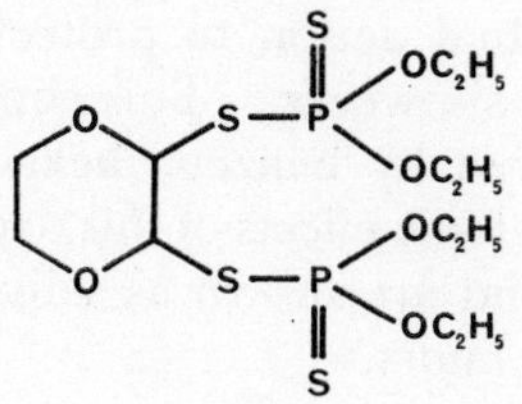

Dioxathion

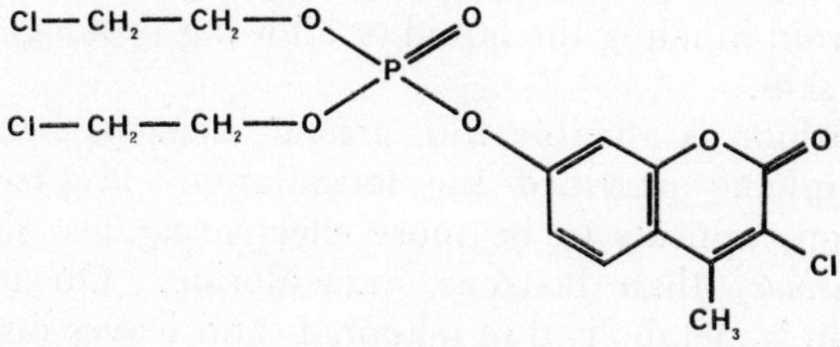

Haloxon

FIG, 24.3
The formulæ of three organophosphorus compounds,

developing a specific esterase which hydrolyses malathion very rapidly. Malathion is used in animal houses and dairies but not on animals. Since this substance is an anti-cholinesterase the toxic effects in mammals include salivation, depression, bradycardia and muscular tremors. The antidote is, of course, an injection of atropine.

However, in recent years several more specific and less toxic organophosphorus compounds have been developed, some of which have been introduced into veterinary practice.

Dioxathion

This organophosphorus compound has insecticidal and acaricidal properties. It is often effective against insects which have become resistant to the halogenated hydrocarbon insecticides. Dioxathion is used mainly against cattle ticks but is also active against ticks of other species, mites, keds and the sheep blow-fly. It is applied as a spray or dip and has sufficient residual action to protect against re-infestation by ticks for five to six weeks. This compares favourably with the protection given by benzene hexachloride which is only three weeks. The toxic effects of this drug are due to inhibition of cholinesterase and are shown as salivation, diarrhœa, colic, lacrimation and tremors.

Atropine in doses three to four times the normal therapeutic dose is a specific remedy for toxicity due to cholinesterase inhibition, because the lethal effects are cardiac inhibition and vascular dilation and these are prevented by atropine. It is important that the person operating the spray or dip should avoid inhaling the liquid or allowing prolonged contact with the skin.

Dioxathion is miscible with arsenic, benzene hexachloride and toxaphene provided the formulations are compatible. Dioxathion, appears to be more effective against sheep ticks (*Ixodes ricinus*) than benzene hexachloride. On absorption dioxathion is metabolised in mammals and leaves insignificant residues in the tissues.

Metriphonate

This organophosphorus compound has both insecticidal and anthelmintic activity, the latter properties have been discussed (p. 283). It is used against parasites which do not multiply in or on the host and is effective either when applied directly to the skin or given orally. The most valuable action of this drug is in the treatment of warble fly (*Hypoderma* species), screw worms (*Cochliomyia* species) and nuche (*Dermatobia hominis*). It is usual to apply Metriphonate locally as a 2 per cent solution at 500 ml./200 kg. body weight by means of a brush so as to ensure a thorough wetting of the skin. This drug does not persist on the skin hence it has no residual effect. It is rapidly decomposed in the body so that residues in the tissues from the use of this compound do not constitute a hazard. Cattle should not be treated for warble fly during the months of December, January and February because at this period the migrating larvæ are in the region of the spinal cord and if killed in this situation may give rise to local tissue changes which may involve the spinal cord. Metriphonate may be given by mouth for the treatment of bots in horses and also given by this route may expel the larvæ of *Œstrus ovis* from the nasal cavity of sheep. It has been claimed that the larvæ of the warble fly when killed in the host tissue may act as an antigen and produce a degree of immunity. There have been reports of allergic responses resulting from sensitisation of the animal by the killed warble fly larvæ. The rapid absorption of Metriphonate from the alimentary tract may, in certain animals, give rise to toxic effects. These are due to inhibition of cholinesterase and can be treated by atropine.

Fenchlorophos is an organophosphorus compound which can be applied locally or given by mouth for the treatment of infestation by *Hypoderma* species in cattle and screw worm (*Cochliomyia* species). Sufficient of this drug is absorbed even after local application to kill the migrating larvæ of these insects. It is effective also against infestations by lice, mites, ticks and fleas in dogs and cats. Given orally and applied topically to dogs infected with demodectic mange at intervals of three days it has affected a cure in a number of cases. When used in cats this drug should only be given as a local application, oral administration usually causes toxic effects in this species.

Residues of the drug have been found in the mesenteric fat, heart and brain seven days after administration hence it is advisable that animals treated with fenchlorophos should be allowed a longer interval than seven days between the time of last treatment and slaughter. Fifty per cent of the drug administered can be accounted for as various metabolites excreted in the urine. Fenchlorophos has an anthelmintic action against certain species of nematodes in ruminants.

Coumaphos and *Crufomate* are organophosphorus compounds of value in the treatment of warble fly (*Hypoderma*) in cattle, and ectoparasites of sheep, pigs and poultry. They are applied externally but are absorbed from the skin; residues persist in the tissue for over seven days after administration. These drugs can also be shown in the milk during the first twenty-four hours after treatment. It is recommended, therefore, that milking cows should not be treated with these drugs, and, with animals intended for slaughter, at least seven days should elapse between the last treatment and slaughter. Coumaphos has some anthelmintic action against sheep nematodes.

Dimpylate is a phosphorothionate hence it is only active after conversion in the body. With phosphorothionates both the chemotherapeutic and the toxic effects, if any, may be manifest only after a delay due to the time necessary for this conversion. Dimpylate is absorbed through the skin to some extent after local application; however, toxic effects are rare. The main use of this drug is as a spray or dip in the treatment of infestations of cattle, sheep and dogs with lice or ticks. It exerts a residual action for as long as twenty weeks after the application and is particularly useful in the treatment and prevention of infestations of sheep with the blow-fly (*Lucilia*). This drug should not be used in the treatment of dairy cattle.

OTHER INSECTICIDES

Pyrethrum

Pyrethrins are the active principles of pyrethrum flowers, which have long been known to possess insecticidal activity. These substances are resins which dissolve in fat solvents. The most important property is their rapid action or " knock down effect ". House flies are paralysed on contact. The pyrethrins stimulate the insect's nervous system causing muscular excitement, convulsions, paralysis and death. They have no residual effect nor do they act as stomach poisons, but they are more

expensive than most other insecticides. Sunlight rapidly inactivates the pyrethrins, but this inactivation is decreased by
the use of an oily vehicle such as kerosene.

There are a number of substances which act synergistically
with pyrethrum such as piperonyl butoxide. These synergists
appear to act by inhibiting the detoxication of pyrethrins in
the insect. They not only potentiate the effect of pyrethrum
but in those insects in which pyrethrum resistance is due to
increased detoxication the use of a synergist enables pyrethrum
to be employed against these insects. The pyrethrins possess
another important advantage in that they are the least
toxic to mammals of all insecticides.

Derris

Derris eliptica, a plant grown in the East Indies and Amazon
basin, has been for many years the source of an important
insecticide. The powdered root of the plant is used as the
insecticide and owes its action to the active principle *Rotenone*.
Derris was probably first used to catch fish by poisoning them.
As an insecticide the powdered root is mixed with a suitable
inert diluent such as talc to give a 1 per cent powder. Derris
is only active against certain insects, and in veterinary practice
was used mainly against the larvæ of the warble fly. However,
for this purpose it has largely been replaced by the organophosphorus compounds. It acts on insects as both a contact
and a stomach poison.

Rotenone inhibits the oxidation of pyruvate and glutamate
and its activity may be due to this inhibition although it does
not explain why rotenone is so toxic to fish and insects and not
to mammals. Derris is usually harmless to mammals, but
the fresh root may be toxic. It is not absorbed through the
skin, but small amounts taken by mouth or inhalation cause
vomiting in dogs and cats. When dissolved in oil it is more
likely to be absorbed and cause poisoning. Derris is less
rapid and more persistent than the pyrethrins, but it is less
stable and readily destroyed by light, oxygen and alkalies.

Carbaryl (1-naphthyl N-methyl carbamate) is one of the
more popular members of the *carbamate* group of insecticides.
The carbamates are generally considered to be more specific
insecticides than the organochlorine or organophosphorus

compounds. These drugs appear to act by inhibiting the cholinesterase of the insects' nerve cord. Carbaryl is useful in the treatment of poultry infested with mites and is active against other blood-sucking arthropods. Even after oral administration carbaryl does not appear to leave residues in the tissues. House flies and cockroaches possess a carbamate esterase which enables them to resist the action of these insecticides. However, it has been shown that by using a mixture of two carbamates even these insects could be killed.

Benzyl benzoate is used to control sarcoptic and follicular mange in dogs and cats and sarcoptic mange in man and horses. It is a clear oily liquid, insoluble in water but soluble in fat solvents. An emulsion containing 20 or 30 per cent or a solution in alcohol is available for application externally. A local anæsthetic to alleviate itching, dicophane or gamma benzene hexachloride, may be added to these preparations. Benzyl benzoate produces toxic effects if too large an area of skin is dressed too often. These toxic effects include nausea, vomiting, purging, and respiratory and cardiac depression.

Monosulfiram (tetraethylthiuram monosulphide) is an organic sulphur compound used mainly to combat sarcoptic and demodectic mange in dogs, cattle and horses, but is active also against fleas, lice, ticks and mites. It is used as a 1 to 2 per cent emulsion or 25 per cent solution. The pure substance exists as a yellow crystalline solid soluble in fat solvents and containing 37 per cent sulphur.

Sulphur as sublimed sulphur or as lime sulphur was widely used as a dip for cattle, sheep and horses affected with psoroptic and chorioptic mange, and for cattle, sheep, horses, pigs and dogs with sarcoptic mange. The animals treated by these preparations should be dipped or thoroughly washed in a solution containing not less than 2 per cent lime sulphur at 100° F. Two dippings at seven-day intervals are required for psoroptic and chorioptic mange. Sarcoptic mange requires four dippings.

Ointments containing sulphur are used to kill skin parasites of the dog and cat. Inorganic preparations of sulphur have now been replaced by the newer insecticides which are more effective and easier to use.

Arsenic was, until recently, the main insecticide used as a dip against ticks. It is still used in some countries for reasons of economy. Arsenical dips have very little residual action and, therefore, need to be repeated at suitable intervals, depending on the tick's life cycle. Improper disposal of such dips may allow domesticated animals to ingest toxic quantities of arsenic.

SUGGESTIONS FOR FURTHER READING

BEESLEY, W. N. (1965–66). Insecticides in veterinary work. *Vet. A.*, **7**, 284.

BROWN, A. W. A., (1963). Chemical injuries. In *Insect Pathology*, ed. Steinhaus E. A., Vol. I. New York: Academic Press.

DAVIES, D. R. (1963). Neurotoxicity of organophosphorus compounds. *In Handb. exp. Pharmak.*, **15**, 860.

METCALF, R. L. (1967). Mode of action of insecticide synergists. *A. Rev. Ent.*, **12**, 229.

O'BRIEN, R. D. (1966). Mode of action of insecticides. *A. Rev. Ent.*, **11**, 369.

WEST, T. F. and HARDY, J. E. (1961). *Chemical Control of Insects*, 2nd ed. London: Chapman & Hall.

CHAPTER XXV

DISINFECTANTS

THE terms disinfectant and antiseptic are usually regarded as synonymous; disinfectant is commonly employed when referring to a drug used to kill micro-organisms on inanimate objects and antiseptic when the drug is applied to the skin and living tissue. The agents considered here are those which may be applied locally to tissues in the treatment of infections caused by pathogenic micro-organisms. However, it is customary to employ disinfectants to reduce the potentially pathogenic micro-organisms present on the surgeon's or animal's skin prior to surgery and agents used for this purpose are considered.

Bacteria are destroyed by heat, light and osmotic pressure, moist heat being better than dry heat. Steam at 115° C. for thirty minutes destroys all life including spores. The disinfectant properties of sunlight are due to its ultra-violet rays. The disinfectant action of osmotic pressure is used to prevent the decomposition of jam, strawberries and salted fish.

There are a large number of chemical compounds used as disinfectants. The number is large because no single substance is a suitable disinfectant for all purposes. An ideal disinfectant should have a high activity against all organisms, and this activity should persist on dilution. The ideal disinfectant should not injure tissues, otherwise healing might be delayed by attempts to disinfect a wound. Disinfectants should be efficient in the presence of organic matter and should penetrate tissue crevices and infected debris; no disinfectant will penetrate sweat glands. Other properties desirable in a disinfectant include solubility in water, stability and cheapness. Disinfectants should not corrode metallic objects and should be chemically compatible with other drugs. It may be an advantage if the disinfectant discolours skin when used to prepare the site of a surgical operation.

The effectiveness of a disinfection is usually tested by finding the dilution which has the same effect as a 1 per cent solution of phenol on a test organism. If the disinfectant under test killed the bacteria in a concentration of 0·1 per cent whereas with phenol 1·0 per cent was required, the disinfectant would be said to have a phenol coefficient of 10.

The test organism is usually *Salmonella typhi*, although sometimes *Bacillus subtilis* is used because this latter organism sporulates and thus presents a more severe test organism. The result of this comparison is called the Phenol or Rideal Walker Coefficient of the disinfectant under test. The determination of the Phenol Coefficient was studied by Chick

TABLE 25.1

The Phenol Coefficients of some Common Disinfectants	
Compound	Phenol Coefficient
Phenol	1
Chlorocresol	12
Phenylmercuric nitrate	250
Cetrimide	150
Benzalkonium chloride	130

and Martin, who found that it was affected by factors such as temperature, duration of action, species and number of bacteria and the presence of organic matter. They devised a more elaborate test in which autoclaved fæces were added to the disinfectant under investigation, but this did not remove all the sources of error and the ideal test remains to be discovered.

Tests such as those described give only a rough idea of the potency of a disinfectant and are most useful when comparing disinfectants of a similar chemical series, for example the phenols. An example of the results of such tests are shown in Table 25·1. They give no indication of the suitability or otherwise of the disinfectant for application to tissues. The activities of disinfectants are sometimes compared by means of the D value. This is taken as the time required for a particular concentration of the disinfectant under test to kill 90 per cent of the test organisms.

The effect of organic matter on a disinfectant is important

X

as some disinfectants such as the halogens are inactivated by it. The activity of most disinfectants is also influenced by the pH of the solution. The concentration at which a disinfectant acts influences the choice, since any substance which kills bacteria is likely to have some damaging action on tissue cells. For example, the caustic action of strong acids and alkalies makes them useless as disinfectants to apply to tissues. Some tissue damage is caused by phenol and cresol when used in bactericidal concentrations, and superficial damage is produced by the disinfectants which precipitate proteins, as these substances do not discriminate between bacterial protein and tissue protein. Alcohol, formaldehyde and mercuric chloride are examples of the latter type of disinfectant. It is desirable, therefore, for a disinfectant to act in low concentration, and in this respect the salts of heavy metals are better than the derivatives of coal tar such as phenol.

It is important to appreciate the time taken by a disinfectant to kill bacteria. The quickest-acting are the oxidising and reducing agents and the halogens. In contrast the heavy metals are amongst the slowest, for example, $\frac{1}{2}$ per cent mercuric iodide or chloride does not kill staphylococci in fifteen minutes. The dyestuff disinfectants act slowly.

The bacterial cell membrane acts as an osmotic barrier and the osmotic pressure within the organism is quite high. The bacterial cell wall of Gram-positive organisms is comparatively rigid and more resistant to rupture than that of Gram-negative organisms. The cell wall is also the location of many important enzymes hence damage to the membrane can result in the inhibition of important enzymes and/or changes in the permeability of the wall causing leakage of metabolites and thus interfering with the metabolism of the organism.

Halogen Disinfectants

Chlorine and *iodine* are widely used as disinfectants. Chloride and iodide ions have no antibacterial action. Chlorine has a phenol coefficient of 200 and is used to sterilise water. It is quickly inactivated by organic matter and alkaline solutions, whereas ammonia increases its activity. The disinfectant action of chlorine is due to the formation of hypochlorous acid. Bleaching powder disinfects by releasing chlorine and a solution of bleaching powder and boric acid, " Eusol ", was used to disinfect wounds. The boric acid buffers the solution, preventing it becoming too acid. These simple sources of chlorine have been replaced by substances such as *Chloramine T* and *Dichloramine T*, which liberate chlorine slowly until they come in contact with protein.

The chloramines are less potent than chlorine but exert a more prolonged action. In addition to its oxidising action on bacterial protein, chlorine probably also acts by halogenating amino groups on bacterial protein. Chloramine T can be used to irrigate wounds and does not retard healing. Dichloramine T is much less water soluble and is used in ointments. *Iodine* is as efficient a disinfectant as chlorine, has a counter-irritant effect and is the best disinfectant for catgut. Iodine acts quickly but is quickly inactivated by tissue and other protein. Solutions of iodine in alcohol and potassium iodide are used to disinfect the skin. These solutions impart a yellow colour to the skin which disappears as colourless iodides are formed.

Iodophors are substances in which iodine forms a complex with a suitable carrier so that free iodine is liberated in solution. These preparations are used mainly as skin antiseptics although it has been shown that a 1 per cent solution of iodine in 70 per cent ethanol is better. When applied to wounds and abrasions iodophors are less painful than simple solutions of iodine. Undecoylium chloride-iodine is such an agent which has potential value as a skin antispetic.

HEAVY METAL DISINFECTANTS

Simple salts of *mercury*, and *silver*, are used as disinfectants. Their action is mainly bacteriostatic. They act slowly and in high dilution, probably by reacting with sulphydryl groups on bacterial enzymes. *Mercuric chloride* has the greatest immediate action and was a widely used skin disinfectant. The *nitrate* and *oxide of mercury* are used as disinfectants in the form of ointment. Mercurous nitrate gives an active, irritant, antiseptic effect whilst the oxide of mercury is so mild an antiseptic as to be quite suitable to apply as an ointment to the eye. An ointment of the red iodide of mercury is a very active blister or counter-irritant. Various organic compounds of mercury act as disinfectants without liberating mercury ions. *Thiomersalate* (merthiolate) and *phenyl mercuric nitrate* are active substances suitable to use as disinfectants on the skin, wounds and instruments. The latter compound of mercury is sometimes used as a preservative in solutions intended for injection.

The salts of silver used as antiseptics fall into two groups, those liberating free silver ions and the non-ionising preparations. The latter are non-corrosive, non-irritant and non-astringent. The silver salt liberating free silver ions which is usually employed is silver nitrate but it tends to be rather irritant. The non-ionising preparations are compounds of silver with protein; these are non-corrosive, non-irritant and non-astringent.

Oxidising and Reducing Disinfectants

Various oxidising agents have disinfectant properties. Chlorine, although an oxidising agent, has already been discussed. *Hydrogen peroxide* releases oxygen when in contact with the enzyme catalase. The effect is increased by the presence of copper or iron. It kills most bacteria, *E. coli* being killed in sixty minutes by a one-in-ten dilution of a ten-volume solution of hydrogen peroxide. The mechanical effect of the bubbles of oxygen released by hydrogen peroxide when applied to tissues is valuable in breaking up scabs and in removing dressings. Liberated oxygen, unfortunately, does not affect all organisms.

Potassium permanganate is an oxidising agent whose germicidal powers are selective. The purple crystals of this substance give a pink-coloured solution in water. It is used as a deodorant.

Formaldehyde is an irritant gas which, as a 40 per cent solution in water, is called *Formalin* and kills most organisms when diluted one part in eighty parts water. It is unaffected by organic matter and disinfects by combining with amino groups on the surface of the bacterial cell. Formalin is used to make toxoids from bacterial toxins. In acid solutions formaldehyde is liberated from *Hexamine*. When this drug is given by mouth it is excreted in the urine, and, provided the urine is acid, disinfects the urinary tract.

DISINFECTANT ACIDS AND ALKALIES

Caustic soda and *quick-lime* are used to disinfect buildings but corrode tissues.

Mandelic acid is a bactericidal agent in acid media and is sometimes used as a urinary antiseptic, for which purpose it is given by mouth either as the calcium salt or as *Methenamine mandelate*. It exerts its action in the urinary tract and bladder provided the urine has an appropriately low *p*H.

PHENOL AND DERIVATIVES

By using phenol as the principal agent in antiseptic surgery, Lord Lister ensured this drug's popularity for many years, despite many surgeons and their patients developing phenol poisoning. It is no longer used except as a comparison for other disinfectants.

Phenol acts quickly : a solution of 2 per cent phenol kills *S. typhi* in ten seconds. Concentrations below 0·5 per cent have no disinfectant properties and bacteria can grow in them. Phenol is more soluble in fats than water and probably acts on bacteria by dissolving in the lipoids of the cell surface. Sodium chloride increases the disinfectant power of phenol solution by making the phenol less water-soluble and so increasing the rate of solution in the cell lipoid. Alcohol, by increasing the solubility of phenol in water, has the opposite effect. Phenol probably kills bacteria by combining with their protein. It is unaffected by organic matter. The main disadvantages are its toxicity and loss of activity on dilution.

Phenol is absorbed from mucous membranes, wounds and intact skin. It is partly oxidised in the body to hydroxyphenols and hydroquinone. Phenol is excreted in the urine as these oxidation products and in combination with sulphuric and glucuronic acids which give the urine a dark colour. Strong solutions are caustic and cause necrosis of all tissues with which they come in contact.

The addition of a methyl group to phenol gives *cresol* of which there are three isomers. These are less water-soluble than phenol and more powerful disinfectants. A mixture of cresols dispersed in water with the aid of soap, " Lysol " is useful for disinfecting instruments. It is less toxic than phenol, more powerful and unaffected by organic matter; however, it is unsuitable for application to living tissues.

Chlorocresol is made by the introduction of chlorine into the cresol molecule. This gives a disinfectant similar to cresol but ten times more powerful. It is sometimes used as a preservative in solutions intended for injection. *Chloroxylenol* dispersed in water with soap makes a very effective disinfectant, less irritant than cresol in soap and suitable for application to the intact skin. This solution has a phenol coefficient of three and is effective in a dilution of 1 : 50.

DISINFECTANT DYESTUFFS

Various dyestuffs are important for their disinfectant properties. Basic dyes are more active antiseptics than acidic dyestuffs. The dyestuffs used as disinfectants are usually derivatives of triphenylmethane or of acridine. The triphenylmethane dyes act by interfering with the glutamic acid metabolism of the micro-organism whereas the acridines inhibit synthetic processes of the micro-organisms by intercalating with the DNA molecule.

Brilliant Green and *Gentian Violet* are triphenylmethane derivatives which both stain and kill Gram-positive bacteria but are inactive against Gram-negative organisms. Serum decreases the activity of these dyes and streptococci resist Gentian Violet.

Acriflavine is a mixture of variable composition derived from acridine and existing as a water-soluble orange powder. It has a phenol coefficient of several hundred and is not inhibited by serum. Acriflavine acts slowly in low concentration and does not affect phagocytosis. However, prolonged applications of this drug delay healing.

Proflavine hemisulphate is the most important acridine disinfectant, being a pure substance of constant composition and less irritant than acriflavine, a 1/1000 dilution has no effect on the exposed rabbit brain. The solution of this salt is acid and requires to be neutralised. It is active in the presence of pus. The acridines appear to act as cations which compete with hydrogen ions for receptors in the tissues of bacteria.

NEWER ORGANIC ANTISEPTICS

The Nitrofurans are a group of compounds which possess antibacterial activity against a wide range of organisms. *Furazolidone* has particularly marked activity against *Salmonella* sp. and *Shigella* sp. *Nitrofurazone* is bactericidal to both Gram-positive and Gram-negative organisms; both *Furazolidone* and *Nitrofurazone* have activity against coccidia (p. 254).

The Nitrofurans are used for their antiseptic properties either by local application or given systemically. The latter route is used mainly for the treatment of infections of the urinary tract. Their activity as local antiseptics is reduced in the presence of plasma. Resistance to the *Nitrofurans* is rare: however, they may exhibit some toxic effects such as depression in growth, neurotoxic actions and inhibition of spermatogenesis.

In the body these compounds are metabolised by reduction of the nitro group and subsequent acetylation. They inhibit a number of enzymes such as pyruvic oxidase and aldehyde dehydrogenase.

The nitrofurans are preferentially reduced by the micro-organisms and thus deprive the bacterial cell of the energy required for its growth.

Nitrofurazone is a potent bacteriostatic in a concentration of 1 : 200,000; higher concentrations are bactericidal to both Gram-positive and Gram-negative organisms. The activity of this drug is reduced by the presence of plasma and blood. The bacteria which are resistant to the sulphonamides and antibiotics usually remain sensitive to nitrofurazone.

Propamidine isoethionate, a drug used in treating babesiasis, is also a useful antiseptic for application to open wounds and burns as a jelly or cream. It is not antagonised by para-amino benzoic acid. Propamidine causes the release of histamine.

Chlorhexidine as the hydrochloride or gluconate is a

potent bactericide against both Gram-positive and Gram-negative organisms and is unaffected by serum or other body fluids. Chlorhexidine appears to act by causing the leaking of intracellular material from the bacteria. An aqueous solution of 0·02 to 0·05 per cent is used to disinfect wounds and burns and a 0·5 per cent solution in alcohol to disinfect the skin before surgical operations and to disinfect instruments. This substance is used as a pessary or in suspension as a uterine antiseptic.

Disinfectant Detergents

A number of anionic and cationic detergents have antiseptic properties and, as with the dyestuffs, the cationic compounds are the more active.

Soaps are bactericidal to some organisms but not to others, *Staphylococcus aureus*, for example, is not affected. Washing with soap alone, therefore, cannot be relied on to sterilise skin. Soaps are the sodium or potassium salts of large anions. The chlorides or bromides of certain large cations have detergent properties similar to soap, and are better disinfectants.

Cetrimide is a cationic detergent. It is obtained by replacing three hydrogen ions of ammonium bromide with three methyl groups and the fourth hydrogen by a long chain of $-CH_2-$. This compound is used to cleanse the skin and is also antiseptic but not strongly so; it is bactericidal to Gram-positive micro-organisms but relatively ineffective against Gram-negative bacteria. It is non-irritant and does not stain. The skin may become sensitive if detergents are used continuously because they remove the normal fats. It is essential to rinse well with water between using ordinary soap and cationic detergent as they are incompatible. A hydrophobic ion of the quaternary ammonium detergent has a positive charge, whereas that of the soap has a negative charge and so they neutralise each other.

Benzalkonium chloride is a cationic detergent with bactericidal properties similar to those of Cetrimide. This activity is reduced by serum, and spores are unaffected. It has the same incompatibilities and disadvantages as the other cationic detergents. The continuous use of the detergent type of antiseptic may cause defatting of the skin which may give rise to irritation and render the skin more susceptible to infection. Protection may be provided by application of a cream containing a suitable oil or fat.

FUNGICIDES

Fungi are killed by many bactericides, but often these drugs lack other desirable therapeutic actions. The fungi causing ringworm are sometimes treated with solutions or ointments of *Phenylmercuric nitrate* or *acetate*, *Dichlorophen* or *Iodine*, *Iodides* have no direct disinfectant action but *potassium iodide*, given by mouth, or *sodium iodide*, by intravenous injection. are the traditional remedies for *actinobacillosis* and *actinomycosis* in cattle. However, these remedies have been replaced by various preparations of penicillin.

Griseofulvin is an antibiotic which, when given orally, is an effective treatment for ringworm. It is ineffective as a local application. This antibiotic appears to act by competing with purine nucleotide for the synthesis of nucleic acids. The fungal cell wall loses its integrity and hyphal growth is decreased and distorted, actively metabolising cells being mainly affected. Griseofulvin is well absorbed from the gut and evenly distributed in the tissues. It appears to be nearly completely metabolised in the body in that less than one per cent of the total dose is excreted unchanged in the urine. Very large doses of griseofulvin cause the arrest of mitosis in the bone marrow and testes although no such effect has been observed when the drug is given at normal therapeutic levels. In man, gastro-intestinal upsets have been caused. It does not appear to be effective in all cases of ringworm, although some cases may require prolonged treatment. Its use in veterinary medicine is somewhat limited because of the high cost of the drug.

Nystatin is an antibiotic with activity against yeasts and fungi; it is poorly absorbed from the gut and finds its main use as a local application, being incorporated in dusting powders, creams and ointments. In veterinary medicine it is most useful in the treatment of mastitis caused by yeasts for which purpose nystatin is given as a solution injected into the teat canal.

Y

SUGGESTIONS FOR FURTHER READING

BEAN, H. S. (1967). Types and characteristics of disinfectants. *J. appl. Bact.,* **30,** 6.

BOND, J. M. (1966). Antibiotics used in the chemotherapy of bacterial and fungal infection. In *Experimental Chemotherapy,* ed. Schnitzer, R. J. and Hawking, F., Vol. IV. New York: Academic Press.

Br. med. J. (1967). Griseofulvin, **4,** 608.

GIBBS, B. M. and STUTTARD, L. W. (1967). Evaluation of skin germicides.. *J. appl. Bact.,* **30,** 66.

HUGO, W. B. (1967). The mode of action of antibacterial agents. *J. appl.. Bact.,* **30,** 17.

KELSEY, J. C. and MAURER, I. M. (1967). Choice of disinfectants for hospital use. *Mon. Bull. Minist. Hlth.,* **26,** 110.

SYKES, G. (1965). *Disinfection and Sterilization,* 2nd ed. London: Spon.

APPENDIX I

Equivalents of Imperial and Metric Systems

$1 \cdot 00$ mg $= 1/60$ grains
$10 \cdot 00$ mg $= 1/6$ grains
$1 \cdot 00$ gm $= 15$ grains
$31 \cdot 10$ gm $= 1$ ounce apothecary
$0 \cdot 06$ ml $= 1$ minim
$28 \cdot 4$ ml $= 1$ fluid ounce
1 litre $= 1 \cdot 76$ pints
1 kilo $= 2 \cdot 2$ lbs
10 mg per kilo $= 1$ grain per stone

APPENDIX II

PREPARATIONS AND DOSES OF THE COMMONLY USED DRUGS

Route

Acepromazine maleate	i.m.	Horse, Cattle,
		Sheep, Pig; 0·05–0·1 mg/kg
		Dog, Cat; 0·125–0·25 mg/kg
	oral	Dog, Cat; 1–3 mg/kg.
Acetylsalicylic acid	oral	Horse, Cattle; 10–50 gm
		Sheep, Pig; 1–3 gm
		Dog, Cat; 0·1–1 gm
Acinitrazole	oral	Turkeys; 0·1–0·3 gm.
Amicarbalide isethionate	s.c., i.m.	Cattle; 5–10 mg/kg
Ammonium bicarbonate	oral	Horse; 3–15 gm
		Cattle; 8–30 gm
		Sheep, Pig; 1–2 gm
Ammonium chloride	oral	Horse, Cattle; 10–20 gm
		Sheep, Pig; 1–2 gm
Amphetamine sulphate	s.c.	Horse, Cattle; 1–300 mg
		Dog, Cat; 1–2 mg
Ampicillin	i.m.	All species; 10 mg/kg
Amprolium HCl	oral	Poultry; 0·0125 per cent in feed
Apomorphine hydrochloride	s.c.	Dog; 0·08 mg/kg
Arecoline hydrobromide	oral	Dog; 5–15 mg
Atropine sulphate	s.c.	All species; 0·04 mg/kg
Bemegride	i.v.	All species; 20 mg/kg
Benzyl penicillin	i.m.	All species, 3–6 mg/kg
Bephenium hydroxynaphthoate	oral	Lambs; 5 gm, Calves; 250 mg/kg
Betamethasone	i.m.	Horse, Cattle, 10–30 mg
	oral	Dog, Cat; 0·0125 mg/kg
Bunamidine HCl	oral	Dog, Cat; 25 mg/kg
Butobarbitone	oral	Dog; 50–300 mg
		Cat; 30–60 mg
Caffeine and sodium benzoate	s.c.	Horse, Cattle; 1–5 gm
		Sheep, Pig; ½–3 gm
		Dog, Cat; 15–60 gm
Calcium borogluconate	s.c., i.v.	Horse, Cattle; 60–180 gm
		Sheep, Pig; 6–20 gm
		Dog; 1–5 gm
Calcium copper edetate	s.c.	Cattle, 100 mg copper equivalent
		Calves, Ewes, 50 mg copper equivalent
Calcium edetate	i.v.	All species; 30 mg/kg
Carbachol chloride	s.c.	Horse, Cow; 2 mg
Carbon tetrachloride	oral	Sheep; 1–5 ml
Cascara Sagrada (Liq. ext.)	oral	Dog; 1–4 ml
		Cat; ½–2 ml
Castor oil	oral	Foals, Calves; 60–90 ml
		Pig; 60–120 ml
		Dog, Cat; 5–30 ml

Route

Chalk (prepared)	oral	Horse, Cattle; 50–200 gm
		Sheep, Pig; 8–15 gm
		Dog, Cat; 0·5–3 gm
Chloral hydrate	oral	Horse, Cattle,Sheep; 60–120 mg/kg
		Dog, Cat; 0·2–1·5 gm
Chloramphenicol	i.m.	All species 10 mg/kg
Chlorpromazine	i.m.	Horse, Cattle; ½–1 mg/kg
		Pig; 2 mg/kg
		Dog, Cat; ½–1 mg/kg
	oral	Dog; 5 mg/kg
Chlorpropamide	oral	Dog, Cat; 5–15 mg/kg
Chorionic gonadotrophin	i.m.	Horse, Cattle, 1·5–5000 units
		Sheep, Pig, 3–1000 units
Cinchocaine HCl	local application, s.c.	0·1 per cent solution
Cloxacillin sodium	i.m.	Horse, Cattle, 2–4 mg/kg
		Dog, Cat, 10 mg/kg
Codeine phosphate	oral	Dog; 2 mg/kg
Cod Liver Oil		Horse, Cattle; 15–60 ml
		Sheep, Pig; 4–15 ml
		Dog, Cat; ½–8 ml
		Poultry; ½–1 per cent in feed
Copper sulphate	oral	Cattle, Sheep; 2 mg/kg
		Dog, Cat; 20–100 mg
Corticotrophin	i.m.	Cattle; 4–600 units
Cortisone acetate	i.m.	Horse; 50–250 mg
		Cattle; 1–1·5 gm
		Dog; 2 mg/kg
Curare—see *Tubocurarine*		
Cyanocobalamin	i.m.	All species; 2 μg/kg
Dichlorophen	oral	Dog; 0·2 gm/kg
Diethylcarbamazine	oral	Dog, Cat; 10–50 mg/kg
Diethylthiambutene HCl	i.m.	Dog; 10 mg/kg
	i.v.	Dog; 2–4 mg/kg
Digitalin	i.m.	Horse; 15–60 mg
		Dog; 1–10 mg
Digoxin	oral, i.v.	Dog; Initial 0·05–0·1 mg/kg
		Maintenance 0·025 mg/kg
Dihydroxyanthraquinone	oral	Horse, Ox; 10–30 gm
		Dog; 0·15–3 gm
Ergometrine maleate	oral, i.m.	Dog; 0·2–0·5 mg
	i.m.	Horse, Ox; 10–20 mg
		Pig; ½–1 mg
Ferric ammonium citrate	oral	Horse, Ox; 4–8 gm
		Sheep, Pig; 1–2 gm
		Dog, Cat; 3–600 mg
Formalin	oral	Horse, Cattle; 15–30 ml
Furazolidone	oral	Poultry; 0·015–0·04 per cent in feed
Gallamine triethiodide	i.v.	Horse, 0·8–1 mg/kg
		Pig; 2 mg/kg
		Dog, Cat; 1 mg/kg
Griseofulvin	oral	All species; 10–30 mg/kg
Haloxon	oral	Horse, 75 mg/kg
		Cattle; 40 mg/kg
		Sheep; 35/50 mg/kg
		Pig; 50 mg/kg
		Poultry; 50–75 mg/kg

Route

Hexachloorethane	oral	Ox; 15–90 gm
		Sheep; 15 gm
Hexobarbitone sodium	i.v.	Dog, Cat; 20 mg/kg
Hexœstrol	implantation	Cattle; 15–25 mg—total 45–60 gm
		Dog; 0·2–5 mg
		Poultry; 15–30 mg
Homidium bromide	s.c., i.m.	Cattle; 1 mg/kg
Iron dextran	i.m.	Piglets; 100 mg iron.
Iron pyrophosphate	oral	Pigs; 0·3 gm
Iron, reduced	oral	Suckling pig; 0·5 gm
Kaolin	oral	Horse, Cattle; 50–250 gm
		Sheep, Pig; 20–40 gm
		Dog; ½–5 gm
Leptazol	s.c., i.m., i.v.	Horse, Cattle; ½–1 gm
		Dog, Cat; 25–100 mg
Lidocaine HCl (Lignocaine)	s.c.	½–2 per cent solution
Liquid paraffin	oral	Horse, Ox; 250–1000 ml
		Sheep, Pig; 25–250 ml
		Dog, Cat; 5–30 ml
Magnesium oxide/carbonate	oral	Foal, Calf; 10–15 gm
		Sheep, Pig; 5–10 gm
		Dog, Cat; ½–4 gm
Magnesium sulphate	oral	Horse, Ox; 100–500 gm
		Sheep, Pig; 25–125 gm
		Dog, Cat; 5–10 gm
	s.c.	Ox; up to 100 gm
Medroxyprogesterone	tampon	Sheep; 60 mg
Menaphthone	i.m.	Dog; ½–5 mg
Mepyramine	i.m.	Horse, Cattle; 0·5–1·5 gm
		Sheep, Pig; 0·01–0·25 gm
		Dog; 5–125 mg
Methallibure	oral	Pigs; 1 mg/kg
Methicillin	i.m.	Horse, Cattle; 4–16 mg/kg
		Dog, Cat; 40 mg/kg
Methyl benzoquate	oral	Chickens; 0·001 per cent in feed
Metriphonate	oral	Horse; 30–40 mg/kg
		Cattle; 80 mg/kg
		Sheep; 70–80 mg/kg
	s.c.	Cattle; 20–30 mg/kg
Morphine sulphate	s.c.	Dog; 2–10 mg/kg
Nalorphine HCl	s.c., i.m., i.v.	Dog; 0·2–0·5 mg/kg
Neostigmine methyl sulphate	s.c.	Cow; 30–45 mg
Nicarbazin	oral	Chicken; 0·0125 per cent in feed
Nitrofurazone	oral	Chicken; 0·011–0·02 per cent in feed
Nitroxynil eglumine	s.c.	Cattle, Sheep; 10 mg/kg
Oxytocin, injection	i.m.	Horse, Cattle; 10–40 units
		Sheep, Pig; 2·5–10 units
		Dog; 1–10 units
	i.v.	Horse, Cattle; 2·5–10 units
		Sheep, Pig; 0·5–2·5 units
		Dog; up to 0·5 units
Paracetamol	oral	Dog; 500 mg
Penicillin procaine	i.m.	All species; 0·5–10 mg/kg
Pentobarbitone sodium	oral	All species; 4 mg/kg
	i.v.	All species; 10–25 mg/kg
Pethidine	i.m., oral	Dog, Cat; 5 mg/kg
Phenobarbitone sodium	oral	Dog; 30–120 mg
		Cat; 15–60 mg

Route

Phenylbutazone	oral	Dog; Initial 1–600 mg
		Maintenance 50–100 mg
Phenytoin sodium	oral	Dog; 0·1–0·3 gm
Phthalylsulphathiazole	oral	All species; 0·1–0·15 gm/kg
Picrotoxin	i.v.	Dog, Cat; 1 mg/min
Piperazine hydrate	oral	Horse, Cow; 200 mg/kg
		Sheep, Pig; 250 mg/kg
		Dog, Cat; 100 mg/kg
		Poultry; 2–400 mg
Polyricinate	oral	Cattle; 10–15 ml
		Sheep; 1–3 ml
Potassium iodide	oral	Cattle; 2–16 gm
		Sheep; 1–3 gm
Prednisolone	i.m.	Cattle; 1–200 mg
Pregnant Mare's Serum	s.c., i.m.	Horse; 3–5000 units
		Cattle; 1–2000 units
		Pig; 50–1000 units
		Dog; 1–500 units
		Cat; 1–200 units
Primidone	oral	Dog; 50 mg/kg
Procaine HCl	s.c.	½–2 per cent solution
Promazine HCl	oral	All species; 4·4–11·0 mg/kg
	i.m.	All species; 2·2–5·5 mg/kg
Promethazine HCl	i.m.	Horse, Cattle; ½–1 mg/kg
		Sheep, Pig; ¼–1 mg/kg
		Dog, Cat; 0·2–0·5 mg/kg
Propylene glycol	oral	Cows; 250 ml
		Sheep; 75 ml
Quinapyramine sulphate	s.c.	Cattle, Sheep, Pigs; 1 mg/kg
		Animals under 150 kg; 5 mg/kg
		,, 150–200; 1 gm
		,, 200–350; 1·5 gm
		,, over 350; 2 gm
Quinuronium sulphate	s.c.	Horse; 0·6–1 mg/kg
		Cattle, Sheep, Pigs; 1 mg/kg
Sodium bicarbonate	oral	Horse Cow; 15–120 gm
		Sheep, Pig; 2–10 gm
		Dog, Cat; 0·3–1·5 gm
Sodium calciumedetate	s.c., i.v.	All species; 75 mg/kg
Sodium iodide	i.v.	Cattle; 4–60 gm
		Sheep; 1–3 gm
Sodium propionate	oral	Cattle; 250 gm
		Sheep; 60 gm
Sodium sulphate	oral	Horse, Cow; ¼–1 kg
		Sheep, Pig; 10–30 gm
		Dog, Cat; ½–2 gm
Spiramycin	oral	Dog, Cat; 50–100 mg/kg
Squill, syrup of	oral	Dog, Cat; 1–4 ml
Streptomycin HCl	i.m.	All species; 10 mg/kg
Sulphadimidine	oral	All species; Initial 200 mg/kg
		Maintenance; 100 mg/kg
Sulphafurazole	oral	All species; Initial 200 mg/kg
		Maintenance; 100 mg/kg
Suxamethonium chloride	i.v.	Horse; 0·15–0·25 mg/kg
		Dog; 0·3 mg/kg
Tetracycline HCl	oral	Dog, Cat; 60 mg/kg
	i.v.	All species; 5–10 mg/kg

Route

Thiabendazole	oral	Horse, Cattle; 50–100 mg/kg; Sheep; 50–90 mg/kg
Thiopentone sodium	i.v.	All species; 10–35 mg/kg
Thyroid	oral	All species; 1–2 mg/kg
Tocopheryl acetate	oral	Calves; 200–600 mg Lambs; 35–100 mg
Tolbutamide	oral	Dog, Cat; 10–30 mg/kg
Tribromosalicylanilide	oral	Sheep; 30 mg/kg
Tubocurarine	i.v.	Dog; 0·12 mg/kg
Turpentine	oral	Horse, Cow; 15–60 ml
Tylosin	oral	Dog, Cat; 2–10 mg/kg

s.c. = subcutaneous injection
i.m. = intramuscular injection
i.v. = intravenous injection

INDEX

Printed by Neill & Co. Ltd., Edinburgh

54145